TO
THE
SUMMIT

High cirrus clouds above Ama Dablam and the northwest ridge, taken during an early-morning wander through Dingboche.

TO THE SUMMIT

NICK ALLEN

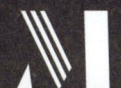
MASSEY UNIVERSITY PRESS

The view from Chukhung Ri, with Ama Dablam poking up through the cloud on the left.

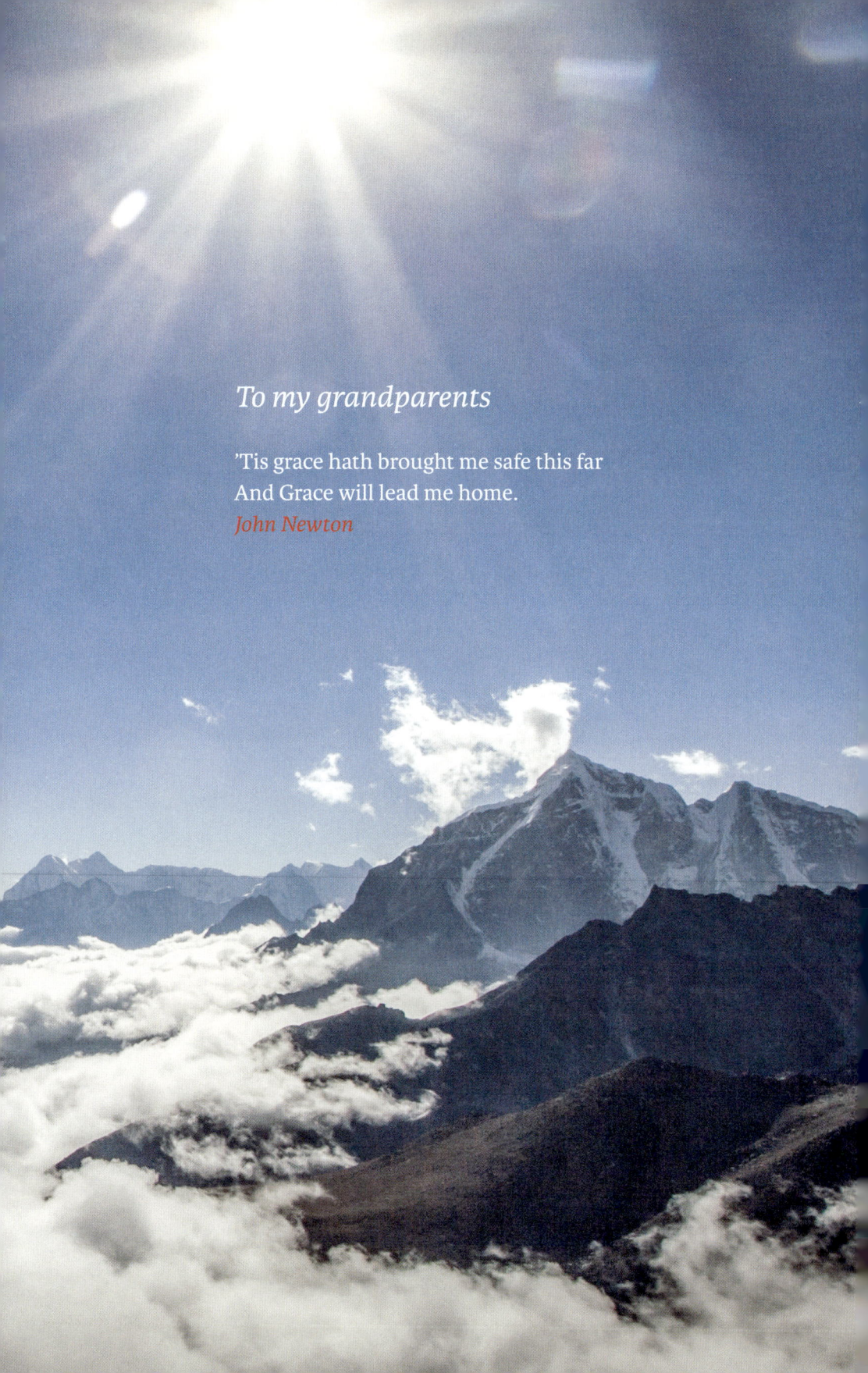

To my grandparents

'Tis grace hath brought me safe this far
And Grace will lead me home.
John Newton

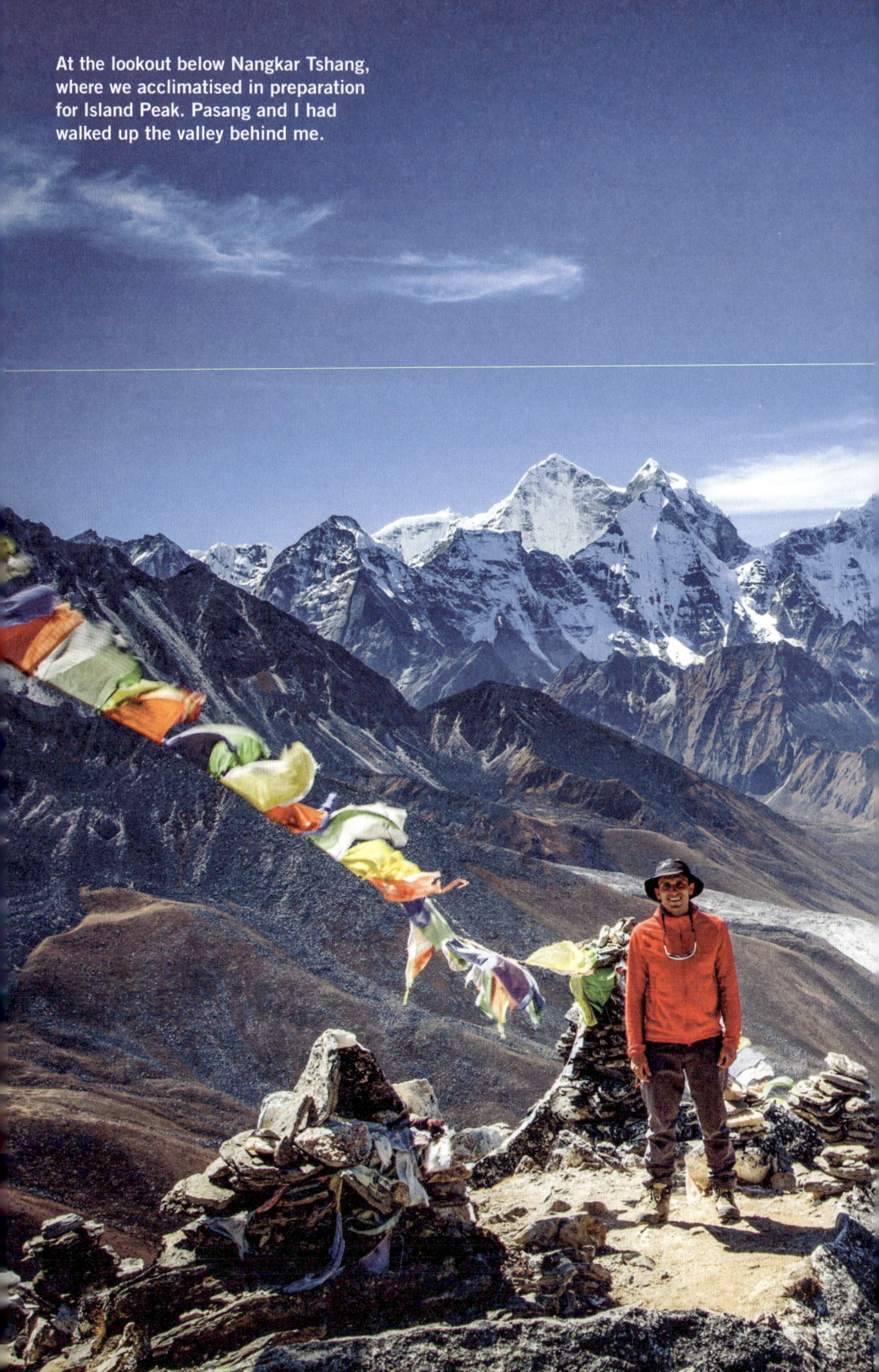

At the lookout below Nangkar Tshang, where we acclimatised in preparation for Island Peak. Pasang and I had walked up the valley behind me.

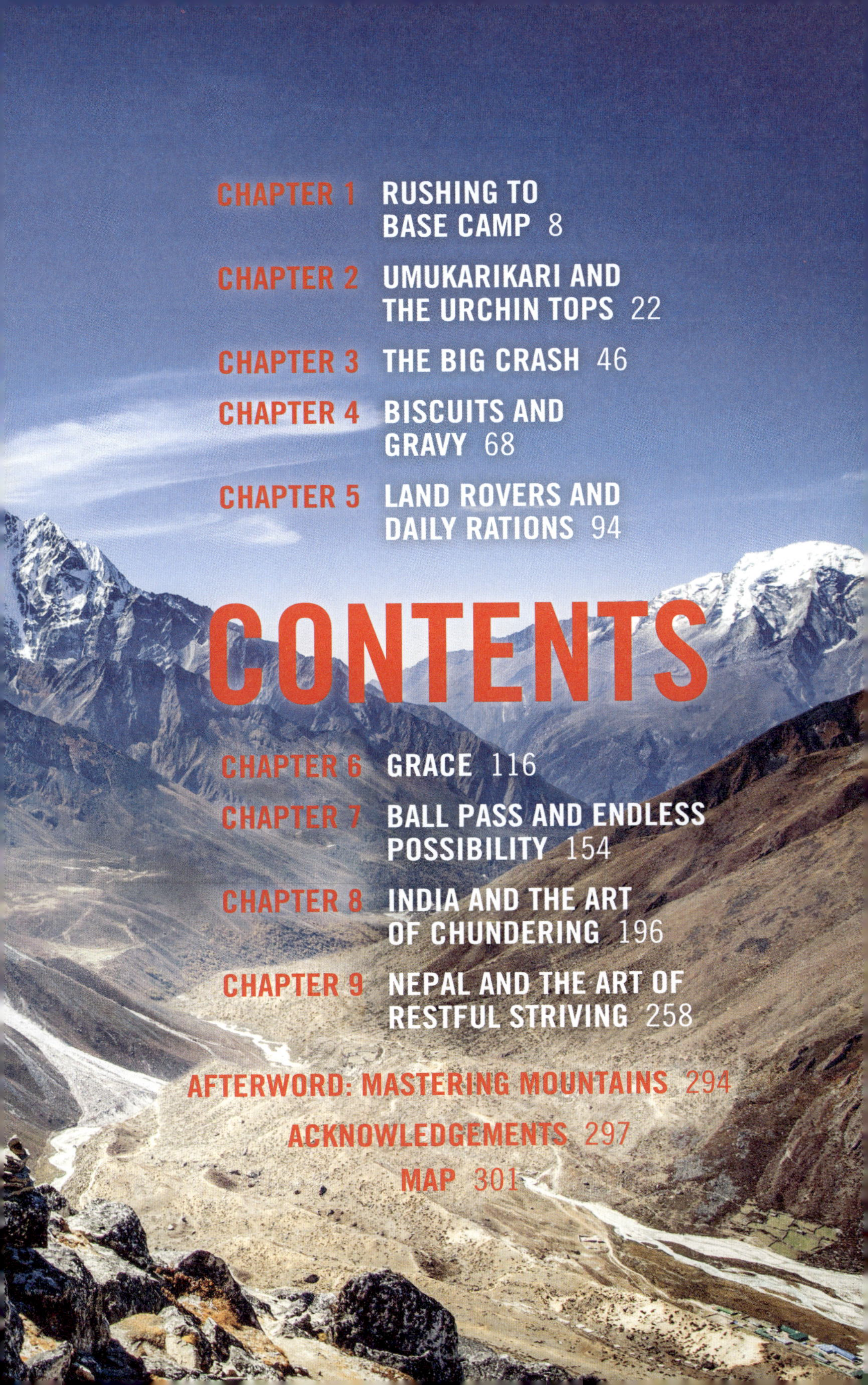

CONTENTS

CHAPTER 1 — RUSHING TO BASE CAMP 8

CHAPTER 2 — UMUKARIKARI AND THE URCHIN TOPS 22

CHAPTER 3 — THE BIG CRASH 46

CHAPTER 4 — BISCUITS AND GRAVY 68

CHAPTER 5 — LAND ROVERS AND DAILY RATIONS 94

CHAPTER 6 — GRACE 116

CHAPTER 7 — BALL PASS AND ENDLESS POSSIBILITY 154

CHAPTER 8 — INDIA AND THE ART OF CHUNDERING 196

CHAPTER 9 — NEPAL AND THE ART OF RESTFUL STRIVING 258

AFTERWORD: MASTERING MOUNTAINS 294

ACKNOWLEDGEMENTS 297

MAP 301

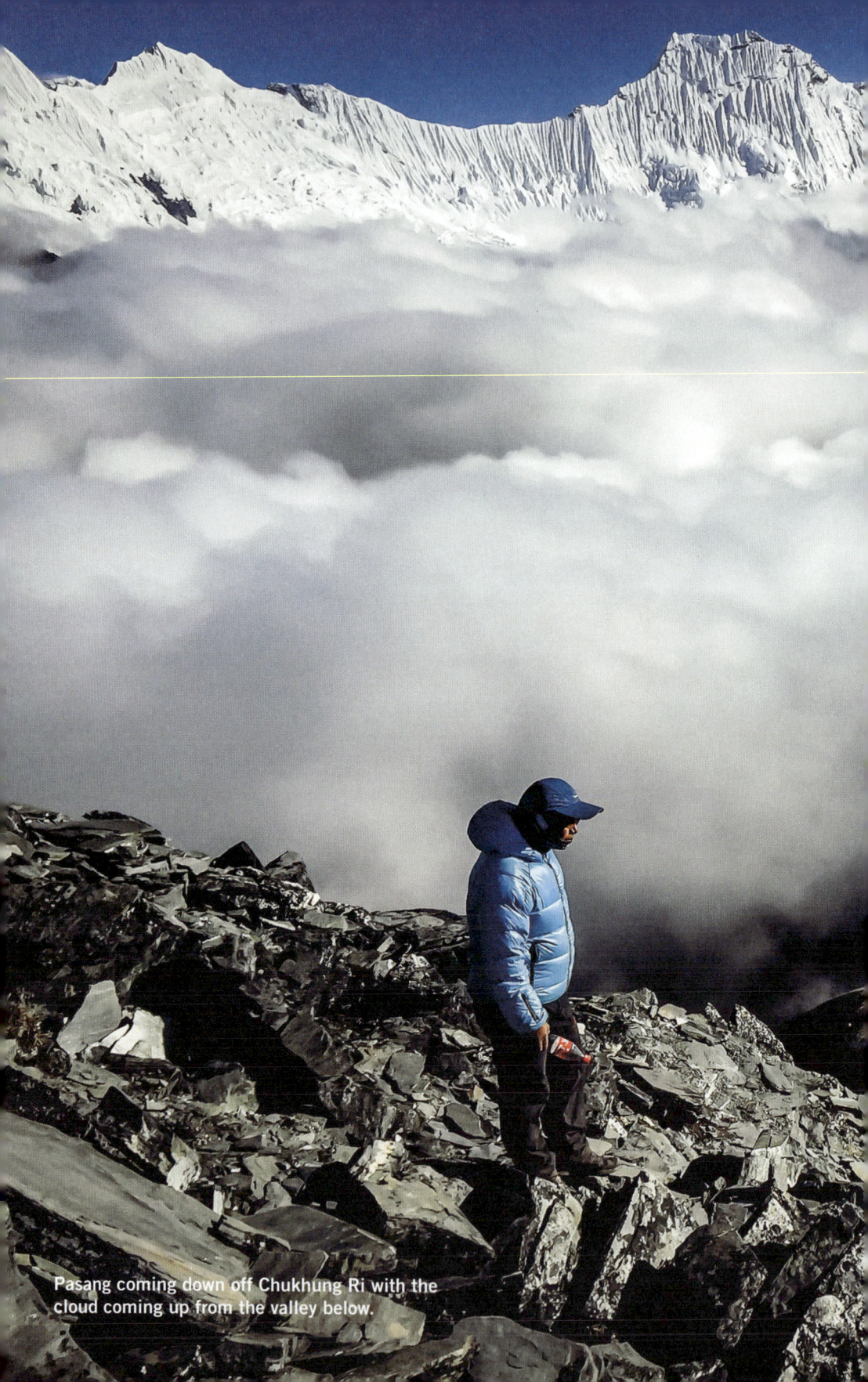

Pasang coming down off Chukhung Ri with the cloud coming up from the valley below.

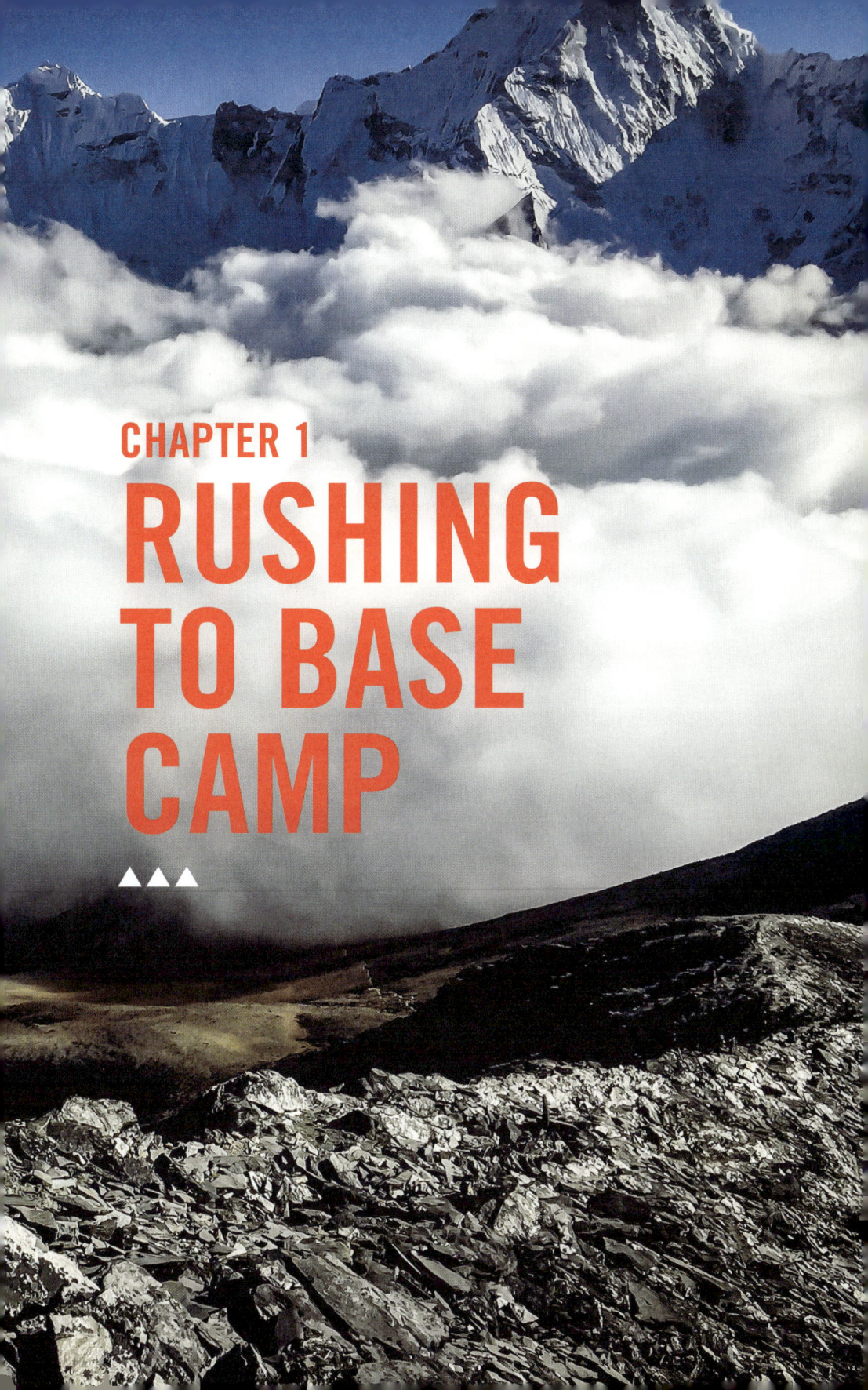

CHAPTER 1
RUSHING TO BASE CAMP

▲▲▲

October 2015
Everest Region, Nepal

'It's too warm,' Pasang shouted over the wind. 'This is very bad — bad weather is coming.' He unzipped his heavy down jacket.

'How far away is the front?' I shouted, trying to make myself heard over the noise of the stiff breeze.

Pasang looked down at the clouds building in the valleys several hundred metres below us. The occasional threatening wisp was cast up towards the barren rock-and-snow summits we stood beneath.

'When the warm winds blow, the storm is coming,' Pasang yelled. 'About one and a half or two days away. It is coming with snow.'

He pointed up to Lhotse (8516 metres) towering above us, seemingly within reaching distance of our position just beneath the summit of Chukhung Ri (5550 metres).

'And see the white trail coming off the top of Lhotse?'

I looked across to the scarred black ridges fringing the thousands of metres of vertical ice and snow that cling to Lhotse's south face. At the top, a sharp-edged wing of cloud and ice was streaming off Lhotse's peak, crowning more nebulous formations swirling off the eastern ridge. The wind was clearly violent.

'Yes, I see it,' I said, trying not to be distracted by the enormity of the view.

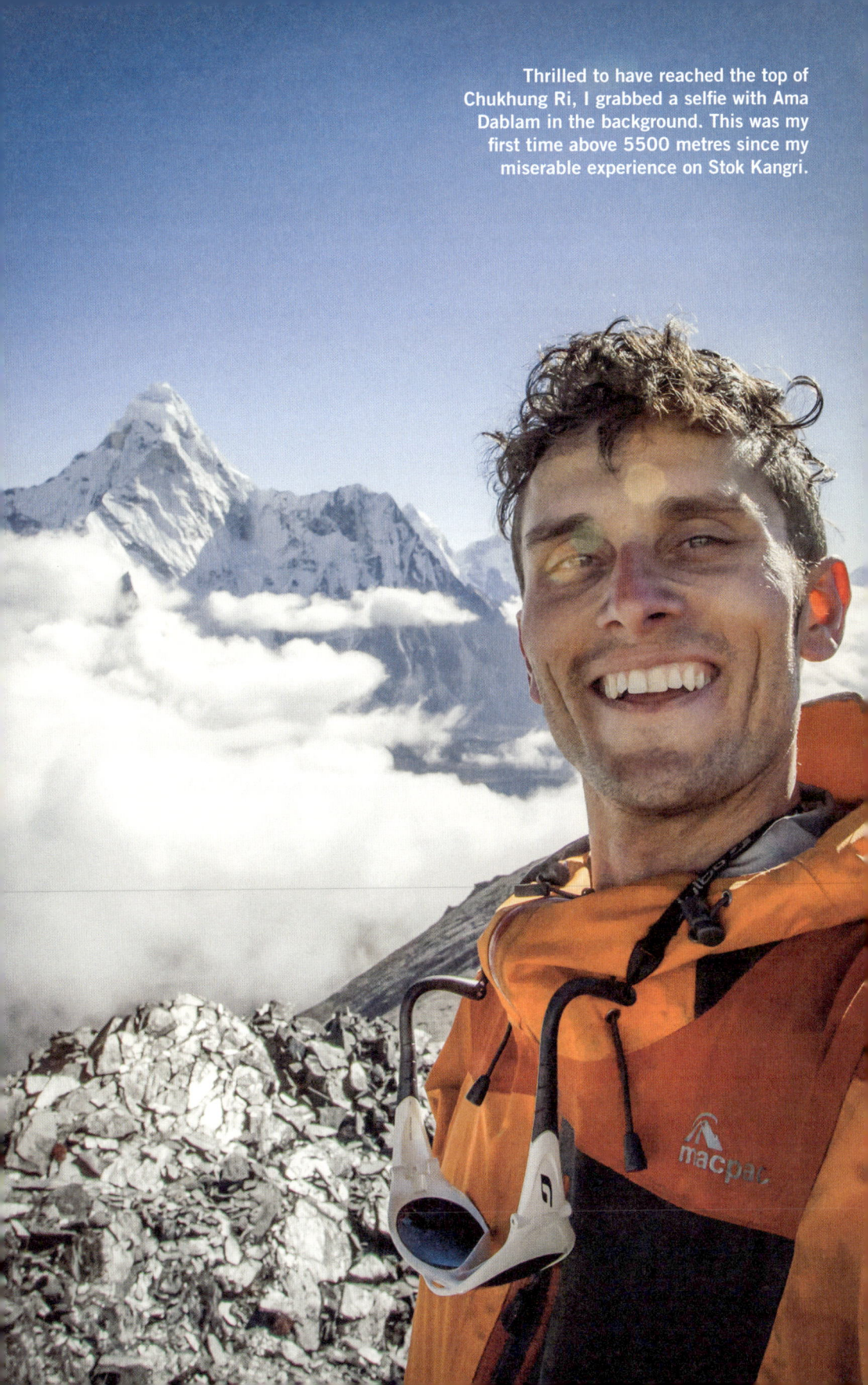

Thrilled to have reached the top of Chukhung Ri, I grabbed a selfie with Ama Dablam in the background. This was my first time above 5500 metres since my miserable experience on Stok Kangri.

Cloud suddenly enveloped us. My focus snapped back to the terrain directly around me. We were scrambling down ledges and slopes covered in loose shards of schist that glistened in the sun. There was no grass or moss at this altitude, just rock fractured by the endless leveraging of the freeze–thaw cycle. It was slow going and I needed to take care, but I quickened my pace so I could catch up with Pasang.

'Sorry, what was that?' I shouted into the wind.

He just kept moving.

When I did manage to catch up, Pasang said, 'Ice trails on Lhotse are very bad sign. The winds have come and it means stronger winds come. Snow and high winds are not good for climbing — we need to reach Base Camp tomorrow, otherwise we miss the weather window.'

The news of an approaching front was hardly surprising. For the last few days we had woken to a sky full of high cirrus clouds, a development that marked a change from the more settled weather patterns of the past week. The clouds were beautiful in the mornings, catching the early light and painting the sky with colour, but they were also the harbinger of an approaching front.

Pasang probably knew this better than anyone; a Sherpa by birth, he grew up in these mountains. His family home was in Khumjung, a few kilometres back down the valley, and as a child and young teen he was responsible for the family's yak herd. Every summer, he would bring the herd up these valleys to graze on the mountain pastures. He slept out in the wild with them, sheltering from storms and during cold nights alone. Yes, he knew how to read these mountains.

The need to get to Island Peak Base Camp the next day worried me. It was a day earlier than we had planned, and I was anxious about rushing our progress up the mountain. Tomorrow was supposed to be a rest day, an opportunity to gain the strength needed for the climb ahead. In view of my traumatic failure to summit Stok Kangri in northern India just three weeks earlier, and considering that our schedule afforded me only one shot at Island Peak, I was worried that forfeiting a rest day could jeopardise my chance to summit. But then I wasn't prepared to surrender to the sky either.

'How long do you think this weather will last? Do you think we could wait until it has cleared?'

I almost slid on the loose rocks as I tried to keep up with Pasang.

'Waiting for the weather is bad option,' he replied. 'It could take one week or ten days to clear, and then there will be much snow on Island Peak, making the walking more difficult. I think we climb as soon as possible. We move quickly, to get back to Chukhung and the teahouse. We have lots to do. We need to do a gear check and pack.'

I tried to think of alternatives, a different solution. 'What if we walked over Kongma La tomorrow, headed up to Everest Base Camp, then came back to Island Peak for a climb?'

'We could do, but another weather window might not come, and we would have no time to do Three Passes trek.'

I was excited about completing the famous Three Passes trek — crossing Kongma La (5535 metres), Cho La (5420 metres) and Renjo La (5465 metres) — and I knew I would be disappointed to give it up, only to sit in a teahouse for days waiting for the weather to clear. And to miss the opportunity to climb Island Peak? Well, that was unthinkable.

I weighed up the options, nervous and uncertain about the best course of action. I felt the burden of my unsuccessful attempt on Stok Kangri. I did not want to lose another peak — to do so would mean writing off the whole trip, and my months of training, as a waste of time. I knew I would kick myself if I missed out on both Island Peak and the Three Passes trek because of a decision to postpone the climb. I need to accomplish something, I thought, and climbing sooner rather than later was probably the least risky option.

We continued our march down the hill to Chukhung village. By now we had moved off the more difficult part of the descent from the summit and on to a sharp but gentle ridge that took us down to a grassy saddle. The ridge was lined with hundreds of small cairns, blackened by the weather, some as old as the town below, no doubt. Sun-bleached prayer flags, tattered and frayed and heavy with moisture, stuck to the rocks or flapped stiffly in the wind. It was much easier to move quickly along the ridge, thanks to the tracks formed over hundreds of years of ritualised prayer offerings. It was easier to think, too, now that I didn't have to concentrate so much on where I was putting my feet.

'I suppose it does make sense to go now,' I said. 'But do you think I am ready for Island Peak? I mean, are you confident that I could summit tomorrow night?'

'Yes, you are ready. Everything's good. Oxygen levels are good, you are fit, everything's good. You just climbed Chukhung Ri with no sign of altitude sickness. You are strong, ready.'

Pasang Sherpa's vote of confidence was reassuring. A six-time summiteer of Mt Everest, Pasang had guided clients up many other significant peaks. And he made a good point: we had been monitoring my blood-oxygen levels every day since our trip began eight days earlier and they were high, consistently matching Pasang's own. My heart rate was encouragingly low, the product of months spent training at the gym. And I did feel strong climbing Chukhung Ri, experiencing not so much as a flicker of a headache or a tinge of nausea. I also now knew that I could reach 5550 metres and function at that altitude, undoing some of the fears that had developed after my abortive attempt on Stok Kangri.

Nevertheless, those conflicting fears still ran deep. My experience on Stok Kangri had delivered a massive blow to my confidence, and I still did not fully trust my body's ability to function at high altitudes. I was plagued by the fear that this was all a pipe dream, doomed to come crashing down around me — that my multiple sclerosis would have the last word. Attempting to summit a day early meant cutting out that important day of rest.

These fears were not new — they had been at the back of my mind even before I left New Zealand — but they had intensified as a result of the struggle on Stok Kangri. For me, 5500 metres represented the point at which you pass into hell. Everything in me wanted to avoid a repeat of that experience, and I was deeply afraid of anything that might increase my chances of failure.

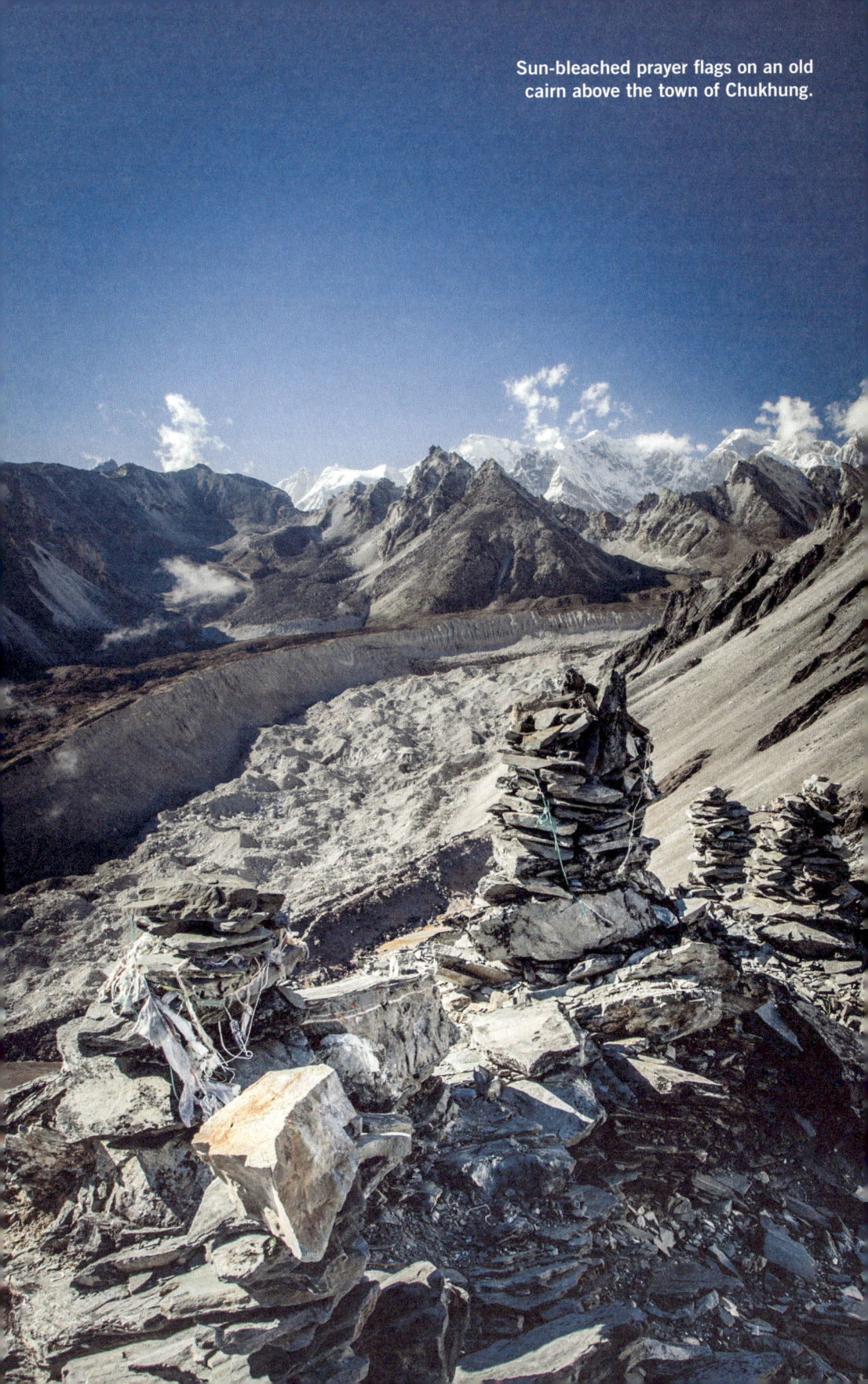
Sun-bleached prayer flags on an old cairn above the town of Chukhung.

On the other hand, I was also deeply afraid of losing the opportunity to climb Island Peak. Although Imja Tse, as it is called by the locals, is a small 6189-metre peak sitting alone beside the towering faces of the Everest Massif, it was the main goal of my entire trip.

I wanted to climb Island Peak for two reasons. The first and main one was to help change the perception of multiple sclerosis as an inevitably debilitating disease, and by extension raise money for the Mastering Mountains Charitable Trust, which I had set up a few months earlier out of a desire to help the MS community. The purpose of the trust is to provide a scholarship for people with MS to help them overcome an obstacle that prevents them from getting outdoors. The public's response to the trust had been overwhelmingly positive and supportive, which was exciting.

The second reason I wanted to climb Island Peak was more personal. I still held the hope of getting serious about climbing, and Island Peak, which is known as the ideal entree into high-altitude climbing, was going to be a toe in the water, a test to see if I could manage something larger.

Stok Kangri and the previous nine months had all been leading up to this moment. So much was riding on my ability to summit — I stood to lose an incredible amount if I failed.

I was also afraid of sounding like a wimp. As Pasang and I talked during the walk back to Chukhung village, I tried to skirt around the issue of my MS, and particularly my fear of fatigue and failure. I did not want to state directly that I was afraid of getting sick. We had spoken about it before, but I did not want to bring it up again.

'Do you think we will lose anything by heading out a day early?' I asked Pasang.

'No, but you will probably lose Island Peak if we stay. Trust me, you will be fine. You are strong. We will go tomorrow.'

We had reached the grassy saddle that fed into the smooth flanks of the mountain. Pasang broke into a jog, gliding down the slope. I followed. This was the easiest way to descend.

We started the following day with a slow breakfast and a final gear check before heading out to Base Camp. We ate breakfast at 7 a.m., as was our routine, then sat in the morning sun drinking black tea and going through the gear again, making sure everything was there. I always enjoy the process of going through my gear a second time — I find it therapeutic. Seeing everything on the ground in front of me, going through a mental checklist again, and arriving at the conclusion that I have everything I need — assuming nothing goes too wrong — gives me a sense of calm.

With all this out of the way, I was ready to finish getting dressed. I love the act of robing up, putting on my technical garments in preparation for the day ahead. The process of getting ready, knowing that I am about to put my gear to its proper use, creates a wonderful feeling of anticipation.

When I was a kid, Dad would take us down to Mt Ruapehu once a year for a weekend of skiing. We would stay at Ohakune in an A-frame and head up to the Turoa skifield. Climbing into my ski pants, pulling on my socks and gloves, putting on my hat and glasses, was all part of an exciting ritual.

Driving up the mountain road, through the snow-laden beech forest and around the ancient lava flows, it felt as if we were flying to a different planet, a new world. When we reached the top of the road I'd open the door of the car, feel the blast of cold air on my face, put on my sunglasses and look up at the sky, a deeper blue. Up the mountain, everything felt innately better than at the lower reaches of the earth — the air and the light purer, closer to the source. Sitting on a chairlift and rising higher up the slopes, I was moving closer to the frozen summit, the dwelling place of climbers, those god-like men who were my heroes.

The track from Chukhung crossed the ice-laced waters of a cloudy glacial stream as it wove its way through the moraine fields, the remains of a glacier long receded. It was a beautiful morning, with a cloudless sky and a heavy chill in the air. I have always loved mornings like this — clear, cool, carrying a sense of exploration, of imminent discovery. This morning, as we walked across the glacier towards Island Peak Base Camp, was no exception.

But the process of dressing and thinking my day through had also brought a sense of unease. As I considered how I would address any problems as they arose, it was easy to become anxious. I could think through the obvious scenarios — a twisted ankle or a graze — and take comfort from the fact that I had what I needed to deal with them. But then there were all those situations that you cannot really prepare for: legs broken in a fall, a collapse from exhaustion, a total loss of strength to a leg, the disappointment of failing to summit.

These scenarios played in the back of my mind, slowly undermining my confidence, as we wound over and around the old moraine mounds, now covered with hardy grass and mosses, beneath the towering peaks. I tried to focus on enjoying the stunning environment — the ravens circling, the impeyan pheasants running along the ground, the movement of ice across the mountain faces, the creaking and groaning of the glacier.

Staying on top of my thinking and remaining unstressed is both a necessity and a battle for me. Stress is one of my primary enemies when I'm trying to manage fatigue, as it quickly leaves me drained and makes me slow to recover. The danger of stress has been reinforced through my many crashes over the last few years, and never more powerfully than at Stok Kangri. But then the benefit of managing stress has also been evident in my many successes. As I walked through the moraine fields I knew I needed to return to basics, settle my thoughts and kill the stress.

I was doing just that as we walked into a beautiful little valley sandwiched between the southern moraine wall of Lhotse Glacier and the peaks towering above. The valley floor was flat — such a pleasant break from the unstable moraine fields — and supported by a braided stream, cloudy white and silver with the fine glacial powder and reflected morning light. The air was still and I felt a sense of the idyllic, of walking into a place that I had always longed for, where there is a view against which you judge all others lacking. For a moment, at least, I felt that childhood sense of wonder, with its pure thrill of being up high among the frozen white peaks.

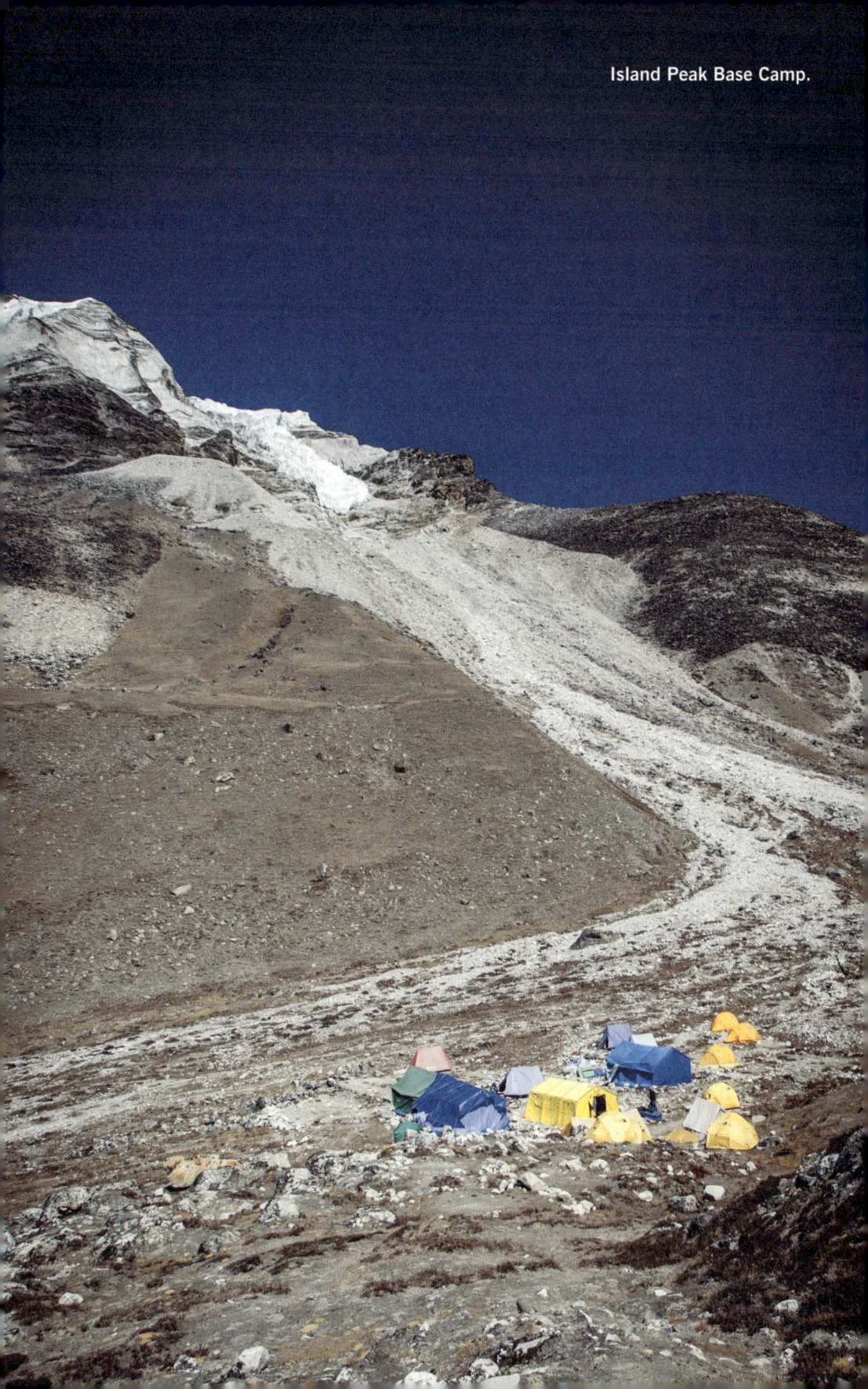

Island Peak Base Camp.

This is what it is about, I thought. Walking along the valley floor, I felt a renewed determination to enjoy the journey, to go as far as I could, and to not let the success of the trip be determined by my ability to summit. I was aware that my concerns about success and failure were reducing my enjoyment of the landscape; a crying shame, I told myself, when I was in one of the most spectacular places on earth. With time, though, I felt a sense of peace and calm, happy to give the peak my best shot and to give away all those things outside of my control.

After we had been tramping for a couple of hours we decided to take a break near the top of the valley before crossing the base of the Imja Tsho glacial lake. We rested in the shade of a massive boulder, facing the stream and the sharply rising peaks. In the distance we could see three men — two climbers and their guide — returning from Island Peak Base Camp. The climbers looked fit and strong, but were obviously tired. The older of the two was relying heavily on his walking poles, while the younger was carrying the pair's ice axes, one in each hand. When they finally reached us they joined us in the shade, dropping their gear, the ice axes clinking as they bounced on the rocks.

'How's it going?' I asked.

The older climber glared at me. 'OK,' he replied, with what sounded like a German accent.

'Did you make it?'

The younger man started digging into his pack, absorbed in the search for his water bottle.

'No,' replied the older man.

I never know quite how to respond to answers like this. You want to acknowledge their frustration and pain, but don't want to devalue their attempt with an offer of pity. After all, in less than 24 hours there was every possibility that I might be replying 'No' to someone who asked me the same question.

'Oh, sorry to hear that,' I said. There didn't seem much more to say. I stared off towards the face that rose thousands of metres up out of the stream in front of us.

Pasang began talking to the men's guide. They spoke quickly in Sherpa. I stole a glance back at the two climbers. The older man looked as if he was about to cry. Raw disappointment was written on his face as he looked blankly at his water bottle, his jaw clenched.

I went back to the little drawing I had begun making with my finger in the dust — a spray of lines, forming a star of sorts.

Pasang shook hands with the other Sherpa and rose to leave. He looked at me and gave a quick nod. Once we were well out of earshot, I turned to him. 'What was up with those guys?'

'They got to Base Camp yesterday and were very sick at night. Vomiting and stuff. Their guide thought that it was acute altitude sickness.'

'Did they climb at all?'

'No, they did not even make a start. The guys were both too sick.'

I felt sorry for them, recalling how devastating it had been coming off Stok Kangri, even though the reason was different. And my sense of calm was now ruffled. Although I was quietly confident that altitude sickness would not be a problem — Pasang had done an excellent job of preparing me — I was still not sure how the altitude would affect my ability to manage fatigue. So far my track record at altitude was not great, and I knew I would be devastated by a second failure to summit: it would be unspeakably, crushingly disappointing.

I had begun to feel tired by now. Moraine is not the easiest to traverse at the best of times, but I was feeling a particular type of tiredness — the type that had proved dangerous in the past — and that worried me. Would I feel like this tomorrow?

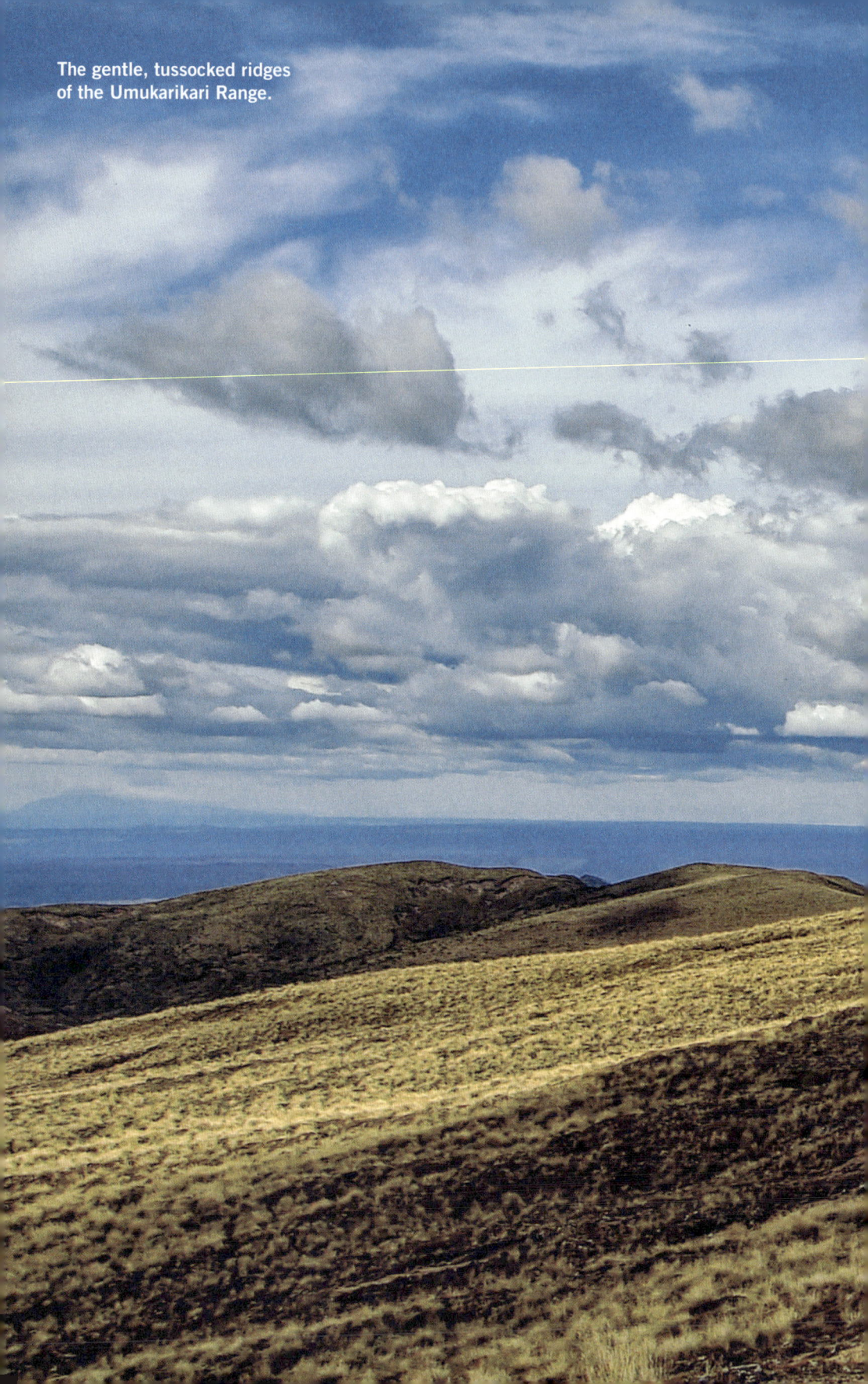

The gentle, tussocked ridges of the Umukarikari Range.

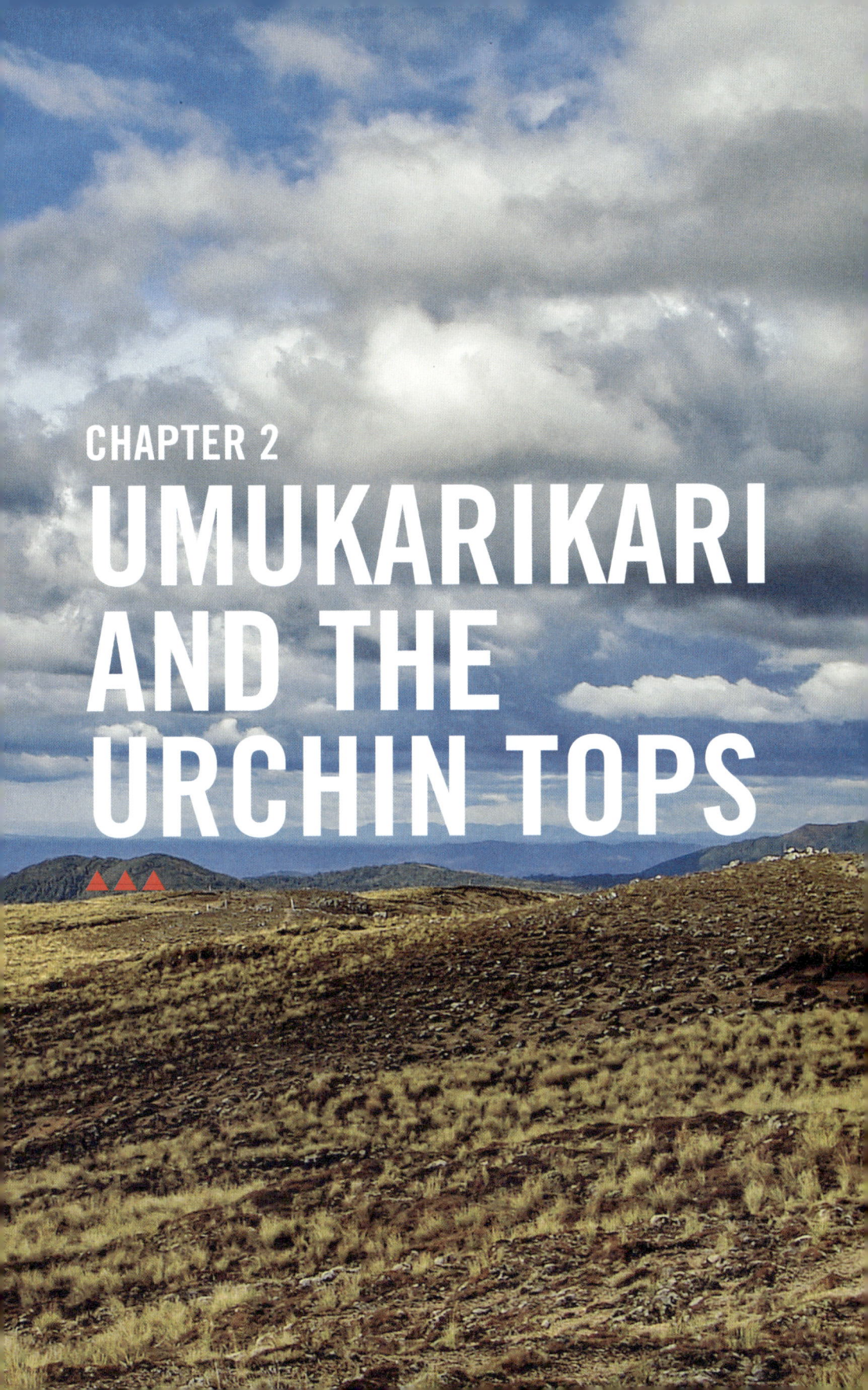

CHAPTER 2
UMUKARIKARI AND THE URCHIN TOPS

January 2006
Kaimanawa Forest Park, New Zealand

The sun beat down as the beech forest became thinner, giving way to alpine tussocks and expansive views of the open tops. Behind us, the cloud-capped peak of Ruapehu, fingers of snow still visible, stood in the foreground, incredibly close, it seemed. To the north was Lake Taupo, blending seamlessly with the blue haze of the humid summer air. Southward, black clouds and grey sheets of rain shrouded the ranges. Ahead of us, a softly tussocked ridge stretched into the distance. The air was hot and still.

I was struggling as we made our ascent out of the bush and up to the ridge line that would take us on to the Umukarikari Range and Waipakihi Hut. My father and my younger brothers, 13-year-old Jonathan and 10-year-old Charles, all seemed to be managing the trek a lot better than I was.

'Hang on, guys. Can we take a quick break?'

'Yeah, let's take a break,' Charles echoed as he flopped down into the tussock. 'It's so hot, and I'm hungry. Have we got much further to go?'

Charles took off his much-loved, ever crooked cowboy hat and fanned his face. It was framed by the shoulder straps of his slightly too large pack, which were pushed up past his ears as he sat down.

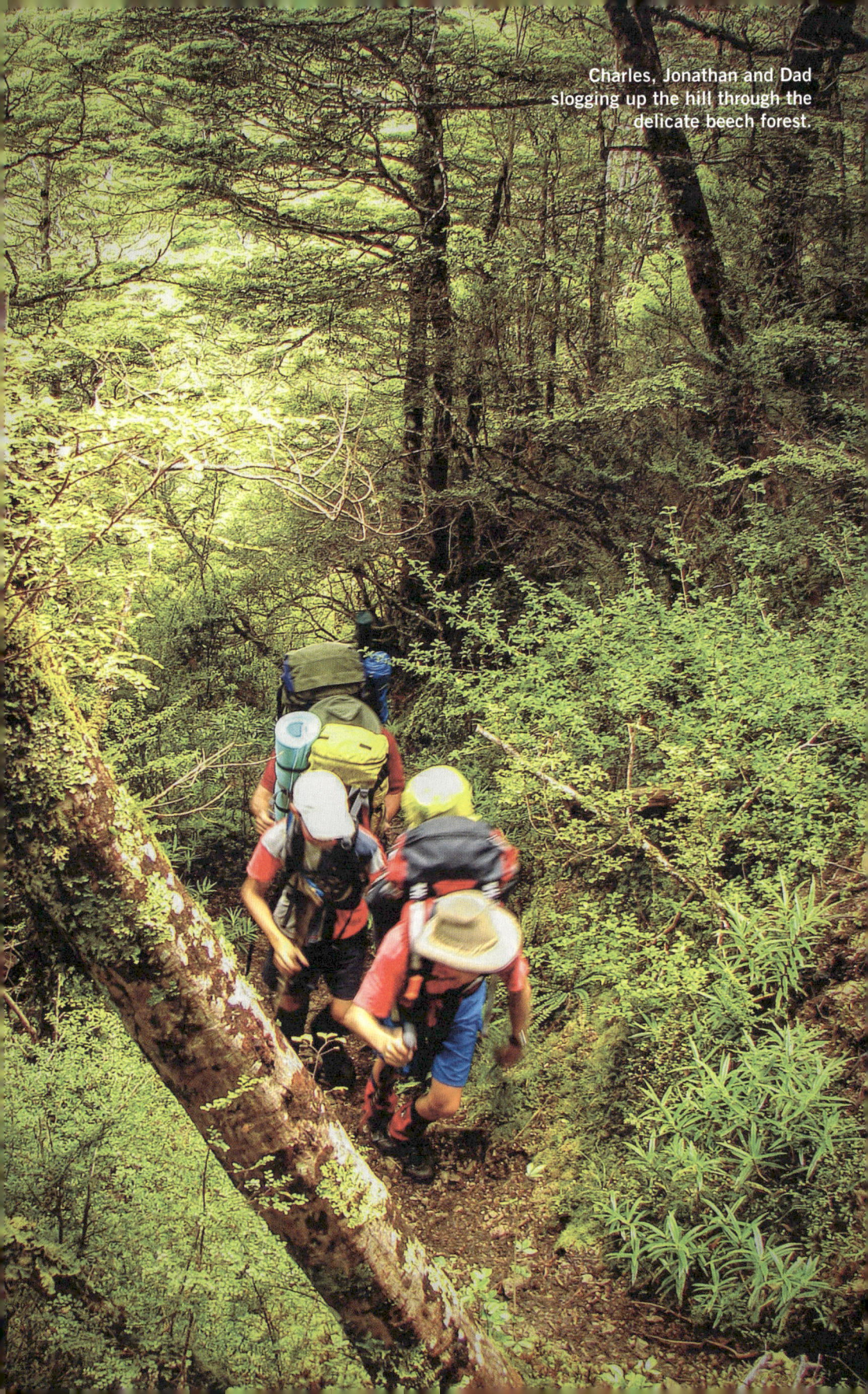

Charles, Jonathan and Dad slogging up the hill through the delicate beech forest.

'Are you OK, Nick?' Dad asked.

'Yeah, I'm fine. Just tired for some reason.' I wasn't sure what was going on, but walking up the hill I'd felt a lack of strength in my legs. As I committed to each step there wasn't enough grunt to carry me upward. It was peculiar and frustrating.

'OK, well, I'm a bit hungry too,' Dad said. 'Shall we eat lunch?'

'But do we have much longer to go?' Charles asked again.

I checked my watch. 'Um, we've been walking for two and a half hours, Charlie, so I think we have another three or four to go.'

'Oh man! It's so hot, and so long! Do we have to come back this way?'

'No, we'll be coming back through the stream down there.' I pointed to the river in the valley beneath the ridge ahead of us.

Charles pushed his head back against the pack and gave an exasperated grunt.

'Charlie, that'll be so much fun!' Jonathan said, reaching for his lunch.

'Come into the shade,' Dad suggested, 'and we'll all have some lunch.'

I sat down in the shade with the others and found myself torn. On the one hand, it was hard to sit still. I was surrounded by spectacular views, and I had my first-ever digital camera at the ready — I'd got it a few days earlier for my twenty-first birthday. I felt an urge to jump up and take some pictures. At the same time I felt abnormally exhausted, in my legs in particular, and I needed to sit down.

I didn't suspect anything sinister about the weakness in my legs, but it puzzled me. Previously I had always had a lot of energy and had felt an amazing sense of strength and stamina. Even when I was tramping and feeling tired, I always had enough to keep on going. Experiencing weakness was new to me.

Perhaps if the weakness in my legs had been an isolated incident I would not have been so bothered by it — everyone has an off day every now and then, even an energetic young person. But it was not limited to that day. In fact, it had come to characterise the previous year. The summer before this, I had regularly cycled 400 kilometres a week and had done a lot of tramping, all without any significant physical consequences. By the middle of 2005, however, I had become aware of a post-exercise malaise and often experienced weakness in my legs. I had stopped cycling to university every day, leaving my bike sitting largely unused in my room, taking the bus instead. Even then, by the end of the flat 10-minute walk to the bus, my legs would often feel like jelly, sapped of power.

I thought that perhaps the cause of the weakness was simply a lack of training. In November 2005 my friend Thomas and I decided to compete in the Lake Taupo Cycle Challenge as a relay team. I resumed training and enjoyed a period unplagued by fatigue. Nevertheless, my legs still felt weak. Late one afternoon I was out with Thomas, training for the race. Our plan was to do a hill climb on Hilltop Road, behind Manukau City, near Auckland, and head up towards the ridge-running Redoubt Road. The ride up Hilltop Road was always a bit miserable, brutally steep. But, although I rarely enjoyed the ride itself, reaching the top always felt like an accomplishment — the ache in my legs was evidence of progress and growth — and I loved the views of the city and countryside.

As we approached the hill I was determined to push it, to get those legs into shape. I stood up in the saddle to sprint to the top. As the gradient steepened, my legs started to protest, losing strength. I began to feel unstable and wobbly, and my legs struggled to support me as I tried to throw my weight into the cranks. I kept pushing, swerving erratically as I tried to maintain my balance. I reached the top first, unclipped from the pedals and stopped. My legs were so wobbly that I needed the bike to support me. I didn't tell Thomas about this, but hoped the fact of reaching the top first would hide my weakness. Luckily, there was a downhill roll ahead of us.

Despite my best efforts and weeks of training, I could never shake the weakness. The day of the race arrived, and the sprint out of Taupo, across Control Gates Bridge and up the hill to Poihipi Road just about killed me. I wanted to keep up with the pack that led the charge up the hill, to finish my half of the race with the strong riders. Sprinting up the hill, I was thrashing myself, pushing as hard as I could go, but my efforts were not enough to stop me from drifting towards the back of the pack.

Near the top of the hill I realised I had fallen to the back, and that I was going to lose the other riders as they powered on. I wanted to appear strong and athletic, not a straggler. But how could I when my legs were faltering? I thought, slightly panicked. We turned on to Poihipi Road and I knew I wouldn't catch them up — the pack was long gone. I was exhausted, and my legs were already over it. It was a wet day, and a bitterly cold southerly was blowing. I pulled up and stopped, pretending I had cramp, a victim of the weather. Cramp was somehow more excusable than weakness.

I love walking along extended open ridges that offer view lines to distant peaks, all objectives for future trips. I love pulling out the map, plotting routes and identifying features. Engaging with the surrounding topography, drawing your position both from the map and from the landscape, gives a grounding sense of place, of being surrounded and defined by an incomprehensibly large expanse of land. Within this expanse there is a sense of freedom. The sense of your own smallness is thrilling and the world opens up before you, full of possibility and adventure.

But now that sense of possibility and freedom to explore seemed distant, abstracted, as I felt the effects of fatigue and weakness. I felt particularly perplexed by the weakness in my legs. It just seemed so strange.

'What's wrong, Nick?' Dad asked as I struggled to lower myself down the large tussocked steps as we finally descended the sharp little ridge leading to the hut.

'Can you slow down a bit? I'm finding this hard,' I replied. I was frustrated, slightly angry, at lagging behind. It was now late in the day and I just wanted this to be over.

'Sure. It's been a long day, and hot! Perhaps you're a bit dehydrated?'

'Maybe,' I grumped as I put my weight on a fistful of tussock and

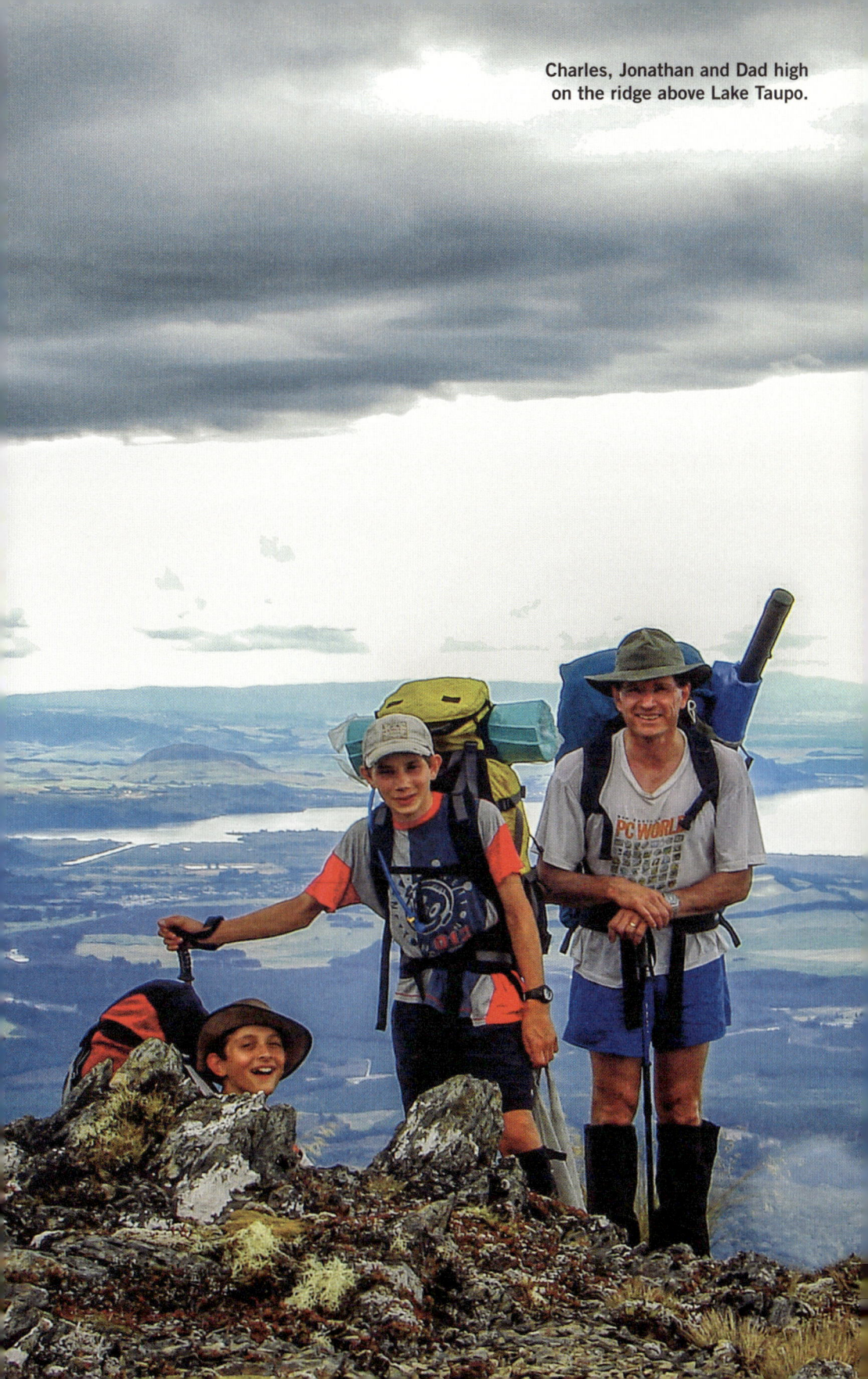
Charles, Jonathan and Dad high on the ridge above Lake Taupo.

dropped, jelly-legged, on to the loose volcanic soil below.

'Do you have a headache?'

'Yeah — a small one.'

'We'll fill up your drink bottle when we get to the hut and I'll dig out a Panadol.'

Several minutes later we crossed a small stream, just a few hundred metres from the hut. The stream was cool and clear, with a deep hole in which you could comfortably swim.

'Oh, Dad! Can we swim here?' Jonathan was bouncing at the thought, his eyes round with excitement. Charles, who had been dragging himself along, suddenly perked up.

'Sure. Let's get to the hut first and get changed,' Dad replied.

The two boys ran ahead, energised by the prospect of a swim. I followed slowly.

The others got into their togs. I knew it would be a lot of fun, but I felt tired. I hardly had the energy to walk back to the stream, much less join in with them. Still, I didn't want to miss out, so I went with them, leaving my togs behind. By the time Dad and I got to the stream the boys were preparing to launch themselves off in a bombing competition. Jonathan was already dripping wet, standing above a bank that dropped deeply into the water.

'Dad! Come and join us! We're doing bombs!' Jonathan shouted, pure joy on his face as he wiped back his long, dripping fringe. Good bombs are, of course, every boy's greatest achievement.

Laughing, Dad joined them on the bank.

'Dad! Watch me!' Charles yelled with great bravado, only to lower himself cautiously into the water with a timid hop.

'Watch out for the sharks!' Dad laughed as he jumped in, grabbing Charles.

Jonathan jumped in beside them, his arms flailing. I watched from my perch on a large boulder, feeling isolated, and sad at not being able to join in.

I pulled out my camera. 'OK, Charlie! Ready? On the count of three: one, two, three!'

Charles launched himself off the edge and I shot a burst, capturing him in mid-flight.

'Now, Joni, your turn! Ready?'

'Yip!'

'Stand closer to the edge! OK? Now: one, two, three!' Another burst.

As it turned out, photographing Jonathan and Charles was fun, a different way to participate in the making of memories. I had them pose, or move, while trying to freeze-frame the action with the click of my shutter.

The next morning the hut was swimming in cloud and the air was condensing on the cobwebs and tussocks. We sat on the veranda in the muted grey light, waiting for the cloud to burn off. I dug a raisin out of my porridge, picked it up and ate it, then looked out into the grey once again.

It was beautiful, even meditative, watching the fog shift. Moment to moment, it moved imperceptibly. However, each time I looked up from my bowl or returned from a snippet of conversation I noticed the grey gaining golden-green fringes with hints of blue as the sun began working its way down the side of the valley.

By nine o'clock we had that blue sky we were waiting for and were ready to get moving. It was going to be a scorching day and I was grateful that we would be walking down the river. There is no track to speak of along the Waipakihi River. At times, in places where the riverbed narrows and deepens, you can find rough tracks that crash through the hardy shrubs and tussock clearings, tracks etched by keen trampers who need to get downstream when the river is running high, or by those who don't want to get their feet wet. We, on the other hand, were all about getting wet, and we used the river as our track, splashing happily as we went.

I enjoyed being in the river — who wouldn't on such a day? Not only was the wet cool a welcome relief from the beating sun, but the Waipakihi Valley was also stunning. The clear mountain water cascaded with increasing force over smooth grey-brown rocks into deep aquamarine pools, shaded by the delicate boughs of the moss-covered beech trees that edge the stream. The beech forest swept upward and on to the peaks of the Kaimanawa Range with a grandeur vaguely reminiscent of the Southern Alps.

As we ambled beneath the peaks, in the water or along the grassy bank, beneath the shade of the beech trees, we passed deep pools where leaves circled slowly, propelled by powerful currents. The increasing force of those currents began to make progress difficult. Stream-walking often requires you to battle the currents, fighting them to stay upright, but as these currents became more powerful we were forced up on the rocky edges of the river flats.

'Damn.' A rock rolled forward beneath my foot. I slipped off, was thrown and stumbled, splashing through the water as I struggled to maintain my balance. I stood knee-deep in the water, dripping, feeling frustrated.

The boys turned round and laughed.

'You all right?' Dad asked.

'Yeah, I just slipped, that's all,' I said. 'Hey, it's twelve. How about we stop for some lunch soon?'

'Good idea. Let's find a nice spot down there,' Dad suggested, pointing downstream to a deeper, slower part of the river where there was a shaded waterhole and a small beach.

It was incredibly hot and I was finding it increasingly difficult both to keep pace and to stay vertical over the rough terrain. Why am I so unfit? I asked myself.

We reached the shaded area beside the river and set down our packs.

'What a spot!'

'I reckon — just beautiful!' Dad replied.

'Can we jump into the water?' Jonathan asked as he took off his shirt.

'Sure! But put on some sunblock first,' Dad told him, digging the tube out of his pack.

I sat and watched the colours on a pool just upstream from our position, enjoying the reflections of the trees on the water. The

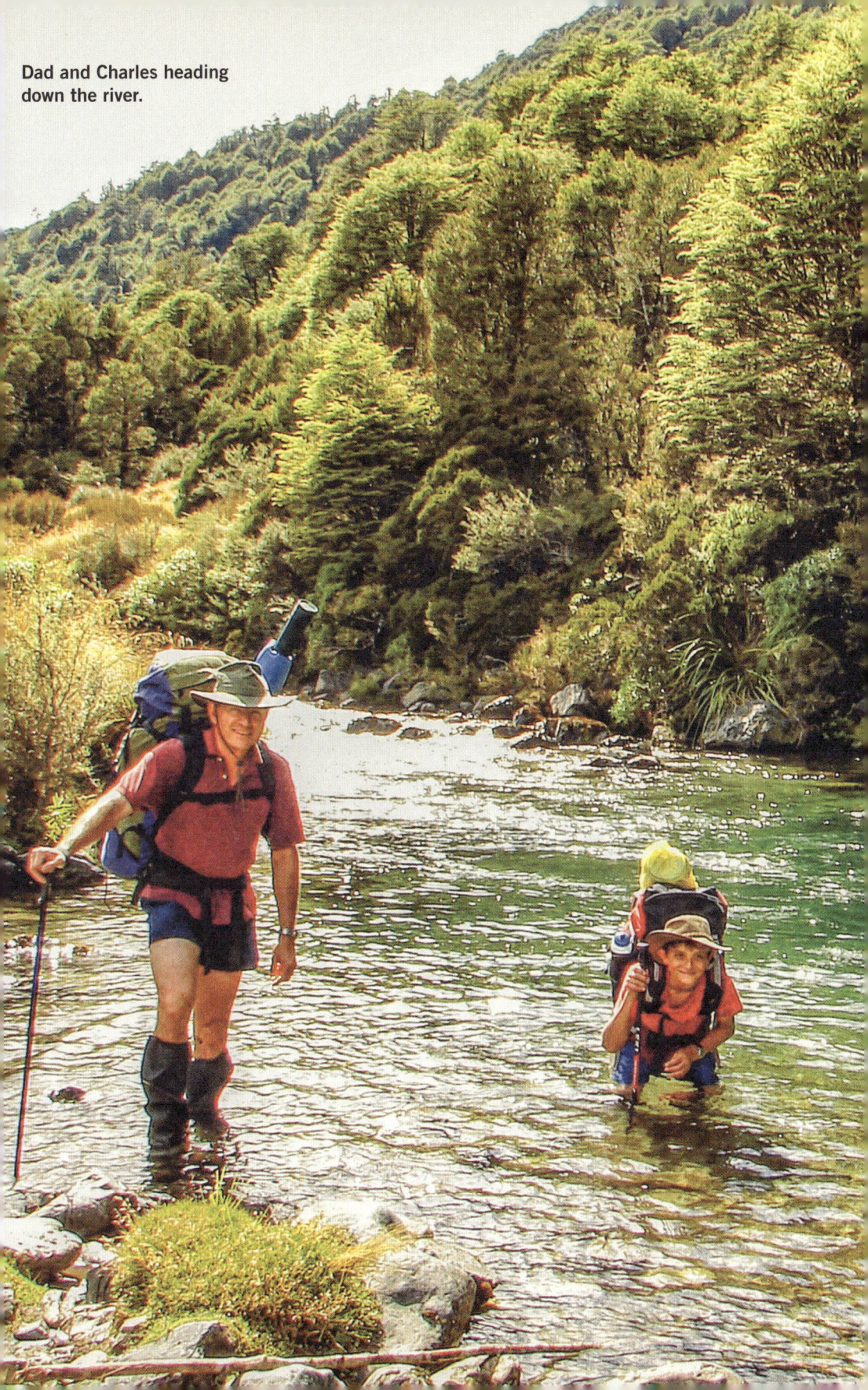
Dad and Charles heading down the river.

moment of peace was abruptly shattered by Jonathan's leaping bellyflop into the water beside me. I jumped out of the way, trying to avoid the wash, and looked downriver. The view downstream was as lovely as the reflections on the water upstream.

There was something profoundly uplifting about that moment, in that particular environment. I am not talking about the superficial sense of pleasure gained through the mere acknowledgement of beauty, but a deeply spiritual sense of peace and contentedness, of wonder and renewal. I knew that this was something I never wanted to stop doing, and that enjoying these reflections of beauty would be key to my continued spiritual and mental wellbeing. I pulled out my camera to capture a sense of the wonder I felt: the subtle ripples of the pool; the movement of the water over the rocks; the softness of the moss on the forest floor, its gentle contours slowly enveloping fallen branches and the tops of the less-worn river rocks.

We ate our lunch and swam, cooling off in the water between mouthfuls, then set off again down the river. There is a point in the valley where the Waipakihi River passes through a narrow gorge, impassable except via a small track that runs over one of the low bluffs. The track was steep and slightly exposed, necessitating a firm grip on the bushes alongside it. My legs felt wobbly and insecure, and the exposed section of the track felt particularly precarious.

After the gorge, the river plains widen, leading to larger areas of loose, rocky riverbed. It was mid-afternoon by the time we reached that point, and again I was feeling increasingly tired. Dad and the boys were often a long way in front of me. The frustrating thing about being behind is that you get caught in a downward spiral of exhaustion. Those who are ahead go for a while then have a break while they wait for you to catch up. You struggle along, pressing on through the fatigue, using the hope of a rest as your motivation. When you finally manage to catch up with them, they have been able to use the rest time to recharge and are raring to go. The moment you sit down beside them they start gathering up their gear and putting on their packs. This affords you only a few seconds of rest before you too have to carry on, still exhausted.

When we were kids, tramping with Dad up to Daly's Clearing Hut in the Kaimai Mamaku Forest Park, or to Pinnacles Hut in Coromandel Forest Park, my sister Fleur and I would often run ahead with our friends. Dad would allow us to go a short distance, to a stream or a track junction, at which point we had to wait for him to catch up. Waiting for Dad at these assigned points was always hard. Fleur and I were invariably bursting with energy and busting to get to the hut, particularly if we had friends with us. We would wait impatiently, then the moment we saw Dad we would bound off to the next point — unless Dad pulled out the scroggin, in which case we were happy to stop. It never occurred to me that Dad, burdened with an 80-litre pack, filled to the brim with everything but our clothes, would need a break.

As a younger man Dad was a successful sprinter, competed internationally, and could run a marathon. As a boy I thought this was the most amazing thing ever, and I found great security in the way he seemed to have an indefatigable endurance. Whether he was working long hours in the office, splitting firewood at the weekend, or taking us for a tramp with a massive pack on his back, Dad always seemed to be unflappable and untiring. To my child's mind, he also seemed to have an amazing way of shouldering all his responsibilities effortlessly, being available for each of us four kids whenever we wanted to talk to him. Without doubt, this and the lives of my wider family had shaped my view of masculinity, and it never crossed my juvenile mind that I might not become all that I admired in Dad: muscular and athletic, a machine that could keep going no matter what.

Now, as I struggled along the rocks beside the Waipakihi River, I became incredibly frustrated. Dad and the boys were significantly ahead of me and had disappeared round a corner, obscured from view by a large clump of toetoe. The tramp had transitioned from enjoyable traipsing to unpleasant slog. Why am I so weak? I asked myself. I rounded the corner and caught sight of the others. They had stopped. I felt hurt and a bit annoyed that I had been left behind, and overwhelmed by the distance I needed to cover to catch up with them — crossing the scoured riverbed seemed impossibly

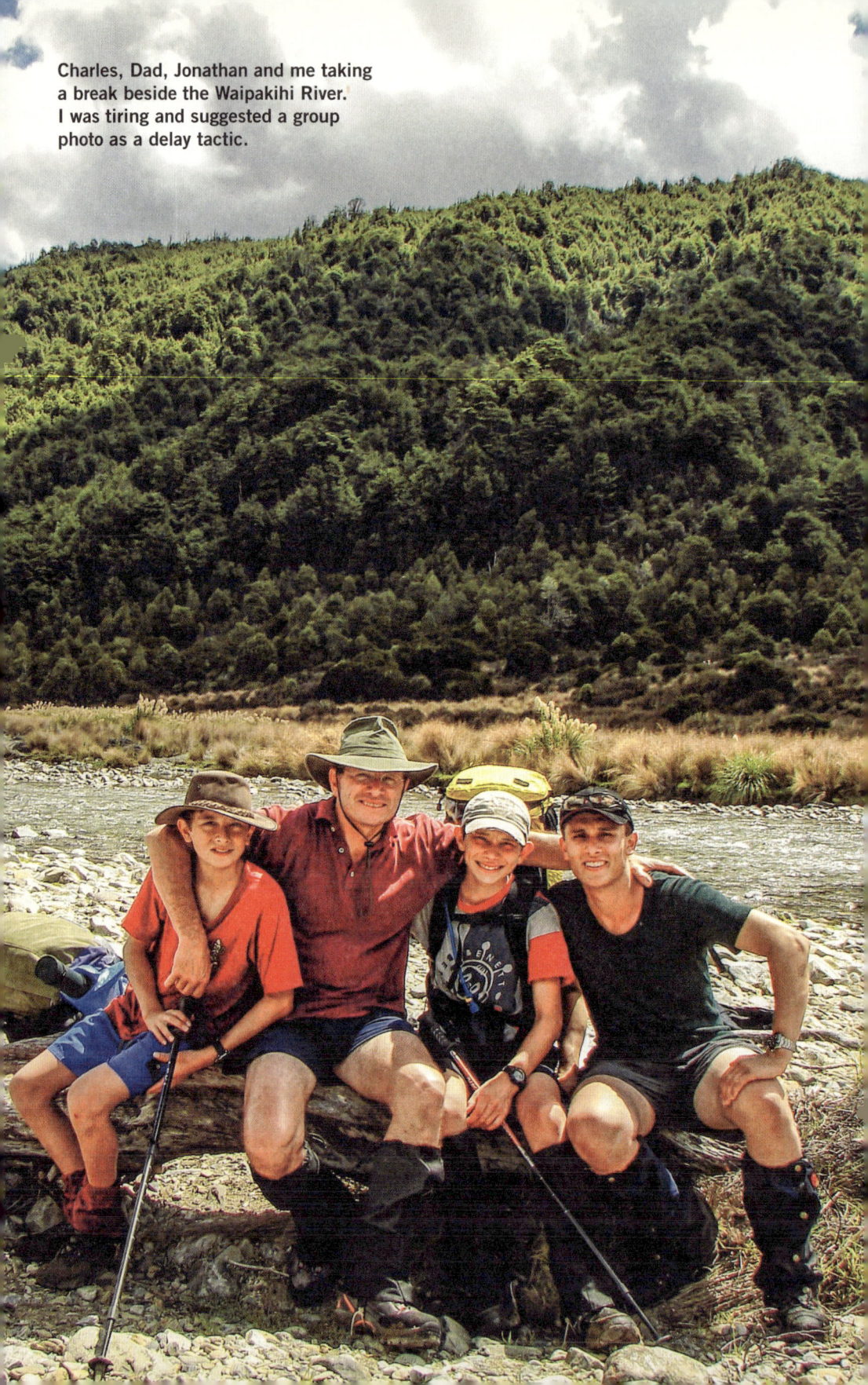
Charles, Dad, Jonathan and me taking a break beside the Waipakihi River. I was tiring and suggested a group photo as a delay tactic.

challenging. I felt like crying, which was alarming and confusing, adding disgust to my feelings of frustration at my lack of performance, for failing to be an unstoppable machine.

I finally caught up with the others. Jonathan started putting on his pack. Charles was evidently a bit tired as well, and seemed determined to sit for as long as possible.

'Yo, Pa, can we take a break? I just need to rest for a few minutes.'

I wanted to appear strong, unperturbed, unemotional. I knew that Dad would not have thought any less of me if I had admitted my weakness, and I knew that there were plenty of perfectly valid expressions of masculinity that did not revolve around athleticism and physical achievement. Nevertheless, I had a certain expectation of myself and was desperate to meet it. I was also desperate for an excuse to delay the progress of the group.

'How about we take a group photo?'

'Sure, good idea.'

Relieved at the prospect of a moment's reprieve, I pulled out my camera and tripod, fiddled around for a bit and walked a little way back upstream to find a suitable angle for the shot.

'OK, go over there and sit on that log,' I shouted.

Dad and the boys headed over to the log, Charles dragging himself somewhat reluctantly.

'Great. Now move to the left so that I can fit in! I mean right. Move right, my left. That's it. Great.'

Charles rolled his eyes in protest.

I took a test shot. It looked good. I turned on the timer, poised my finger over the shutter release and shouted, 'OK, and ten seconds from —' pause — 'now!'

I ran across the rocks towards them, reaching my spot beside the log just as the flashing red light blinked to indicate the photo was being taken. I was sitting again, relieved, aching to rest. I left the camera for a few minutes, enjoying the reprieve, before slowly idling over and packing it up again.

'How much further to go?' Charles moaned.

'Not sure,' Dad replied.

'Not too much longer, I hope,' I said as I pulled the mouth of my pack closed, flipped the lid over and dug the map out of the top.

Dad and I examined the map, looking to the landscape for clues.

'I think that big stream we crossed earlier was this one, Thunderbolt Creek,' Dad said, pointing to a line on the map.

'I think so too, so that must put us about here, just before this sharp elbow in the river, next to this tributary.' I planted my finger on the map. 'We have a couple of kilometres to go, Charlie — another thirty to forty minutes then we are done.'

Charles grunted. I knew how he felt. Knowing that the end is near can make everything harder — the legs more tired, the pack straps more painful, and water-filled boots heavier. My entire body ached, from my neck to my fingertips and toes, every muscle totally spent — or so it felt. With this came a sort of cognitive fog, leaving me feeling slightly dazed and unresponsive. Those last few kilometres dragged, and the jolts and knocks of streambed travel made my head ring.

We finally arrived at the large grassy plain that indicated the beginning of the next day's walk, where the track across the river would take us up and over the Urchin tops and back to where we had started. We'd brought a large blue tarp with the intention of setting up a bivvy.

'Pa, I need to sit down for a bit. I want to help, but I'm not feeling so great.'

'No worries, Nick. We can prepare the bivvy. How do you suggest we do it?'

'Why don't we use the big tree over there, the one with the mossy area beneath it? We could string some rope over those lower branches and down to the ground, then use a branch or log as a post to give it a bit of height.'

'Great idea.'

I sat back and watched, exhausted.

Sitting back is something I find hard to do on a normal day, and even more so on a trip that I've organised. I felt a strong sense of responsibility: I was the one who had chosen the track, organised the trip, and convinced Dad and the boys that sleeping in a bivvy would be fun. Rightly or wrongly, I felt as if the success of the trip was up to me, leaving me feeling guilty about my fatigue.

The unfortunate thing about guilt is that it taints everything. My memory of that evening, as Dad and the boys splashed in the river, built a campfire and cooked dinner, then climbed under the tarp to sleep, is still clouded by the uncomfortable sense that my fatigue was transgressive, a failure to perform to some as yet unarticulated standard.

I just need to train harder, I thought, yet again.

The next morning was overcast, a welcome respite from the heat of the previous two days. We were not in too much of a hurry; the trip up and over the Urchin tops and back to the carpark was not that long — only three to four hours.

Dad had brought his fly-fishing rod and stood in the river for an hour or so, attempting to catch something. I felt a bit better that morning and explored the area with my camera, then the boys and I sat on the bank watching Dad cast his fly into the deeper edges of the river — the side that the great roots of the beech trees ran into — in the hope of luring a trout, but without success.

Finally we packed our gear, crossed the river, and a bit before ten o'clock started heading up the steep spur towards the Urchin tops. It was hard work ascending the ridge, the huge steps and rough-rooted path a bit of a cruel start to the day. I think we all felt it in our quads and glutes, but I was determined not to feel tired and forged ahead of the others, attempting to lead them up the hill.

When I graduated from high school my grandmother gave me a book that would become one of my prized possessions: *Mountaineering: The Freedom of the Hills*. I loved the title, as it encapsulated my feelings about the mountains, and I loved the book. It was filled with information on everything from rock-climbing techniques and how to read the weather to instructions on choosing the right type of crampons and performing first-aid. In short, it was a

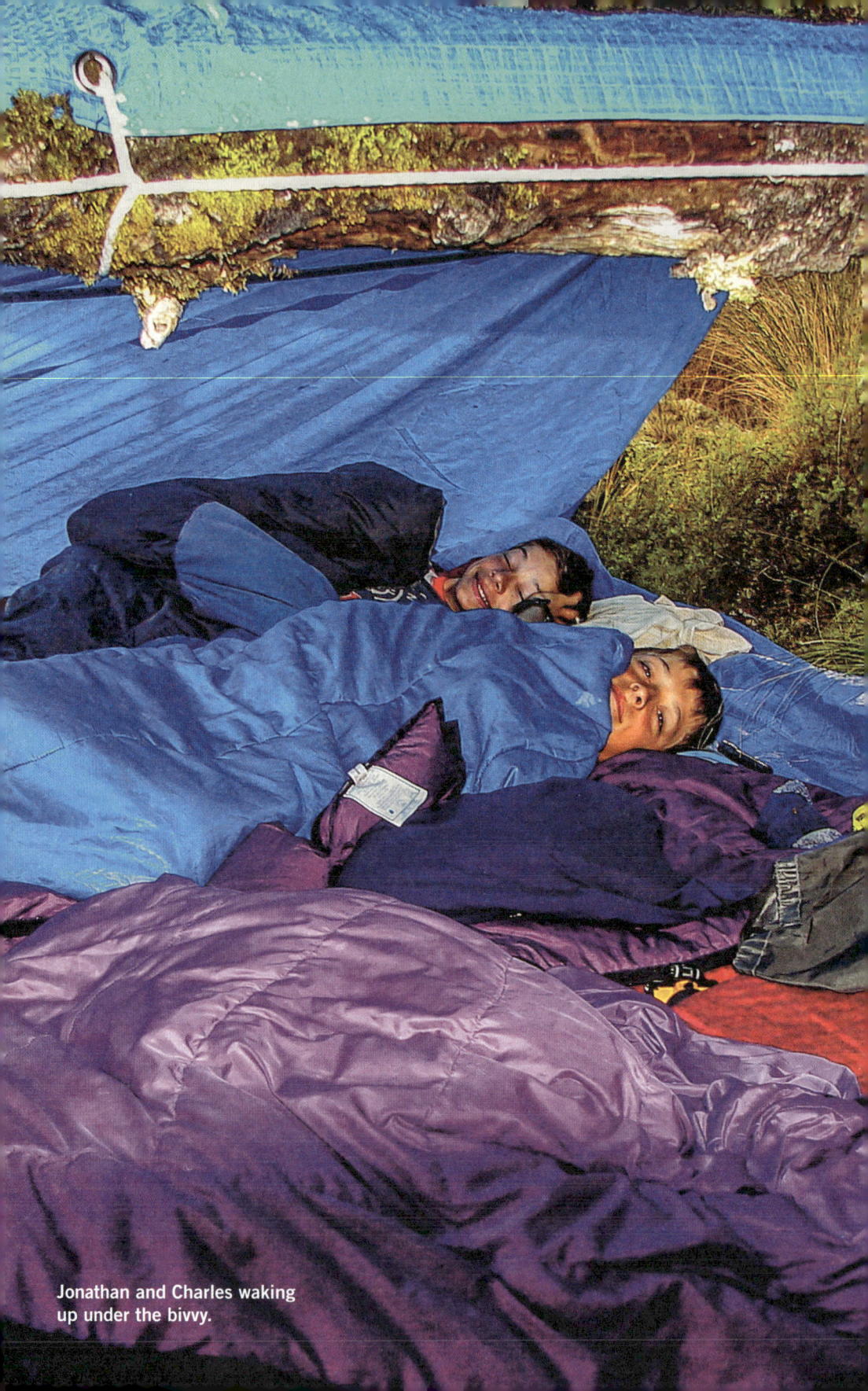
Jonathan and Charles waking up under the bivvy.

climber's bible, and I read it from cover to cover.

On the flyleaf, Granny had written an excerpt from Henry Longfellow's poem 'The Ladder of St Augustine':

> The heights by great men reached and kept
> Were not attained by sudden flight,
> But they, while their companions slept,
> Were toiling upward in the night.

This inscription had become something of a motto for me, and the words remained fresh in my mind as a type of inheritance, a nugget of truth passed down. I had seen Granny just a week earlier, fading quickly as her body lost its battle with cancer. I wanted to be a great man and to achieve those mountain heights. Therefore, I thought, I must toil, I must push on, I must strive. Rest is for the wicked.

After a while the track up the spur towards the Urchin tops flattens off and begins to follow a narrow ridge that leads into the open tops. We had been travelling through beautiful, dense beech forest — my favourite. There is a certain gracefulness about the fineness of beech forest, the way the light filters through the canopy, catching on the tiny leaves. There is a softness, too, particularly when the forest floor is covered with a carpet of fine, bright-green moss. Then you reach that transitional band in the vegetation, the point where the beech trees are stunted, almost miniature, just before your head pops out above the canopy and the incredible views become apparent.

I was blown away by the views that day as the Waipakihi River stretched out 300 metres below us, laced with tussock grasslands and forest. As we stood on the rocky outcrops of the mountain's ridge the base of the clouds was only a few metres above us. We stopped for a few handfuls of scroggin and to admire the spectacular view.

I felt exhilarated and thrilled. But I was also beginning to feel profoundly tired. Again, I pulled out my camera, took some photos, and as a delaying tactic suggested we take another group shot. This always takes a few minutes, between fiddling around with the tripod, getting people organised and setting up the camera.

After grabbing the shot we moved on and up along the ridge, wisps of cloud racing past, onward into the mist. I tried to divert the feeling of excitement and the thrill of walking into the clouds into energy for the ascent. I led the charge again, determined not to let tiredness get the better of me.

It was windy on the tops, we were hungry, and I was still tired. As we neared the summit we decided to shelter behind a small bank in order to secure some protection from the wind. As we sat on the loose scree Dad pulled out the salami and a thickly sliced loaf of slightly stale bread. I felt useless as I watched Dad do all the work. The sense of failed responsibility was strong: I was the one who should be doing this. I know, absolutely, that this sense of responsibility is misguided, that there is nothing wrong with other people helping, but under the weight of a compounding sense of inadequacy it was difficult to relinquish that role.

I pulled out my map and examined it — that, at least, was something I did well.

'We've only got three kilometres to go,' I announced.

Charles let out a huff of air. 'Man! How long will that take?'

'Not too long, bro — only about another hour and a half or so.' Then, turning to Dad, I asked, 'Hey, Pa, so what shall we do about the car?'

'Dunno. What are your thoughts?'

'Well, we could walk back on the road, but that would be another four or five k's. I wonder if, when we get to the top of the final ridge, we could duck down the hill from the point where the track veers left —' I traced the route on the map with my finger — 'go through the bush to the road that runs to the power station, and then, at the Waikoko camping site, cross the river and head up the bank to the carpark. What do you think?'

'Sounds a bit hard,' Dad replied with a grimace.

'But you can follow the power lines through the first section, then there is a nice ridge you can follow up from the river to the carpark.'

'Yeah, but it's pretty steep country! Look at the contour lines as you head down to the river then up the bank.'

'True. But otherwise we have to walk for ages.'

'Well, I'm happy to do that. We might even be able to catch a ride. Would you like me to get the car and you stay with the boys?'

Jonathan and Charles both looked fairly nonchalant about the whole thing.

'No, no. I'm happy to do it.' I refused to lose yet another point of usefulness or purpose.

'Are you sure?'

'Yes.' I was adamant.

Coming down off the tops, I felt a sense of relief. Normally I don't look forward to the end of a tramp; instead, I feel a certain heaviness as I come to the end, knowing that the reality of life will soon crash in on my escapist outdoor paradise. But this time I was looking forward to the end in a shattered, I-can't-wait-for-this-to-be-over kind of way.

As we neared the end of the track, approaching the Urchin tops carpark, an English couple who had been at Waipakihi Hut caught up with us. We could hear them as they approached behind us, fit and fast. We stepped aside to let them pass.

'Gidday!' the guy said.

'Oh, hi! How are you guys going?' Dad asked them.

'Good. We camped at the top of the grass clearing last night — how about you?'

'Yes, we camped up there too, underneath the big beech tree.'

'Ah yes,' the man replied. 'We wondered if someone stayed there last night. Looked like a great spot! We saw it this morning when we walked past.'

'It was a good spot,' Dad agreed.

'And we made a fire!' Jonathan added.

The couple smiled. 'Cool!' the woman said.

'Hey, how are you guys getting back to the Umukarikari carpark?' I asked. I knew they would be facing the same problem.

'We brought two cars and have a car parked here. We'll drive around and pick the other up. Why? Do you need a lift?'

I suddenly felt very relieved.

'That would be great,' I replied, looking at Dad.

'Yeah, perhaps Nick or I could get a lift?' Dad asked.

'Sure. But, I have to warn you, it's a small car and it will be a tight fit with our packs.'

'Oh, I'm sure we can make it work,' I replied, smiling. 'I don't mind squeezing in — it's not too far and it would just be great to get a lift.'

We rounded the corner and the carpark came into view. Dad turned to me. 'How are you feeling, Nick?' he asked quietly.

'Not great. Still pretty shattered.' I needed to be honest.

'Would you like me to get the car?'

I paused. I really did not want to give up my last opportunity to be useful. But I was just so tired.

'OK. I'll stay here with the boys,' I said.

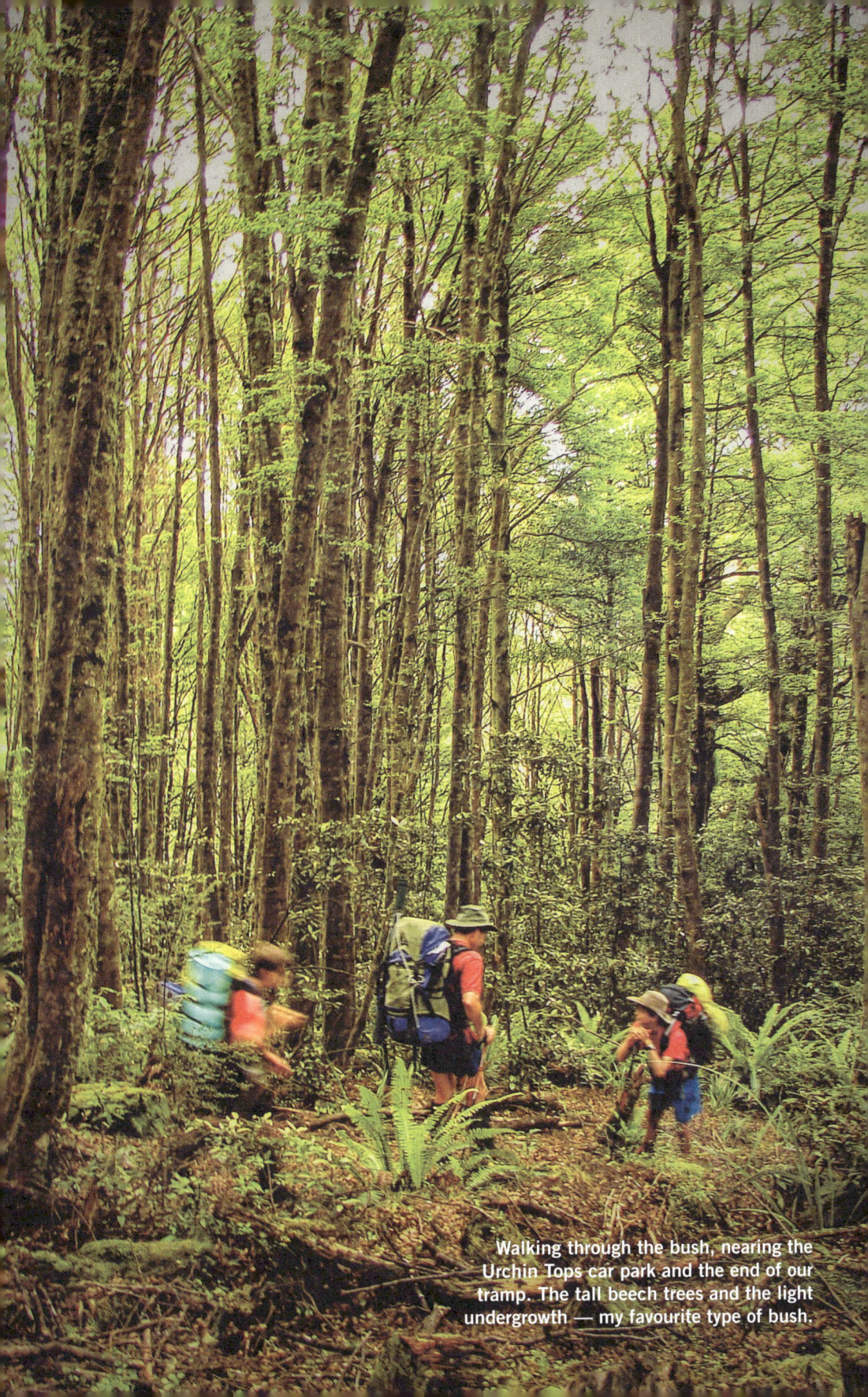

Walking through the bush, nearing the Urchin Tops car park and the end of our tramp. The tall beech trees and the light undergrowth — my favourite type of bush.

Night-time fog over the mouth of the Waikato River.

CHAPTER 3
THE BIG CRASH

▲▲▲

March 2006
Taupo, New Zealand

It was a few days before 24 March, and my alarm was set for 5.30 a.m. It was an old analogue thing with a blaring wail that could be heard from the other side of the house, similar in tone and volume to the alarm you'd expect to hear on a submarine at the moment an attack is imminent. Fleur had given me the alarm about ten years before as a birthday present and it had served me well, never failing to wake me up. Its only downside, however, was that it was difficult to set with precision. It was thus hard to predict when exactly the alarm would go off — much like a naval attack. That was OK most of the time, and I just factored it in.

On this morning the alarm went off and I crawled out of bed feeling particularly tired and groggy, as if I had been woken from a deep sleep. I fumbled for the light and climbed into the cycling jersey and Lycra shorts I'd carefully laid out the night before. My bike, which lived in my room, was all set up and ready to go, with water, lights and pump. I loved my road bike, which I'd custom-built. I'd been working at a bike shop for a couple of years and had been able to amass a collection of parts that together amounted to a really great bike. It was fantastic to ride: stiff, responsive, with a beautifully formed aerodynamic frame.

I was training for the Rotorua–Taupo Flyer, a 100-kilometre cycle

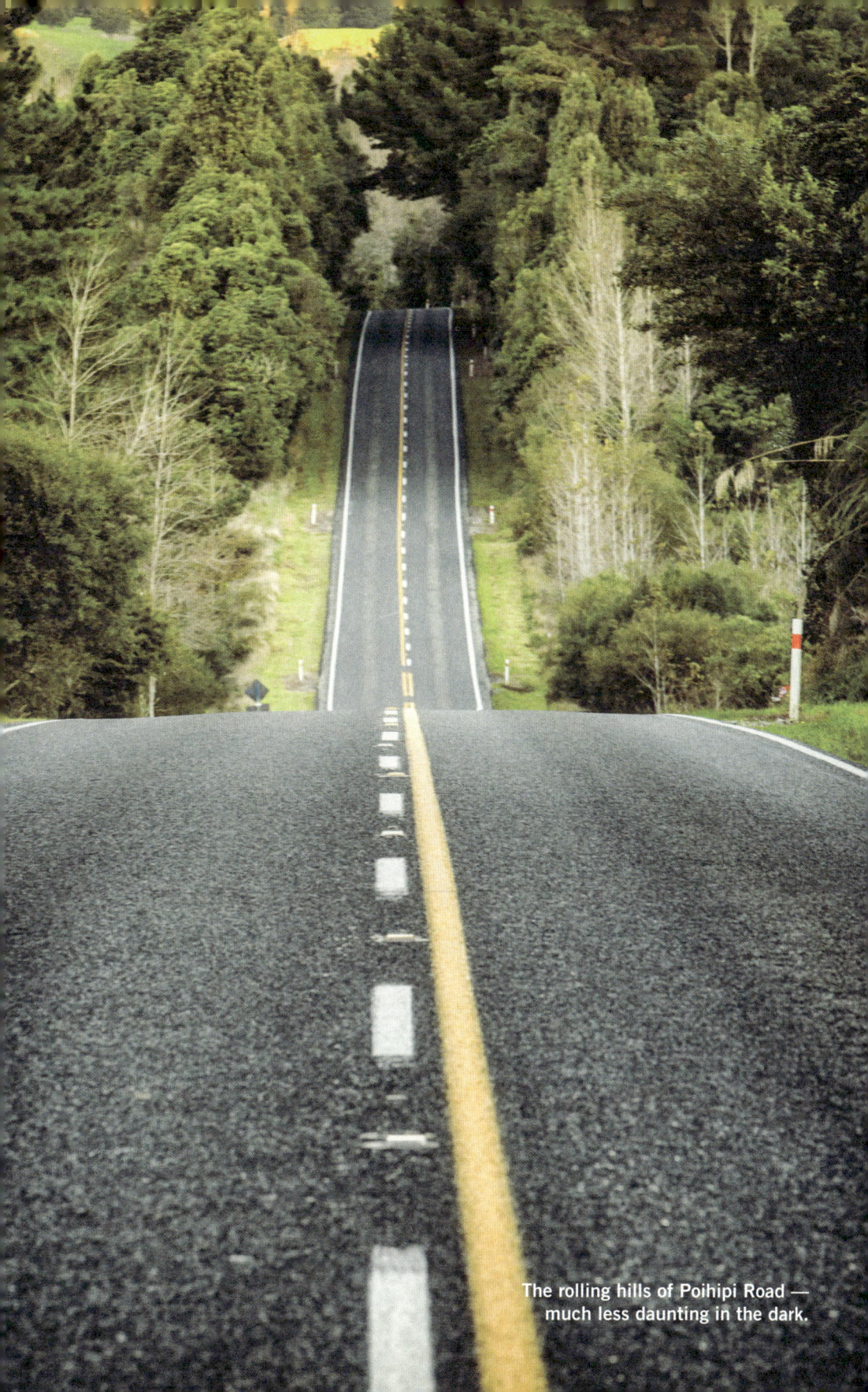
The rolling hills of Poihipi Road — much less daunting in the dark.

race that was coming up at the beginning of April. I often tried to get out early, before work, and get a good ride in. I had every intention of doing this most mornings, but often I would wake feeling oddly fatigued and wouldn't go. As a result I'd given up hope of being competitive in the race, but I also knew I could complete it without too much difficulty. Having set aside the pressure of competing, I was focused more on just looking good, on being able to give a better-than-average performance across the whole course, and finishing strongly, without too much huffing and puffing. After all, I did not want to look like some unfit toff on a fancy bike, nor did I want to be overtaken on a hill by a school kid.

It was a bit cold as I walked out of the front door with my bike. 'If you have a bike, get on it at night / and go to the top of the Brooklyn Hill,' I muttered to myself, quoting a Jenny Bornholdt poem, 'Instructions for how to get ahead of yourself while the light still shines'. I pulled the zip of my jersey up to my chin, drawing my windproof vest tightly round my neck, closed the door quietly and walked carefully down the concrete steps in my cleated shoes.

A light mist hung about, seemingly motionless as it rose out of the Waikato River, blanketing our street in fog. The house sat just above the Taupo harbour, at the mouth of the Waikato River, and mist was a common occurrence on cold mornings. Climbing the hill above Taupo generally takes you above the fog, which you can see snaking along the river valley, leaving a tongue that protrudes out on to the lake.

At the end of the driveway, in the yellow, fog-lit fan of a streetlight, I thought of Jenny's advice:

> *As you come to each light*
> *you will notice a figure*
> *racing up behind.*
> *Don't be scared*
> *this is you creeping up on yourself.*

It was cool, quiet and dark — peculiarly quiet and dark. This would be the morning to get creeped out — ghosts in the dark mist racing up behind. Good thing I'm escaping into the country, I thought, smiling, unwilling to see my shadow. I looked at my watch, the glowing hands indicating 35 minutes past. I'd got out quickly this morning, I thought.

It's a bit of a slog, beginning the ride with a push up Norman Smith, cold legs protesting at the gradient. Once you get on to Poihipi Road it's not so bad. You follow the ridge for a short time, heading out of town, then you are rewarded with a brilliant downhill section that edges the Craters of the Moon thermal area. It's a great little stretch of road, with good views — when it is not so dark — and heavy with the smell of sulphur. There's nothing like a good whiff of sulphur on a cold, damp morning.

There were almost no cars, and I was able to cut the corners down the hill, something I rarely got to do because of the traffic. It's great when you can ride the clean, firm surface of the centre of the road, away from the loose gravel and shards of glass. On a clean surface you can really lean into the corners, taking them hard and fast. And the great thing about doing it in the dark is that the headlights of any vehicles give you good warning, enabling you to get on the right side of the road before they reach you. I would never try cutting corners like that in the light of day — it would be too risky.

Which got me thinking. Normally by this point of my early-morning ride the sky was beginning to light up the horizon. As I hit the bottom of the hill and pedalled quickly in an effort to maintain as much momentum as possible on the next uphill, it also struck me as odd that the lights on the geothermal drilling rig beside the road were so bright beneath the pitch-black horizon.

I looked at my watch again. I could see the faint glow of the minute hand: 45 minutes past the hour. Earlier, I had assumed it was after 5 a.m., but now, as I slogged up the next hill, I realised that I had not paid attention to the hour hand. I was standing, out of my saddle now, plugging my way up the hill on a high gear, choosing a gentle cadence. Forty-five minutes past what, I wondered. I dropped a few gears and put my watch in front of the light attached to my handlebars:

4.45 a.m.! Damned alarm clock!

The idea of turning round and going back to bed did cross my mind. But I was well awake now, and I decided that I might as well continue, enjoying the cool and quiet. There is a special, slightly magical, aspect to riding in the pitch dark. The moist morning air is refreshing as it fills your lungs and glides over your face.

The light from my single halogen bulb provided me a bubble of brightness of around 10 to 12 metres. Operating out of a bubble of light is great, especially when there are lots of hills; being unable to see the top when you are slogging up a long, steep section of road is a huge psychological help and makes the ride feel less daunting, more enjoyable. When you can't see much more than the road and the subtly illuminated grass or bush verge, you fall into a kind of trance, following the thick white line as the light dances to and fro across the road, punctuated by the lichens and mosses, colourful interludes on the less trodden edges of the black tarmac. To my tired mind — and it *was* tired that morning — the rhythm and blur of the line and lichen were most hypnotic, lulling me into a slightly dazed plod. But it only took a bump or a small fallen branch to jolt me out of it, making me pay more attention to the road.

Getting to the top of a hill, it was hard not to pull over, turn off the light, grab a drink, catch my breath, and look up at the stars. A good few kilometres out of town and away from the light pollution, the stars were increasingly defined, sharper and brighter.

When I was a bit younger, riding at night had been one of my favourite things to do after a long day studying. I would often go out at 10 or 11 p.m. and cycle for a couple of hours before going to bed. Back then, I had loads of energy and that kind of activity never fazed me. We lived in Drury, South Auckland, and one of my favourite spots was the top of the Ararimu hills, up to the old macrocarpa tree, just past Otto Road. Ararimu Road travels for a time along a ridge that gives you sweeping views of Auckland and the Waitemata Harbour. On a clear night I would look out on a field of fiery stars, flickering above and below in the innumerable street and house lights. It was generally pretty quiet up there, and it was a great spot to rest for a

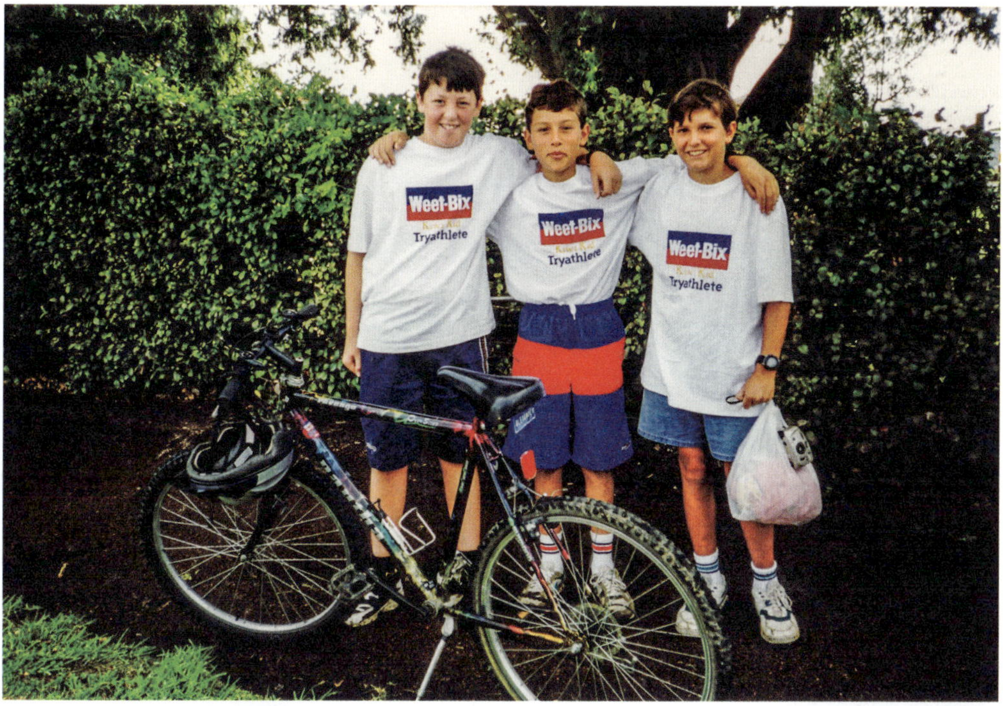

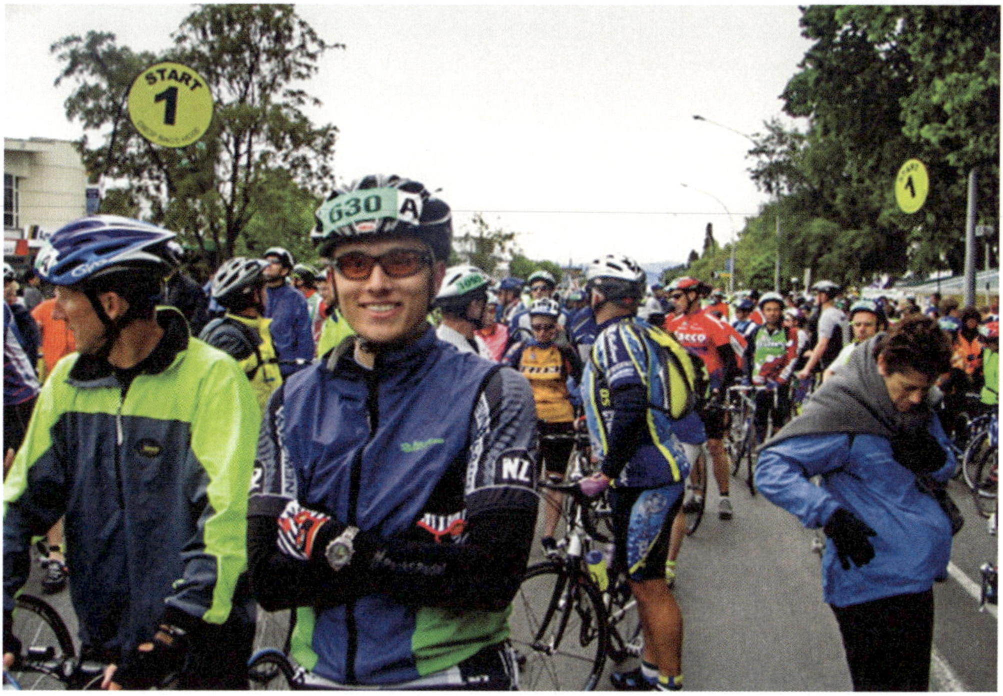

Top to bottom: Me with my mates Alexander and Joshua after completing the Weet-Bix Tryathlon in 1997, when I was 12 years old; Me in my favourite New Zealand Cycle Team jersey, waiting to start the Lake Taupo Cycle Challenge in 2005, aged 20.

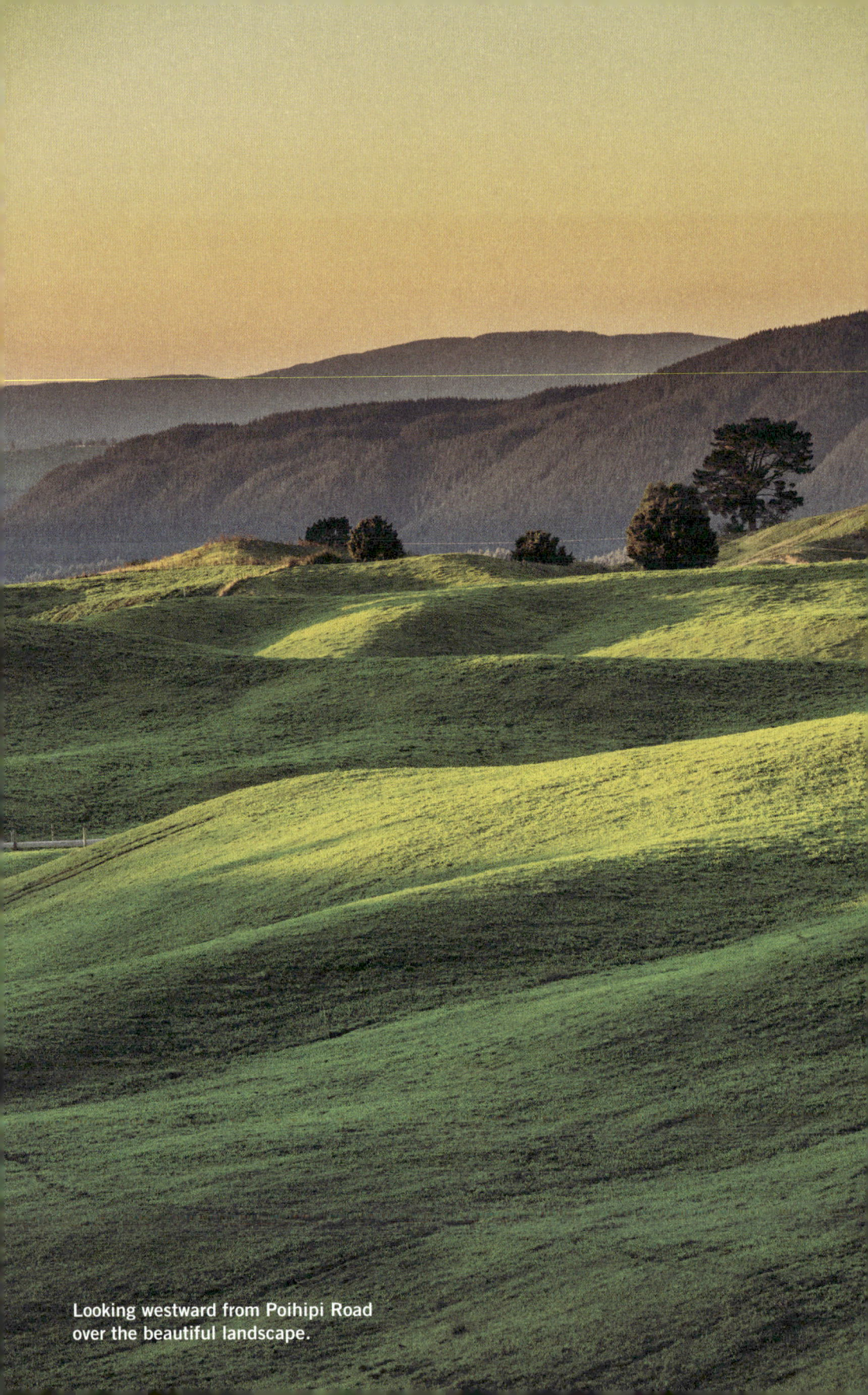
Looking westward from Poihipi Road over the beautiful landscape.

moment, gather my thoughts, and prepare for a fast, eye-watering descent back down the hill.

I continued in the silence of the early morning, enjoying the ride. I was pushing it up the hills, driving my legs to what seemed the point of total fatigue, trying to work my body into shape, but then I would take it easy going down, coasting, in an effort not to wear my body out too much. It was around the 25-kilometre mark that I started to feel really tired. I slowly wheeled over into the tungsten glow of the streetlight near the lonely red-brown farm shed that sits on the corner of Poihipi and Tirohanga roads, at the turn-off to Mokai Marae.

The sky was just beginning to brighten, the horizon sitting below a lighter blue, just enough to give definition to the surrounding landscape and ridges that lay to the west, stretching out for miles. I had never stopped there before, but I had driven past it often enough and I'd always liked it as a stretch of road. I unclipped my feet from the pedals and stopped. My legs were hammered, jelly. I decided to rest for a few minutes, and pulled out a muesli bar to have a quick snack.

By this stage I was deep into dairying country, with its shelter belts and bush blocks. I love this kind of landscape. I find the openness of the land inviting and engaging, imbued with mystery, hints of its past greatness signalled in the massive grey logs that lie rotting on the edges of some of the bush blocks. I also find those hints of the past slightly melancholic, a fading echo of a landscape cleared by our ancestors for gain, calling to be rescued from its decay.

But now wasn't the time to muse on such things. I was getting cold. I stuffed the muesli-bar wrapper into my back pocket and rubbed my gloved hands together. I thought about continuing for another few kilometres to reach State Highway 32 and the end of Poihipi Road — I had plenty of time — but I felt tired. The road would be mostly downhill, and the thought of having to come all the way back up was not appealing. I felt bad that I was contemplating the possibility of turning back. Had I been cycling just 18 months earlier, my younger self would have jibed me with a friendly tease, pushing me to just do it, to finish it off, to complete the road.

'Just think how pleased you will be to have reached the end of the road. It will bug you forever if you don't finish it: you know it will. Come on, just do it,' he would have said.

I knew that it would bug me — it still does, just a bit — but I had a day's work at the prawn farm ahead of me and I knew I would need energy for that. But then, I had woken up at around 4.20, I reasoned. Let's not forget that.

▲▲▲

'Hi, Mum, could you come and pick me up from work? I'm not feeling great — I think I might have a tummy bug.'

'Darn. Do you want me to come over now and get you?'

'No, it's only an hour until the end of the day and I should be able to finish it off. I really want to tidy up before I leave anyway. The mess will be enormous tomorrow if I don't.'

'Are you sure?'

'Yeah, I'll be OK. But can you bring the four-wheel-drive when you do come? I have my bike with me.'

'Yip, sure. I'll see you at four.'

I put my phone back in my pocket and took another bucket of water from the pond. I was working at the Huka Prawn Park, supervising visitors as they fished for prawns in the large geothermal pools — as silly as it sounds, it was quite a fun job.

It had been a beautiful day. The sun was out, and every now and then tufts of low cloud rolled across the sky, helped along by a light breeze. Clouds were a godsend on a day like this, giving moments of reprieve from the sun that reflected off the glaring surfaces of the water and the white pumice soil. Still, the best thing about a bright day was that it guaranteed more people — and I enjoyed a busy day with lots of people. Visitors would rock up to my little hut and show me their tickets, at which point I would present them with the tools of the trade: a bamboo rod with a tiny hook and a couple of metres of trace, a pottle of finely cut squid pieces for bait, and a bucket of ice in which they could collect their catch. I loved the interaction with the clients, particularly showing them the art of catching prawns, which actually involves a fair amount of technique. From there, they would drift slowly along the edges of the pond or sit beneath the umbrellas as they waited for the first bites on their lines.

It was the desire for more people contact that had taken me to the Huka Prawn Park in the first place. The previous year, 2005, I had been studying electronic and computer engineering at the Manukau Institute of Technology (MIT). I was two years into my degree but I was not enjoying it as much as I had hoped. I wanted to do something different. I would often talk to Dad about my frustrations, asking him what he thought I should do.

We'd had one memorable phone conversation about nine months earlier, on a wet and blustery June evening. I'd just walked home in the rain from the bus, I was cold, and my shoes were wet. My legs hurt, and they felt like jelly as I walked up and down the footpath outside the house where I was boarding with family friends, Val and Trevor. I wanted to sit down, to rest. I was confused about the state of my legs, and by the fact that I was crying as I spoke to Dad.

It was dark, and I looked over the front gate towards the living-room windows. I knew the fire would be burning in the hearth, that I could get warm and dry, sit on the couch and rest. Yet at the same time I felt profoundly alienated from that warmth and rest. I loved Val and Trevor, and I knew that if I had walked into the living room right then they would have tried to help me. But I felt too ashamed of crying to go back inside. And how could we even begin to look for a solution when I could not articulate the overwhelming sense of agitation that I felt inside. I seemed to be caught up in a process of physical and emotional change that I was unable to control. Something was definitely wrong, but I had no idea what it was, and that scared me.

I thought that perhaps Dad could help me.

'I just can't do it anymore, Dad! I just can't! It will kill me.'

There was silence as I sobbed.

'I understand it must be hard, Nick.'

'Dad, I don't love it anymore. I mean, it's a great place to study and I enjoy engineering, but only as a broad intellectual pursuit. All the nitty-gritty details and circuit theory is just so boring.'

'I can see that, but all courses of study have parts that are boring. I mean, I didn't enjoy the tax law paper I took, but I needed to do it to become a qualified accountant. Sometimes we just need to learn these boring things to get qualified.'

I knew Dad was right, but I had not reached a point of resolution. I dived deeper.

'But it's not just about that. Engineering crushes me relationally and spiritually. And life should be so much more than that, you know? If engineering was my thing, shouldn't this be feeding and exciting me? And it's not doing this. That's why I want to change and do something else.'

'In what way do you feel it is crushing you spiritually and relationally?'

'Well, designing, constructing and diagnosing electronic circuits for the rest of my life will be soul destroying. I just can't do it. Ugh! I feel so frustrated right now!' I was finding it hard to breathe. 'I need to be working with people — and I don't mean people who design, construct, diagnose electronic circuits. I can't tell you how much I wish that a circuit could talk, that I could diagnose something that was living, dynamic. In engineering you only design and work with dead stuff!'

'Nick, I understand,' Dad tried to reassure me. 'But who's to say that those things won't come with time, once you get a job? I think you'd be best to finish your degree and then look at moving into a field that involves lots of people contact. And, Nick, you are a gifted problem-solver — that is where your skills clearly lie. And your interests have always been in the sciences. I just don't think you would enjoy a job in marketing, human resources, or some role like that.'

'Look, I totally agree. That's why I want to do medicine. There is that guy, Mavs, in my class who is transferring to med school next year. He is exactly like me — fed up with circuits and stuff. And people are systems — living, talking systems — that I could use my problem-solving skills on. And it is still a science. I don't see why I wouldn't be good at that too?

'I mean, let's say you walk into the room coughing. Imagine how cool it would be to read all your vital information, listen to your chest, and be able to say, "Your problem is this; take that and you will get better." Can you imagine how gratifying that would be? People would actually appreciate it, and as a GP you would form relationships with people. It would be technically challenging, relationally stimulating, and gratifying. That's the kind of stuff I want to be doing, instead of farting around with bloody circuits, replacing resistors or blown capacitors, trying to get the stupid thing to work. You know, I thought I could change lives as an engineer. But you just can't! In medicine you can, though.'

'I do understand what you mean, Nick,' Dad said. 'That's why I can't do pure accounting. The numbers bore me and I need to have people contact too. But I still had to study boring old accounting to get to this point.

'At the end of the year you will be halfway through your degree, and Mum and I think it would be best if you completed it. That will give you a great base to fall back on, if you need to. And then you can always do a graduate diploma in something. Anyway, medicine is going to be a whole ton of nitty-gritty information too: think about having to memorise all the names of bones, all the names of drugs, and all the information about chemical pathways and stuff.'

I knew Dad was right, but I did not feel as if I understood my situation any better. In fact, I felt more confused. If my current course of study was not the root of my problems, what was? The prospect of another two years like this was crushing. I felt trapped and powerless. Then there were the tears. What 20-year-old guy cries to his dad? But I couldn't help it. I just seemed to be driven to tears so easily. What was going on?

It was a few months after this that I became aware that it might be possible to study cheaply in the USA. As a teenager I had dreamed of studying nuclear physics and mechanical engineering at the University of Illinois, and the prospect of a change of scenery was exciting. I thought that maybe the added dimension of overseas travel would make the rest of my engineering studies more enjoyable — or, at the very least, bearable. I decided to apply for a student visa for the US, with the aim of beginning my studies there the following September, the start of the American university year.

When it came to choosing a university, I didn't really think through the process very carefully. I thought, somewhat naively, that wherever I went the experience would be pretty much the same. In the end I chose a university in Greenville, South Carolina. I'd met a few people who went there, it sounded a fun place to be, and the tuition fees were cheaper than in a lot of other places. After completing the final semester of 2005 at MIT, I decided to take a break from study and get a job to pay for my US adventure. This was how I came to be working at the Huka Prawn Park.

At the end of each day, as the fishing wound down, I had to clean the fishing areas — my least favourite part of the job. I would clear off the grime, dust and bird poo that had accumulated over the day, and collect any buckets that had been left empty. Then there was the job of picking off all the sun-baked squid bits that had been distributed over the decks and tables surrounding the pond. This was often a challenge after a nice hot day. I would then repair any rods that had been broken, replacing lost hooks and traces. I had been just about to begin this process when I called Mum to ask her to pick me up.

I sloshed the bucket of water over the deck around my little hut. The water shot along the grooves in the wooden decking, off the end of the deck, and back into the pond below. I picked up the big hard-bristle broom and scrubbed, the water splashing brown against the pickets supporting the safety bannister, loaded with a day's worth of shoe-borne dust and dirt. I felt sick but I kept scrubbing until it was clean. I'd lower the bucket on a rope into the water, fill it and draw it back up again, ready to rinse off the section of deck I had just cleaned.

Another wave of nausea came over me. They were increasing in intensity but I wanted to complete the job. I was annoyed at suddenly feeling so ill, and frustrated that it was impeding my work. Not only that, but Dad's parents were down from Auckland, and I had been looking forward to hanging out with them after work.

As I walked round the edge of the pond, taking down umbrellas and picking up buckets, I wondered what was wrong. Maybe I'd succumbed to some sickness because I was now dealing with so many people each day, and was perpetually tired. I was working seven days a week, attempting to hold down four jobs: I worked at the prawn farm from Thursday to Sunday, as a draughtsman and designer at an engineering firm from Monday to Wednesday, I had just picked up a job as a waiter, doing a couple of evenings a week at a local restaurant, and then, in between all that, I had a freelance job developing a commercial website.

I felt suffocated by the awareness that something was not right, but I was convinced that round the next corner, beyond the next goal, everything would come right and I would be able to find that state of restfulness I longed for. I knew that I was struggling to keep up physically, but I figured that if I pushed myself until I got to the States then perhaps everything would work out and I would be able to rest and recover once I got there. This mindset was driving me into the ground, pushing me to a constant state of exhaustion and stress. I relied heavily on energy drinks to get myself through the day.

As if trying to keep up with four jobs was not enough pressure, there was also the stress of applying for my US student visa and sitting the standardised university entrance exams. The visa application was a headache: all the different statements, letters and photocopies that you had to supply in triplicate; all the forms you had to fill out by hand; all the criteria you needed to meet. In addition to all of this, and working to earn the $20,000 needed to meet the application criteria, there were the exams: the SAT tests that are required for admission to most undergraduate programmes in the US, and an English proficiency test. It was an incredible amount of work, and I hoped it would pay off.

Perhaps if I had cared less about my academic and physical performance I would not have reached this point. I felt as if both my self-worth and my socially defined worth were determined by my ability to achieve. For this reason, I could not tolerate weakness in myself and could not bear the thought of being perceived to be stupid, weak or non-athletic. I felt compelled to excel at everything I put my hand to. For example, I had to excel in my entrance exams, otherwise I felt as if I would lose legitimacy as a person. I had to cycle long and hard, even if I was dying on the inside.

Previous levels of performance had become my accepted norm, the bar to which I compared myself. I struggled to be content with a 50-kilometre bike ride along Poihipi Road, or a 50-kilometre round trip up and over the famously gruelling Hatepe Hill. When I was younger I used to cycle 100 kilometres on a Sunday afternoon just for fun. I always felt as if I should be performing better, pushing harder, and that my weakness and fatigue was a flaw, something to be kept hidden, something to feel ashamed of.

Meanwhile the silent but aggressive undertow of physical deterioration was dragging me towards breaking point. During my first year of study, in 2004, I had begun wetting my pants. I could not understand why my bladder was not working properly, and I reasoned that perhaps it was just part of growing up. I had not told anyone about this: I was 19, and it was far too embarrassing to even broach such a subject. Initially the wet spots were the size of a 50-cent coin, but they had grown to the point where I had to pad my undies with a wad of toilet paper to absorb the spillage. Then there was the worsening weakness in my legs, the tremor in my hands, and the increasing levels of fatigue. It was a storm waiting to happen. I just did not realise it.

I had just finished cleaning up when Dad arrived at 4 p.m. on the dot. I walked down towards the car and saw that Grandma and Papa were with him. I tried to appear upbeat as I greeted them. They were obviously concerned, and while it was really great to see them I felt self-conscious, even slightly embarrassed, about having to be picked up. I knew they would be entirely understanding, nevertheless the process of putting my bike in the car, an action that implicitly

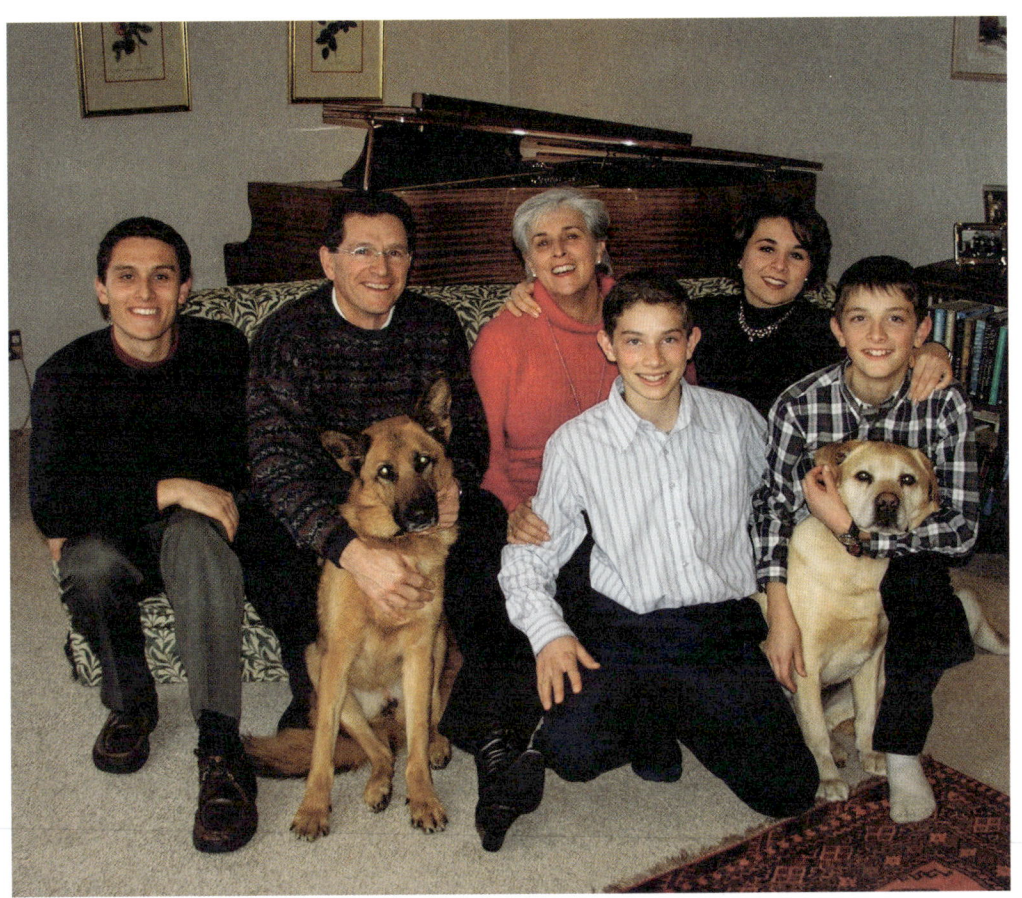

The family, just before I left for the USA. In the back, me, Dad, Mum and Fleur.
In the front, Xena, Jonathan, Napoleon and Charles.

admitted a failure of strength, bothered me.

Dad was standing by the boot, ready to help me to get the bike in. I pulled off the front wheel, handed it to him, then put the bike in the back of the car as quickly and discreetly as I could.

I felt utterly shattered, but I wanted to enjoy Grandma and Papa. When we got home I blobbed out on the couch for an hour or so, talking with them. And then came the shivers, the stupor and the desire for sleep.

It was Wednesday morning when I finally got out of bed, dehydrated, nauseous and profoundly weak. I had slept for almost four days, waking for three or four hours each day, just long enough to take in a little bit of vegetable soup or something similar. Now Mum was taking me to see my GP, Penny Crocker.

I explained to Penny that I thought I had picked up a tummy bug on the Friday, and that I was still feeling really bad.

'OK, tell me about Friday,' she said. 'Where were you and what were you doing?'

'I was at the prawn farm. I felt fine in the morning and I rode my bike to work, like I do most days, and I was fine. Around mid-morning I began to experience stomach cramps and low-grade nausea. After lunch I started getting diarrhoea and feeling really nauseated and slightly feverish. I didn't think I could cycle home, so I called Mum.'

'Any vomiting?'

'No.'

'Sore throat, cough or chest pain?'

'No.'

'How is your appetite?'

'Not great. I haven't really eaten much over the last few days.'

'Any problems with the waterworks?'

'Um . . . no.' I didn't think my bladder problems would be related, so I decided not to tell her about them. It would be too embarrassing.

'Right. In what ways are you feeling unwell now? Tell me about that.'

'I feel so incredibly weak. My legs feel wobbly. This morning, when I showered, I felt like I hardly had the energy to rinse my hair.

Afterwards I felt totally wiped out. And then, walking upstairs to the kitchen, I had to use the handrail because my legs felt so weak, and I find it hard to balance — it's kind of like I am super-dizzy, I suppose. And I feel like my mind is in a total haze.'

'OK. Could you pull up your shirt.' She gave me a general examination, tapping my chest, feeling my throat, testing my abdomen for pain, measuring my weight, height, pulse and blood pressure.

'This sounds like a stomach bug,' Penny said, 'so I will prescribe you some rehydration salts and medication to help with the nausea. And how about I write out a medical certificate, giving you until the end of the week off to recover?'

Three months later I was again in Penny's office, the latest in a series of visits.

'Hello, Nicholas. Have a seat. How is it going?'

'Still not great, which is frustrating.'

'So there is still no improvement?'

'Not really.'

'I see. Tell me about it.'

'Well, fatigue, dizziness and balance still continue to be a big problem. I feel so tired all the time, and still find it hard to balance, particularly as I tire doing anything mildly exerting. I still have great difficulty focusing — in fact it is probably getting worse — and I almost constantly feel like I am walking in a haze. I don't feel I can safely drive at the moment. It's really weird — the traffic and motion of the car is really confusing, or disorientating, and I feel like I get overwhelmed and it's all too much to take in. No matter how much I sleep, I still feel exhausted.

'Oh, and I forget things all the time. My mind is just a sieve and I find it hard to hold a conversation. And I find it hard to get work done. It takes such a long time to think things through. Also, I feel like I want to cry all the time. It's just so stupid. Like, the other day, I dropped a pen on the floor and then had to choke back tears. It's so dumb.'

Penny replied sympathetically then turned to record all this in her notes. When she'd finished typing she ran both hands through her hair then cupped her head in her hands, elbows on the table.

'To be honest, Nick, I am at a bit of a loss as to what is going on. We did all that blood work over and over, and those faecal samples at the beginning, and at no point has there been anything that would even slightly suggest a viral infection. We stuck you on antibiotics, just in case it was giardia or something. That didn't work. The blood tests from last time continued to rule out the possibility of a continued viral illness. I am clutching at straws here — I can't think what else we can test or do.'

'It's weird, isn't it?' I said. 'And it's just frustrating because I am still feeling so smashed. You know, I can't walk up the hill at DeBretts anymore. We go to the hot pools there a couple of times a week but after the hot water I feel so weak I can hardly stand. Mum and Dad have to drive down the hill from the carpark to pick me up. I cannot, for the life of me, walk up the hill from the pools to the carpark.'

'How is the exercise going generally?'

'Well, I did go for a bike ride a couple of weeks ago and probably pushed it a bit hard. But I only went twelve k's! It's so dumb. And it took me forty minutes, too, so I was taking it slowly. But it was still too much! I was totally smashed for two whole days afterwards. I could hardly move. It's really frustrating.'

I paused, sighed and looked at the ground.

'In fact, I've decided to sell my bike. I just can't handle riding anymore. It's too hard and it's smashing me. I feel super-gutted at having to sell it, but I just can't hack riding anymore. It's too much.'

'I'm sorry to hear that about your bike,' Penny said. 'I can imagine it must be frustrating and sad — although twelve k's is still pretty good. But are you keeping up with other exercise?'

'Yes, I am trying to walk a bit, to keep up fitness.'

'Good. And how is work?'

'Well, I had to quit my job at the prawn farm. It was too physical, unfortunately — it's a shame, as I really enjoyed the work. And I gave up the waiting job, so I am just continuing with the engineering and constructing this website. I'm hoping this will allow me a bit more time for rest and recovery.'

'Good idea. It's important to just take it easy and slowly work at getting better.'

Penny had also sent me off to see a specialist, Nic Crook, and now she asked how that had gone. 'Oh good,' I said. 'Well, he thought I would get better within six months or so, and suggested that it might be post-viral fatigue or myalgic enceph—' I couldn't remember how to pronounce the unfamiliar word.

'ME,' Penny replied. 'He thought it might be myalgic encephalopathy.'

'Yeah, that's the one.'

'How long until you head overseas?'

'Um . . . about two months.'

'What did he say about the trip? Did he think it would be OK for you to go?'

'Yes. He encouraged me to go, especially since he expects me to make a full recovery soon.'

'How do you feel about that?'

'Well, I'm pretty nervous, actually. I don't think I could cope with it at the moment. But then, at the same time, I would be pretty devastated if I didn't go. I think I will just go in the hope that I will get better, as he suggested. I'll try to take it a bit easy when I'm over there.'

'Good idea — there's no point in killing yourself by loading up with heaps of work, you know.'

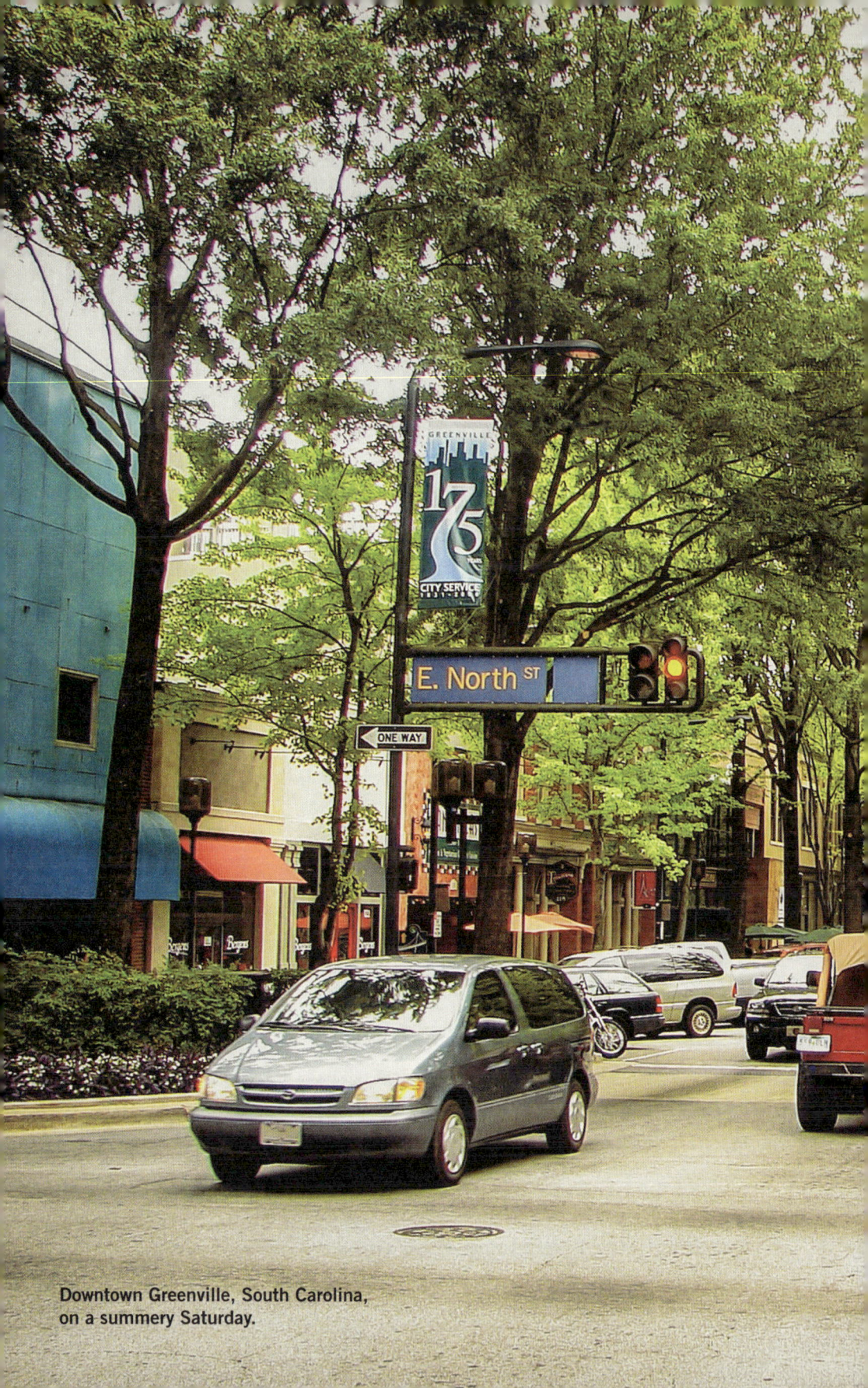
Downtown Greenville, South Carolina, on a summery Saturday.

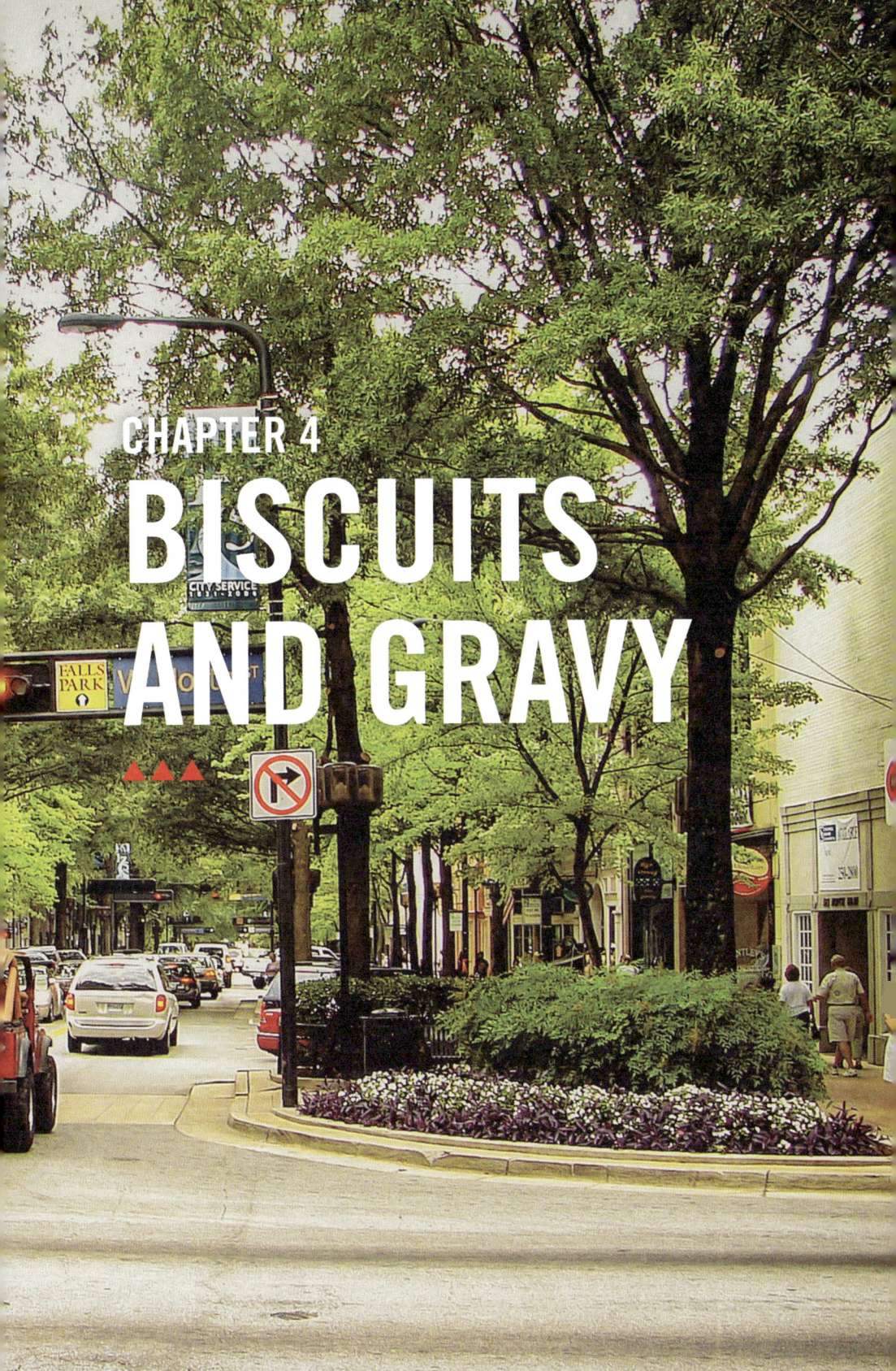

CHAPTER 4
BISCUITS AND GRAVY

August 2006
LAX, United States of America

'What size would you like your Big Mac Combo meal, sir?'

'Um, large, please,' I replied. I was too chicken to go for a super-sized meal.

'Very good. That's five dollars and sixty-nine cents, thank you, sir.'

I handed the server a $10 note and smiled with anticipation. It was my first purchase in the USA.

'Thank you, sir. Please wait over there. Your meal won't be long.'

I was eager to try an American Big Mac to see if the meal was any different from the New Zealand version. It had been on my mind ever since I left Auckland and the cross-hatching of streetlights had disappeared beneath the blackness of the night sky. Flying Air Tahiti, I'd had a layover of several hours at Faa'a International Airport, but the only food available in the transit lounge had been snacks. I'd had to settle for an overpriced Mars bar, which barely put a dent in my appetite, confirming my desperate need for a Big Mac.

As I waited in the queue to go through customs at Los Angeles International Airport thoughts of tomato sauce and mayonnaise oozing out of the side of my mouth, the feeling of the hot, moist slabs of bread cupped in my hands, and the smells of salt, fat and deep-

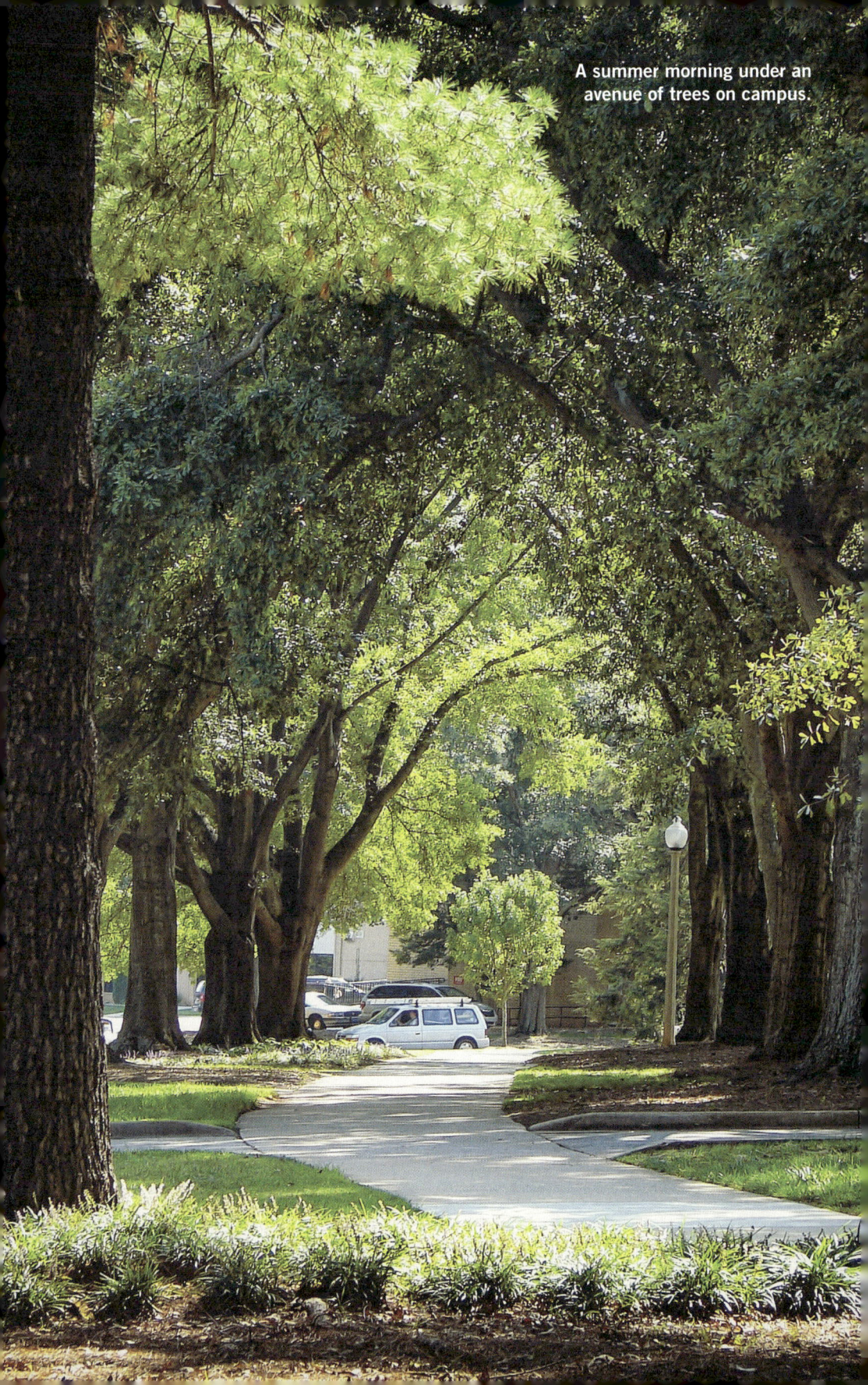

A summer morning under an avenue of trees on campus.

frying oil kept filtering through my mind. I was looking forward to this meal so much.

'Here you go, sir. Here's your meal.'

'Wow! Thanks heaps. Oh, can I have some tomato sauce?'

'I'm sorry, sir, what was that?'

'Oh, um, ketchup — could I have some ketchup?'

'Certainly, sir.' A pile of tomato-sauce sachets was added to the tray.

'Thanks!' I said as I ogled my meal. As it turns out, large Big Macs in the USA are ginormous. The fries overflowed from a massive paper carton, and the Coca-Cola came in a huge plastic cup. As I walked away in search of a table, I reckoned this would have to be the most epic McDonald's experience ever.

I was pretty excited about being in the US. Perhaps it was the legacy of all the American movies I had seen and all the other cultural artefacts the country exports, but I had the sense that America was a place that hummed with opportunity. I felt it would provide me with the freedom to master my fate and steer my course towards a new and greater self. I believed that everything would be better — and that I would get better — in this land.

I also assumed that there would be shared cultural values that would grant me the freedom to fit in, to be loved as a fellow journeyman, to be strengthened, and to enjoy the country's riches, eventually perhaps allowing me to retire early. To this end, I secretly hoped that I would complete my engineering studies and get a job doing something awesome, something I thought you could only do in America — stuff like designing rockets, satellites or fighter jets. Perhaps if I could work on cutting-edge projects like that I might actually enjoy engineering.

I polished off my meal and sat back in my chair, ready to evaluate my first American Big Mac experience. I had to admit, in fact, that the Big Mac had been a bit underwhelming. The beef was dry and tasteless, the fries exactly the same as those in New Zealand, and the drink sickly sweet.

Nevertheless, despite feeling tired, bloated, sticky and generally gross after umpteen hours of travel, I was satisfied and ready for the next few hours of travel to Greenville, South Carolina.

I sat next to a very friendly and somewhat drunk young sailor on the flight to Greenville. He was heading home on leave to see his family in a town called Gaffney.

'I is a barber, my daddy is a barber, and so is my grand-daddy: I come from a long line o' barbers. And when I get out of the Navy, I'm gonna take over da family business,' he said proudly, his very thick southern drawl made even thicker by alcohol.

'Wow, that's cool! How long have you been in the Navy?'

'I been serving my country proudly for six years, and I have done one tour o' duty. I'll do one more tour, then I'll leave the Navy after that.'

'That's awesome.' I smiled. 'I bet you must be looking forward to seeing your family.'

'Say what?'

'Are you looking forward to seeing your family?'

'Dawg, I can't wait! We're goin' to have a mighty fine feed when I get home.' He paused, an idea brewing. 'Dawg, you should come to my home for dinner! My mama makes the best fuckin' bar-bee-cue in the whole state of South Ca-row-line-a.'

'Wow, thanks heaps for the offer! How far is Gaffney from Greenville?'

'Oh, it will take ya under an hour,' the sailor said dismissively.

'Gotcha. I won't have a car, unfortunately, so that might be a bit too far for me. But thanks anyway.' While grateful for his generosity, I was not so sure I wanted to accept the invitation. I was acutely aware of the cultural gap between us. What would we talk about for a whole evening? I also wondered how he would feel about the idea when he sobered up. Perhaps another time, I thought, once I had this whole American thing a bit more sorted out.

'I c'n pick you up, dawg.'

'Thanks heaps, but you really don't have to — that's a long way to drive,' I told him, trying to wriggle out of the situation gracefully.

'Bro, you playin' right? It ain't no hassle, aight?' He looked at me wide-eyed. 'I've never meet someone from fuckin' Middle Earth before, dawg! What's your country called 'gain?'

'New Zealand.'

'Yeah, dat's the one. Noo Zee-land. And where's that at?'

'It's in the southern hemisphere, next to Australia.'

'Throw a shrimp on the bar-bee, mate!' He laughed, slapping me on the shoulder. His teeth glinted gold. 'You come to my house and we will have a real bar-bee-cue. We'll have bar-bee-cue sauce and pulled pork wi' corn bread, sweet po-tada pie, fried okra, and collar' greens.' He closed his eyes. 'Mmmm-mmm, it will be a migh-tee fine pig pickin'! 'Cause dat is how we do things in South Carolina: southern hospitality!'

He smiled again and ran his hand across the flat rim of his baseball cap, which had all the labels and stickers still attached.

'That sounds amazing!' I tried to sound enthused, even though I didn't know what half the stuff was. He was very enthusiastic, but I felt as if I was being embraced only because I was something exotic, a stranger from a world of hobbits and dragons.

'Dawg, it will be outta this world,' he said, smiling again, his yellow-gold teeth on clear display.

I laughed and then paused, wanting to change the subject. 'Bro, if I may ask, are your teeth all gold, or just gold-plated?'

'Dawg, I just got this done yesterday.' He took out the gold plate that wrapped around his teeth, hugging them front and back. 'Dawg, ain't dese sick?'

'It's cool! What's it called?' I asked.

'What dat?' He put the plate back in, working it into place with his lips.

'What is this thing called?' I asked, pointing to my own front teeth.

'Ah, it's called a grill, dawg. It's genu-ine twenty-four carat gold. I got it and my gold neckless wi' my last pay cheque. My brothers is gunna be wanting my stuff and I gunna be struttin'.' He smiled smugly, wiggling his shoulders as if walking with a swagger, and waving his gold necklace, complete with a large diamante-encrusted dollar sign.

At that moment the voice of the captain interrupted our

conversation, announcing our imminent arrival in Greenville.

'Dawg, how about I gi' you my number, and then you come o'er to my place for dinner?'

'OK,' I said. 'I don't have a phone, but I'll grab it just in case.' With a final attempt at noncommittal politeness I acknowledged the gift of his hospitality, even if it was the result of his inebriation.

Pop-Tarts were the first American food that mystified me, and the main element in the first American breakfast I ate. I had met Carrie, a young woman from Greenville, when she was travelling through Taupo. She lived in a small apartment near the university that I was going to attend, and we had kept in touch through email. Carrie and her mother were away at a wedding and she had offered me the use of their flat for a few days. I was very appreciative of this generous offer, and of the unexpected gift of a hamper of food, with instructions scrawled on a piece of paper: 'The Pop-Tarts are for breakfast — they go in the toaster.'

I stood at the kitchen bench in front of the toaster and read the text on the box: 'Frosted Strawberry Flavour', 'Made with Real Fruit', '8 Toaster Pastries'. OK, I thought, fruit and pastries. That's not too bad — no different from croissants and jam for breakfast.

I opened the box and drew out two Pop-Tarts, which were topped with a thick layer of sugary icing. They looked more like something you would serve a child for dessert, or as a treat on a wintery Saturday afternoon after they had cleaned their room, dusted the house, and washed all the dishes without being asked. It felt wrong to be eating them for breakfast but I was ready to try something new, so I quickly stuck them in the toaster to avoid thinking about it any longer.

I moved down the kitchen bench slightly and rested on my elbows, catching the cool draught that was coming from the air conditioner. Carrie's note included an apology for the air conditioning: 'Sorry about the jet engine. To turn it off . . .' At this point I was too tired to care about the noise: it was too hot without it, the breeze was soothing, and I slipped into a tired, time-zone-confused daze as I waited for my Pop-Tarts.

I felt exhausted. It had taken around 24 hours to fly from Auckland to Greenville and I had slept very little of that time — long legs and economy-class seats mixed with long layovers at busy airports, are never a good combination. But it was not just the sleep deprivation that had worn me down; there was also all the standing and dragging that you do as you crawl your way through immigration, customs, different terminals and security on the way to the departure lounges. What's more, it was hot.

I used to deal with the heat without any problems. However, over the last few months I had begun to find heat difficult, making me feel generally worse and physically drained. When I arrived in Greenville it was just before midnight, the temperature was in the low thirties (degrees Celcius), and it was incredibly humid. The air felt thick and syrupy. I felt smashed.

But I was here now, and that was the main thing, I thought. I had overcome the hurdle of getting here, so I should be able to have fun, regain strength and recover. The difficulty was behind me, I reasoned; it was onwards and upward from here.

The toaster popped up, giving me a fright. The Pop-Tarts were ready.

I cautiously bit off a small piece of one corner. The fruit filling was hot and I juggled the dry, crumbly pastry on my tongue as I tried not to let the contents burn my mouth. I waited a moment before taking the next bite, blowing on the Pop-Tart, and then took a larger chunk, getting some of the icing this time: more sickly sweetness. It made me feel slightly ill, left a weird oily film on the roof of my mouth, and tasted nothing like real strawberries. Nevertheless, I enjoyed it as something new — something that challenged my notions of normality and nutrition. I waited for the sugar rush.

'Breakfast: Biscuits and gravy, scrambled eggs, fruit jello,' the menu read. Oh no, not again, I thought as I dragged myself unenthusiastically towards the servery.

The first time I had biscuits and gravy I thought they were pretty cool, albeit utterly confusing. I had just arrived at the university — everything still new and exciting — when I encountered them on the menu board in the foyer of the university's 'dining common', as it was known.

'Excuse me,' I had asked the woman operating the student-ID scanner.

'Yes, sir?'

'Is it still breakfast time?'

'Yes it is, sir.'

'Biscuits, gravy, eggs and jello —' I hesitated for a moment — 'for breakfast?' I was bewildered at the thought of such a combination.

'Yes, sir. Grab a tray and walk right through, please.' She pointed to the open door leading to the servery.

This time, though, I scanned my card without comment, barely cracking a smile as I walked past the woman and into the massive dining hall. It was filled with 1980s faux-wood, Formica-topped tables and seats for 2700 people. At this time of the morning, with no more than a handful of people eating breakfast, the space felt absolutely cavernous. Later in the day it would be swarming with people and it would be hard to find a seat.

The first time I joined the queue leading to the servery I had attempted to get a look at this perplexing food combination, wondering what it would taste like. The more I thought about it, the more wrong it seemed. If Americans do Pop-Tarts for breakfast, I thought, I guess it's not too much of a logical step to do biscuits and cookies as well. But gravy? Gravy on a chocolate chip biscuit is never right at any time of the day, and certainly not for breakfast. And that's not to mention the inappropriateness of jello — or jelly, as we call it — for breakfast. And served with scrambled eggs? It sounded horrific.

I was hoping to be horrified, that first time, to experience the rush of encountering something inexplicably strange. Which is probably why I was disappointed when I reached the front of the line and discovered that biscuits and gravy were nothing more than scones with a slightly spicy white sauce that tasted vaguely meaty. The guy in front of me filled up his glass with Coca-Cola, which flowed freely at one of the many drink stations. Biscuits, gravy, jelly and Coke for breakfast — it was still a pretty strange mix. I decided to go for an orange juice, bringing some normality to the craziness on my plate. It was with a slightly subversive thrill that I dug into my meal that first time. It reminded me of when I was a kid and our favourite babysitter would let us eat ice-cream for breakfast when Mum and Dad were away.

Now, five months after that first breakfast, I found the biscuits sat like stodge all day in my stomach and the gravy, once it cooled, was disturbingly gelatinous — wobbling, congealing as you walked. The jelly was not that great either — some days it was so rubbery you could bounce it on the table and could barely carve a slice off with your spoon. Nevertheless, I comforted myself with the fact that the whole meal probably had more nutritional value than the much nicer coffee cake they served for breakfast on other days of the week.

I walked towards a table, paying special attention as I carried my tray. My hands were shaking uncontrollably and threatened to slosh my orange juice all over the place. I had given up coffee in the hope that the continual tremor I was experiencing would improve, but it had not made much of a difference.

I sat down at the end of a table, alone, several seats away from anyone else. I hated my shaking hands. The tremor made everything difficult and clumsy, particularly when combined with my deteriorating motor skills. I felt stupid as I fumbled with my knife and fork, and had to focus on my grip as I lifted my cup for fear that I would drop it, as I had done before. I felt ashamed of my body and I could not bear for people to see me like this.

More than stupid, I felt angry. I was not angry towards God, but angry at my body. I was losing that unified sense of self I had enjoyed as a child: I now felt fragmented by the growing disconnect between my mind and my body. I knew what I wanted my hands to achieve and where I wanted them to go, but I often felt incapable of making them do what I wanted. Work, you bloody hands! I wanted to scream. Why won't you bloody well work?

I struggled back across the campus to my dorm, breakfast sitting heavy in my stomach. I felt ghastly, completely run-down and in pain. It was a bit after 8 a.m. and the campus was still relatively quiet, a relief from the usual bombardment of activity. As I did on most mornings, in order to block out the pain, I tried to focus on the pleasure afforded by my proximity to nature. The campus was beautiful. The grounds were meticulously kept, and between the avenues of large trees, finely manicured gardens and tastefully designed buildings I could find fleeting glimpses of the wild beauty that I loved in the bush at home. This was particularly true out the back of the campus, past the maintenance sheds and the piles of mulch and soil, in the small enclave of uncultivated woods that had become a haven for me — when I had the energy to get out there.

It was mid January now and we were in the depths of winter. I pulled the collar of my jacket up round my neck, grateful for the cooler mornings, a reprieve from the heat of summer. The journey from the dining common to my room took only seven minutes, but it seemed interminable. I felt as if I had been run over by a train: my whole body ached, my muscles dragged, my balance was poor, my head spun, and my mind was barely able to make sense of the world around me. Every step felt laborious. I finally reached my cold room, closed the door, lay down on the bed, and took a couple of tramadol to manage the pain. I wondered how on earth I could make it through another day.

There was nothing particularly comforting about my dormitory, which had the atmosphere of a 1950s bomb shelter: the door frames were made of steel; all the internal walls were solid concrete block, painted beige and grey; the beds and cabinetry were bolted to the walls; and the old tiled shower blocks were reminiscent of caves, dark and dank, with bare plumbing on the walls.

Some people likened the dorm rooms to slightly glorified prison

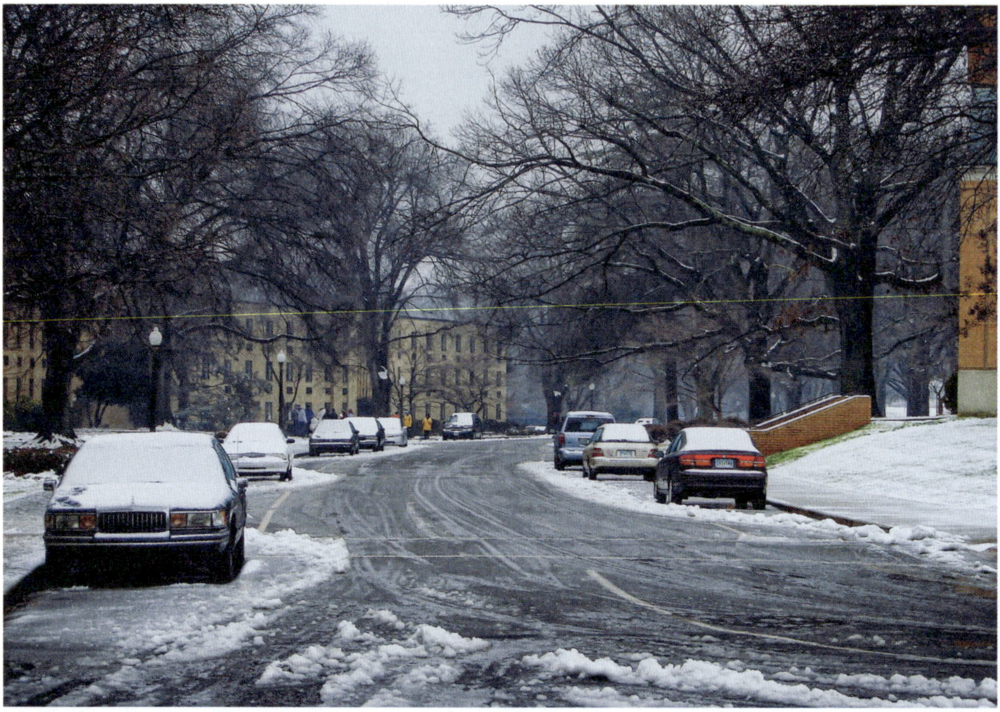

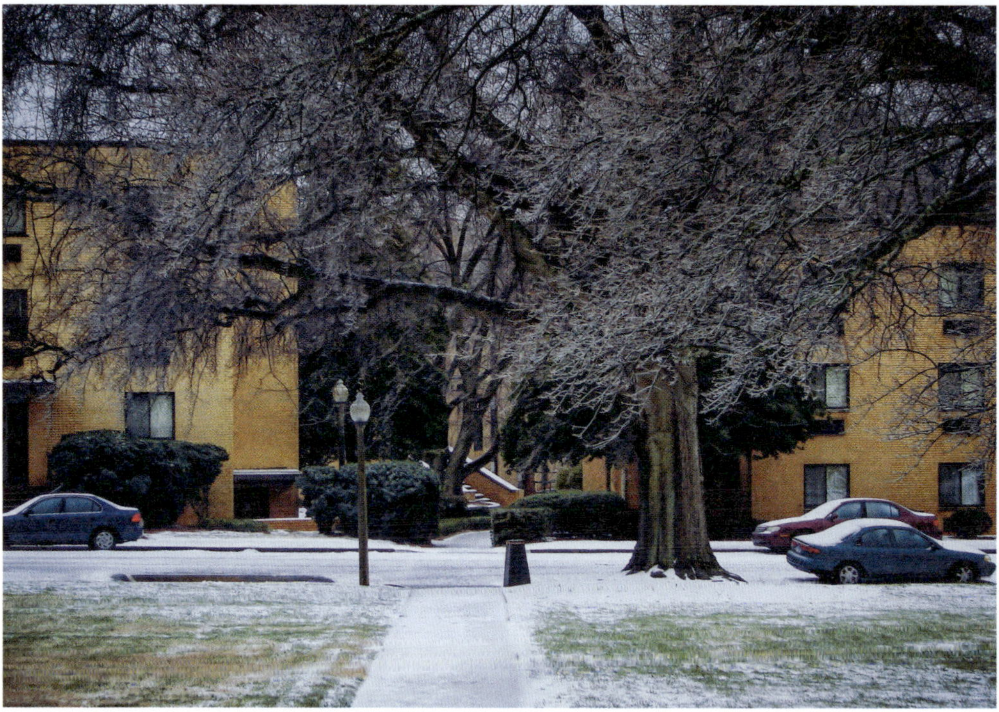

Snow on the guys' side of campus. Snow days were a welcome reprieve from the daily routine, an opportunity to have fun and throw a bit of snow around.

cells, but I begged to differ. Admittedly the small screened window in each room and the drab interiors did encourage comparisons with prison cells; nevertheless, I would argue that they were more bomb shelter than prison cell for two reasons. First, the dorm had been built by GIs who had just returned from the Second World War and were eager to find refuge from the evils of mankind. Second, the science building, which was of the same vintage, had a Cold War-era sign on how to handle a nuclear attack: 'DUCK & COVER. If you see the flash, duck and cover.'

If the room lacked comfort, it also suffered from a lack of privacy. The doors couldn't be locked, so people were able to come in and out at will. There were three of us in my room and my two roommates, Keith and Kittrell, were popular guys, resulting in a steady stream of visitors. To begin with this was a lot of fun, offering me the chance to chat, make friends and observe the hilarious rituals of life in a guys' dorm. One night two friends of Kittrell burst into our room, stood about three metres apart and faced each other in a duel, taking turns at trying to rake their opponent in the gonads with a tennis ball. This concluded, unsurprisingly, with one of them lying on the floor, in tears and struggling to breathe. I was never sure why our room was the chosen venue for such antics. While this type of horseplay was fun to watch, it also meant that study periods and uninterrupted times of needed rest were rare.

But it was not just the people walking in that precluded privacy: the conversations outside the room, in the hall, were also invasive. Sound carried down the concrete hallways rather efficiently, conveying conversations to any rooms with open doors — which was annoying if you wanted to study and have some level of airflow in your room. Even if you had your door closed in an attempt to achieve peace and quiet, the gap beneath the door was enough to allow sound to disturb you.

When I enrolled at the university I hadn't thought through the implications of living on campus. Now, I felt as if every part of my life was public or, at the very least, under threat of being made public. The lack of privacy led to a sense of exposure, of vulnerability, making it difficult to rest. Trying to catch a quick nap, for example, I was always braced for the possibility of someone springing into the room. It was also difficult to have a private conversation, whether you were in your room, in the hall, or even outside, where people could be streaming past you.

I did not expect this vulnerability to be frightening, but it was. In a land that seemed to glow with the promise of freedom and success, I was surprised to find my value as a person measured by my ability to perform. It seemed as though, to be a success, I needed to meet a set of rigid KPIs. There was a lot of self-declaration via form-filling. How many times had I attended church this month? How active was I in the university's community groups? Did I drink alcohol? Did I listen to rock music? They said it was pastoral care; I felt it was intrusive and graceless. I had hoped that in the US I would find acceptance for who I was, but I came to realise that some at the university just wanted cookie-cutter individuals.

Over time, it became clear that I needed to toe the line if I wanted to be free and accepted. Meeting the expectations was exhausting. I also became aware of an ill-defined disdain for anything considered 'un-American'. My perspectives, opinions and experiences — all that is uniquely me — were not socially acceptable (beyond being exotic novelties) unless they fitted the mould. All this was frightening, especially as the extent of my cultural difference dawned on me.

I had learned the importance of keeping my mouth shut and toeing the line quite early on. One Saturday afternoon I walked into the dorm with a friend after I'd been to a gun show.

'Man, that gun show was totally nuts,' I said. 'I don't think I have ever been so freaked out — like, for real.'

My friend laughed. 'Why was it freaky?'

'Well, for starters, you join the queue to get in, and there are all these guys standing there with guns slung over their shoulders! I looked around and the bolts were still in the rifle chambers, the shotgun barrels weren't broken, and it looked like some of the people had automatic weapons. And they were all standing there in the line! It felt so unsafe.'

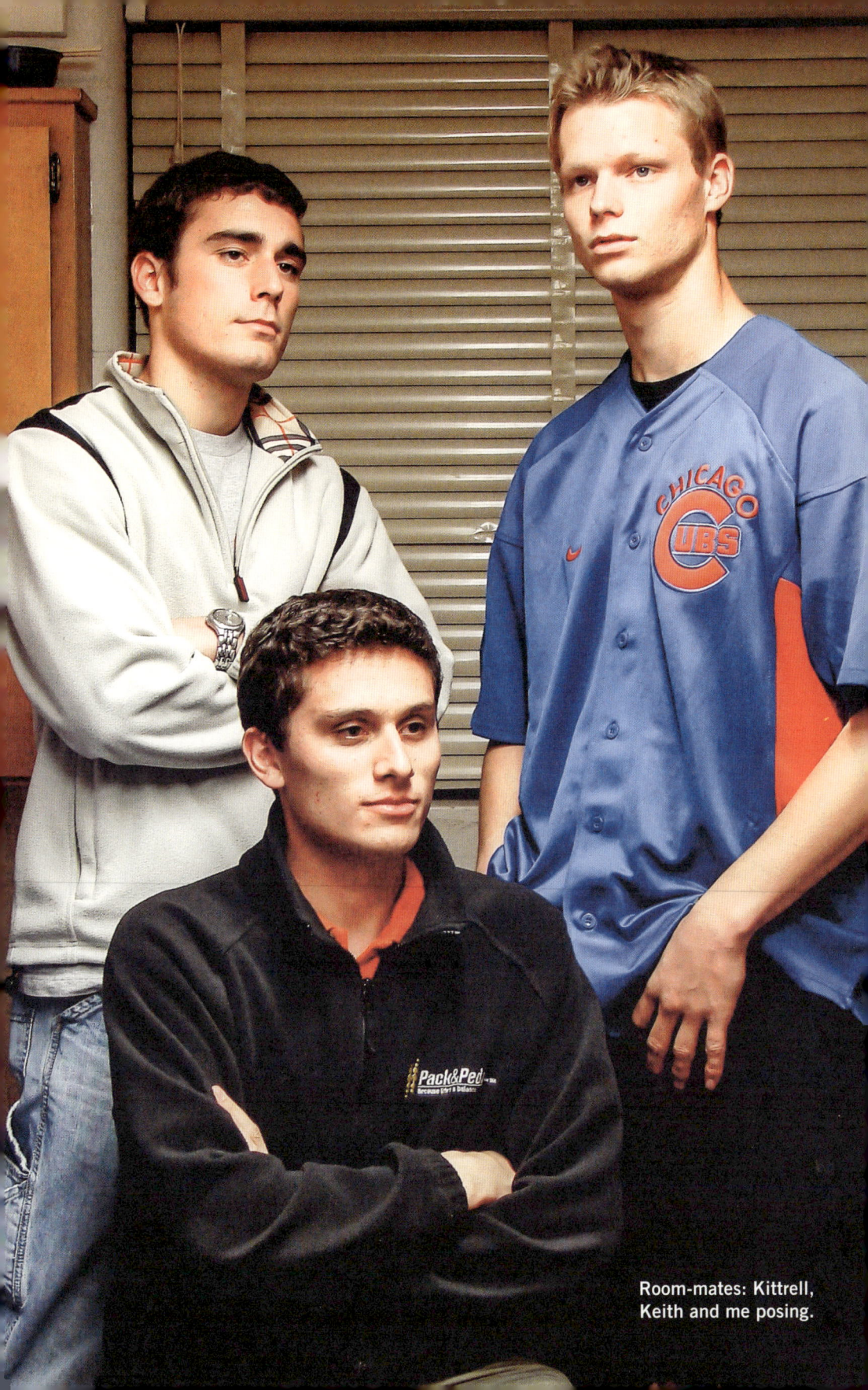

Room-mates: Kittrell, Keith and me posing.

'You were surrounded by guns — why would that be unsafe?' my friend asked, surprised.

'Ever since I was a kid, Dad has drummed into me that you always treat a firearm as loaded, and that you should never point a gun at a person. The guy in front of me, with his M16 rifle slung over his shoulder, would have shot me in the chest if the gun was loaded and had gone off. I mean, there were guns pointing at people everywhere, which is pretty scary if you treat them as loaded.'

'But none of them would have had any ammo,' he said sceptically.

'Maybe, but when you walk inside, there's ammo everywhere. And more people waving guns around, without police checks! I could have bought a massive fifty-calibre sniper rifle or an AK47 if I had wanted, grabbed some ammo, and mowed down a ton of people. It was just so nuts — well, terrifying actually. I think that was one of the most unsettling experiences of my life. It's no wonder there are so many shootings over here. I think the government should impose gun restrictions like we do in New Zealand.'

I had just entered the hall as that last sentence left my lips. People heard. One guy leapt out of his room, right in front of us. He was a strange fellow, this one. He had a large Confederate flag above his bed and always wore a black trenchcoat. On another occasion he had come into my room and shouted at me because I was (unknowingly) whistling 'a damned Yankee marching tune'.

'The government must never control guns! It is a fundamental human right to be able to own a firearm and it is an essential part of maintaining our freedom. Gun control is a part of the liberal agenda to rob us of our freedom and I will not have it!' he shouted. His aggression left me momentarily speechless. Other people peered out of their rooms.

'I am not sure that gun ownership is a fundamental human ri—'

I was quickly interrupted. 'It is too! The Second Amendment makes it clear, and I quote, "the right of the people to keep and bear arms shall not be infringed". End quote. Notice that it is a right. It is a part of the natural right to self-defence and is necessary for our freedom — a freedom liberals want to rob us of.'

Someone else pitched in. 'Yes! And not just for self-defence. Everyone should carry concealed weapons — it is proven to prevent crime.'

'I agree! The liberal agenda is going to ruin our country,' the first guy said, with a crazed look on his face.

I quickly realised that nothing I said, no amount of arguing, would change his mind.

More people appeared in their doorways, listening, curious. Given my opponent's unwillingness to entertain any perspective but his own, I thought I would go all out and express what I thought was the heart of the matter, a closing pushback.

'But isn't there something fundamentally hollow, I mean, isn't there something profoundly, deeply hollow and selfish about your sense of freedom if it requires you to carry a concealed weapon for safety and allows you to take another person's life in order that you might maintain your own personal freedom? That doesn't sound much like freedom to me.'

Well, that did it. I may as well have thrown a match at a petrol can. Guys appeared from everywhere and a heated debate ensued, with arguments coming from different sides. I quickly slunk away to my room and shut the door, trying to block out the sound. As the argument continued I lay down, my head beneath my pillow. I just wanted to be left alone. This was not what I had expected, not what I was prepared for.

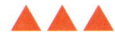

Now, my biscuits-and-gravy breakfast still felt heavy in my stomach as I turned on to my side. I tried to relax, but rest didn't come easily. The mere prospect of being watched, heard or intruded upon makes rest elusive. This vulnerability felt deeply frightening, particularly as it was not just my ideas and opinions that were being pushed out into the open. My body was changing and new symptoms were appearing, a process outside of my control that was leading to a sense of intense isolation.

Rightly or wrongly, I didn't want others to know I was struggling. I wanted to be cool, to be part of the in-group, and not to be sidelined as the sickly foreigner, weak and unsuccessful. I couldn't properly express what was going on, and I felt that I needed to keep it, and all the accompanying fears and emotions, bottled up. I knew I was losing my strength and ability, but I refused to acknowledge it in public. In order to talk to my parents about my symptoms and struggles I would seek the least populated places, often talking late at night, moving through the shadowy fringes of the campus.

So now I continued to toss and turn on my bed, grateful for the gradual onset of sleepiness. Lights almost never went out before 12.30 a.m., which meant five or six hours of sleep each night if I was lucky. And my sleep was often interrupted by the increasingly intense tingling in my hands and face. I need a solid eight to nine hours of sleep per night to function properly, and I knew this lack of sleep was unsustainable. However, I felt powerless to do anything about it: the rhythms of university life created an entirely rigid structure within which I and all other students had to operate or be penalised.

As I felt myself on the edge of sleep I contemplated setting the alarm, just in case I overslept, but I figured it was unnecessary — I rarely slept for long. Suddenly I woke, startled by the sound of the bell ringing in the hall. Life on campus was ruled by bells: the bell that rang on the hour, signalling the start of a class period, and the bell that rang 50 minutes later, signalling the end. The first bell was at 7.50 a.m. and the last at 4.50 p.m. The only way to escape the tyranny of the bell was to check in to the university's hospital — the only building in which no bell rang.

I looked at my watch: it was 10.51 a.m. I bolted upright. I had missed my 10 a.m. class. I swore under my breath. I could still make my 11 a.m. class if I hurried, but I didn't have much time. I quickly put on my shoes, brushed my teeth and hair, straightened my shirt, gathered the relevant books and stuffed them into my backpack, and started a quick walk down the hall.

I was on the second floor and halfway down the steps when I heard his voice. It was Dwight, the Vietnam veteran who hung out in the dorm's foyer, desperate for friends. I stopped dead in my tracks. Every time I walked past he would ask me how my day was going, invite me to his house for dinner, and talk for ages.

I found these conversations draining and I clearly did not have time for one right now. I had three options: (1) continue as planned, run out of the door, and hope that Dwight didn't see me; (2) ignore him as I walked past; or (3) run back upstairs, go back down the hall, and exit out one of the back doors.

The first option rarely worked and the second seemed exceptionally rude, leaving the third. Of all the days, I thought as I turned round, went back up the stairs and down the hall. My class was in the science building, on the other side of the campus. It was 10.56 a.m.

I knew I could not run for more than a few metres, so I walked as quickly as I could. I still felt really tired, despite my sleep, and my legs were killing me. In my hurry, the toe of my left foot caught the curb and I tripped, staggering as I tried to stay upright. So much for impressing the group of preppy girls who were walking past.

I did not have time to stop, and I knew I could not afford to be late for this class. I was worried enough about the consequences of missing the previous class. Attendance rolls were called before every class, and lateness and absence were not tolerated, earning demerits and even the threat of expulsion. Absences were also treated with the additional punishment of a visit to the student discipline committee. The DC, as it was known, was in the centre of one of the busiest buildings, right across from the main staircase. I had seen people standing there before a panel of university staff, explaining their actions, some for small misdemeanours such as mine, others for much more serious offences such as plagiarism. I had never been summoned but I felt sure it would be a humiliating experience as I waited my turn along the 'walk of shame', as it was known. The very prospect of a summons arriving in my email inbox created a pit in my stomach.

It was now 10.58 a.m. I tried to run the last hundred metres, rushing past the hospital, in order to arrive in my seat before the hour-bell rang. I felt as if my legs were going to give out. My head was reeling and I felt as if I was going to collapse, but I kept running — it was not far now. I looked through the glass doors of the campus hospital, to the nurses' station, as I walked past and remembered the first time I had checked in there, in November, about three months after my arrival.

It had been a moment of real struggle as I walked through those swinging doors. On the one hand, I was desperate for relief. I was in a huge amount of pain and felt incoherent after weeks of sleep deprivation. I badly wanted to remain in control of my situation, to appear strong and on top of life — I did not want to acknowledge my weakness. But I wasn't strong, and I was no longer in command of my situation. Life was spinning out of control. I finally had to admit this as I found myself kneeling on the ground, pounding my fist into the floor, groaning through my clenched jaw as I fell defeated beneath the overwhelming weight of pain, assignments and the unknown trajectory of my illness.

Walking through the hospital doors was to admit failure to everyone, it seemed, but it was with a sense of relief that I had climbed into my hospital bed. The ward was quiet, no one could visit me, and I was able to rest completely, without fear of interruption. Better than that, I was not required to go to class and I automatically gained extensions on my assignments. It was a get-out-of-jail-free card.

Now it was January, and I was in my second semester. This one was going even more badly than the previous semester, and it had only just started. In fact, I was spending more time in the hospital than out of it. Being in hospital was the only way to cope, the only mechanism available to me through which I could find grace in the university's otherwise inflexible system of enforced regimentation. But it also meant I was falling further and further behind in my classes, and that I was racking up a fairly large medical bill.

As I ran past those swinging doors to get to my class I knew it would not be long before I was back there again. I was in too much pain, I was too close to collapsing, and I was feeling too disorientated to take anything in.

UNIVERSITY MEDICAL ASSOCIATES, L.L.C.
TONYA N. WREN, M.D.
1809 WADE HAMPTON BOULEVARD, SUITE 120
GREENVILLE, SC 29609

(864) 322-4665 TEL.
(864) 232-4716 FAX

NAME Nicholas Allen   AGE
ADDRESS   DATE 1/29/07

Rx ILLEGAL IF NOT SAFETY BLUE BACKGROUND

℞

Please allow Nicholas to drop his physics course due to medical reasons.

Refill _____ times
☐ Label

DISPENSE AS WRITTEN   SUBSTITUTION PERMITTED
                       6JFP0332016

A slip from the doctor giving me permission to drop a class.

My bum hit the seat just as the bell rang. I was safe. I planted my face in my arms, resting on the desk. I was in class, but I knew that nothing was going to go in. I was too tired for that, but an observed obedience was all that mattered.

▲▲▲

'Hi, Ma,' I said, sitting on the edge of my hospital bed. The nurses had given me special permission to use my phone. This was going to be an important conversation.

'Darling, are you all right? What's been happening?' I could hear the concern in Mum's voice.

'Yeah, I'm OK. But some stuff happened on Friday and the doctor is recommending that I come home.'

'Oh, darling, I am sorry,' Mum replied. 'But you're OK now?'

'Yeah, I'm OK. Just not feeling great, that's all.'

'So, what happened?' Dad asked, joining the conversation on speaker phone.

'Well, on Friday afternoon, I was sitting in the library, studying, and all of a sudden my vision went crazy, all distorted and stuff.'

'How do you mean?' Dad said.

'Everything went double and slightly washed out. It was strange, and I felt like I had no balance whatsoever — I had to hold on to the table just to stand up — and I felt completely disorientated, like the room was spinning beneath me. I just didn't know what was going on.'

'How long did the double vision last for?'

'Well, I had it for the rest of the day. It eased up a bit on Saturday, but then came back again on Sunday afternoon, although not as strongly as on Friday. It's cleared up now, though.'

'Did you see the doctor straight away?' Mum asked.

'No,' I paused, trying to think of a good excuse. The truth was that I had felt too overwhelmed to even begin figuring out how to access the doctor after hours. 'It was late on Friday afternoon and I knew I wouldn't be able to get an appointment. And then it was the weekend and the surgery was closed. But I saw Tonya, my doctor, on Monday. So that was good.'

'Darling! Why did you wait so long? It could have been serious!'

'I don't know,' I replied hesitantly.

There was silence for a moment.

'Nick, how were you feeling before this happened?' Dad asked.

'Just same old, same old. You know, the usual stuff.'

'Tell us about it.'

I never like it when people ask me that question; it means that I have to verbalise and admit to how I am feeling. But I know that Dad only wanted to help, and he couldn't do that until I gave him the necessary information.

'Well,' I sighed, preparing myself for the depressing litany of complaints that were to follow. 'There is still all that weird sensory stuff: the tingling in my hands and face, that thing where stuff feels really hot or cold when I touch it, and all the dizziness — or lack of balance or whatever it is — I still find it so hard to balance. Then there is that damn stupid problem with wanting to cry all the time. And at such stupid stuff!'

Just thinking about my tendency to cry was making me want to cry. I paused for a moment and took a deep breath.

'Then there are my legs, which have given out a couple of times as I was walking down the hall, just recently, and they are always in so much pain. Tonya tested my reflexes when I saw her the other day and apparently the reflexes in one of them are all out of whack. My hands are crazy too. I'm dropping things all the time — the other day I dropped my laptop! And I find it hard to even type on my computer, or use my knife and fork. It's so frustrating. It's like my fingers just won't work. They feel so stiff and slow.

'It's like, you know when you look in the mirror and you have to do something, and it's hard and confusing and you feel like you can't make your hands do what you want them to because everything is backwards? Well, it's like that all the time. All the time! I see my hands but I just can't make them work correctly.'

I was feeling frustrated again, but it was good to be able to rant without fear of being overheard.

'And I'm failing all my classes. In my calculus class, my semester grade is, like, fifteen per cent or something ridiculous. I go to the class and I just don't get it anymore. It's like my brain is so deep in the fog that I can't even get simple equations. It's so weird and frustrating!'

'Have you talked to your lecturer?' Dad asked.

'Yes! But when I go to him for help he gets frustrated with me and tells me to do more practice. The other day I started crying when he said that. So then I excused myself and walked out. I practise and I try hard and I just don't get it. It's like I just can't do maths anymore. And it's March! We are almost halfway through the semester and I am practically failing everything. I just don't think I will be able to recover from this point. The classes and my grades are too far gone.'

'So you are failing your other classes too?'

'Yeah. They're not quite as dismal, but I'm still failing. I'm finding it hard to read, too. I look at a page and the words don't even make sense. I have to read a sentence backwards and forwards to try to figure out what it's saying. It's so slow, and with all the mid-semester assignments coming up I just don't think I'm going to be able to make it. 'And then I feel so incredibly tired all the time. I never seem to be able to get on top of it. I feel so, so smashed all the time.' I was choking back tears.

'Oh, darling,' Mum said. 'So what's the plan from here? What does the doctor think about all this?'

'Well, so I went to see Tonya on Monday, and she thinks that it definitely sounds neurological. She has been saying that my symptoms are probably neurological since the beginning of the year, but now she is pretty convinced of it.'

'OK,' said Mum. 'But where does that leave you now, in terms of a diagnosis?'

'Well, Tonya thinks that I should come home to New Zealand, to see a neurologist and have an MRI scan.'

'I see,' Mum replied. 'Did Tonya give you any hints, suggesting what she thinks it might be?'

'She was pretty guarded, but she did mention multiple sclerosis.'

'Wow!'

'What do you think of her recommendation, Nick?' Dad asked.

'Well, it makes sense. Neurologists and MRI scans are so expensive here and my travel insurance will only pay for so much. I think it makes sense to come home. And I'm going to fail this semester anyway, so there's not a heap of point in continuing. It is time to come home.'

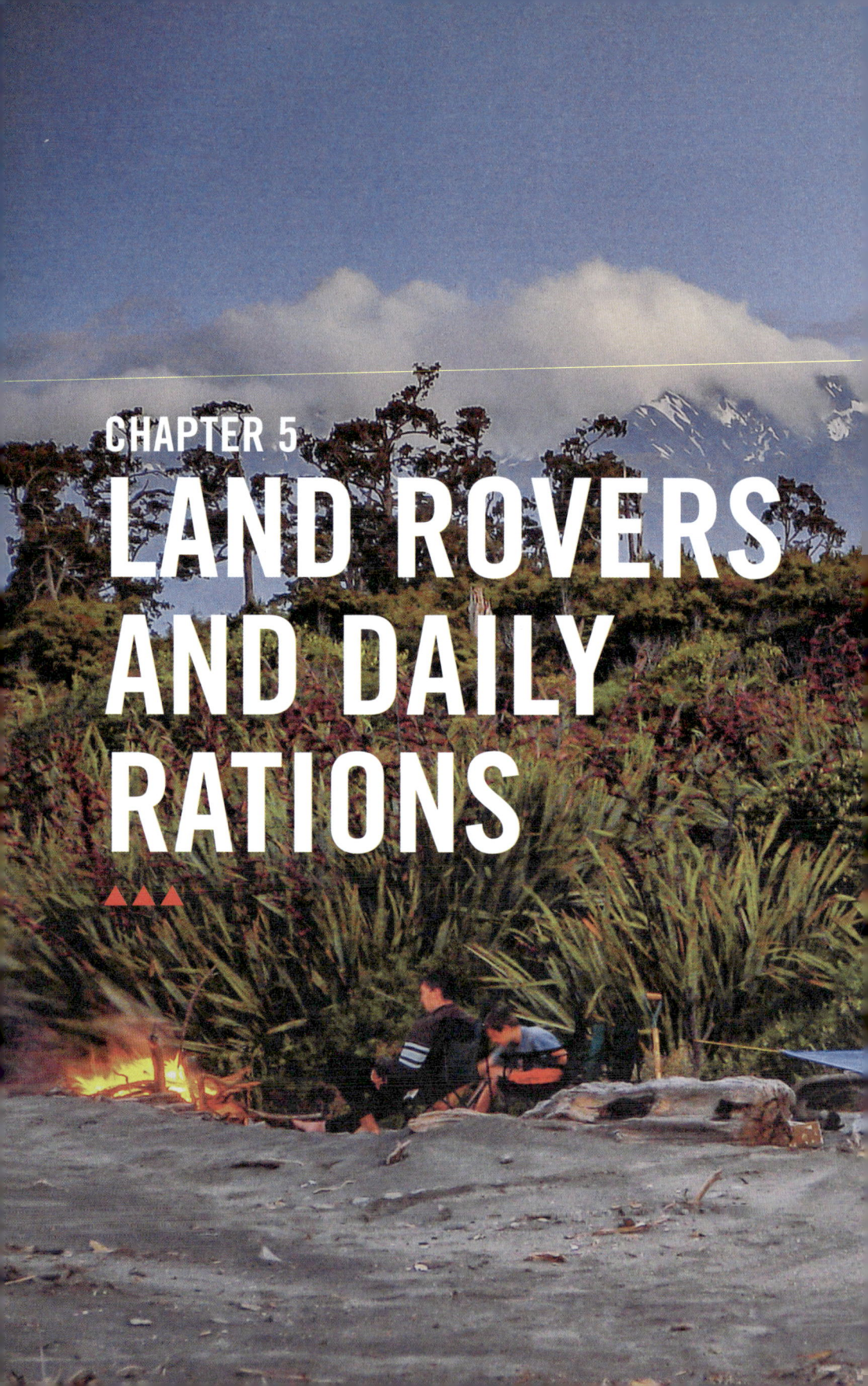

CHAPTER 5
LAND ROVERS AND DAILY RATIONS
▲▲▲

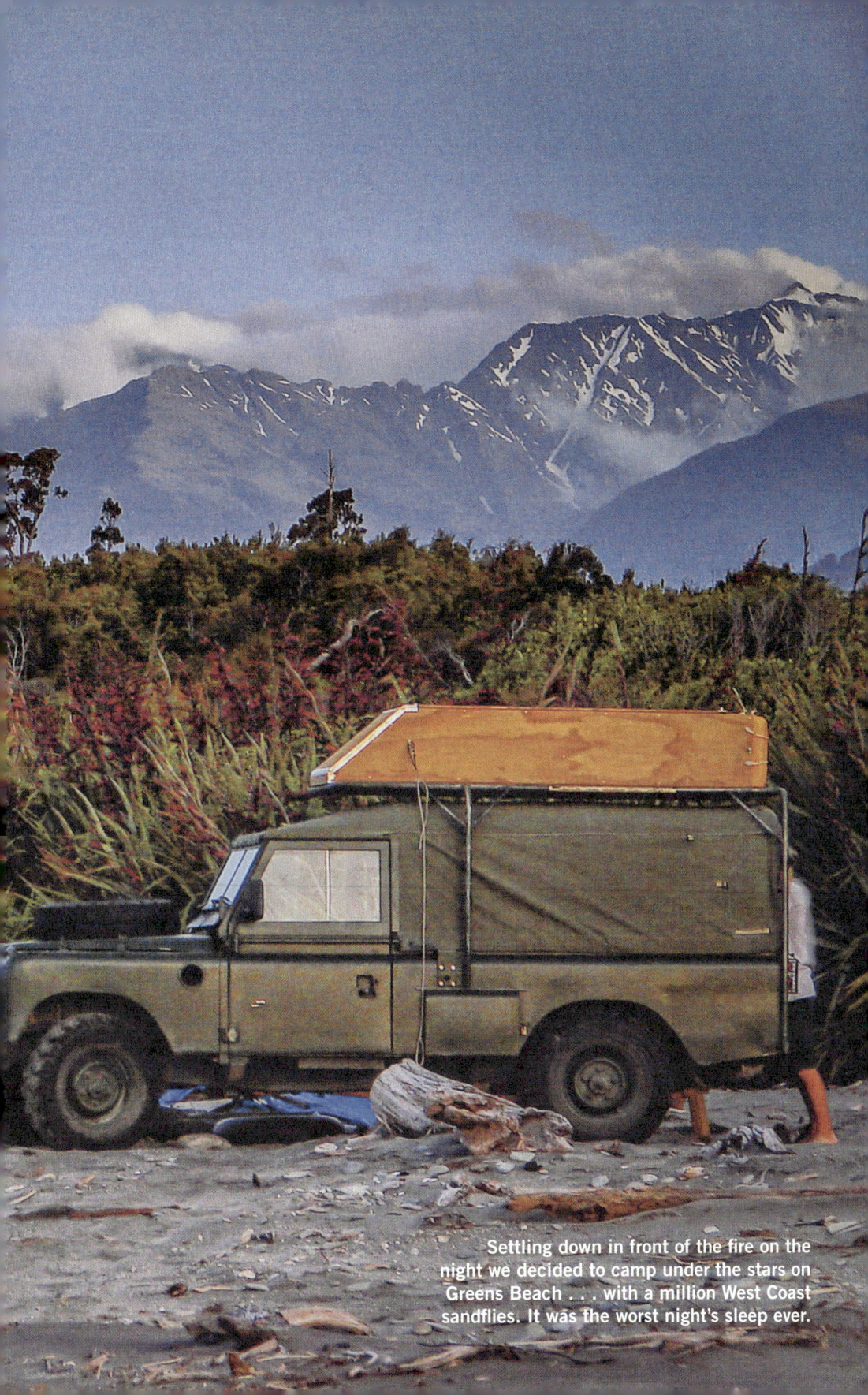

Settling down in front of the fire on the night we decided to camp under the stars on Greens Beach . . . with a million West Coast sandflies. It was the worst night's sleep ever.

December 2007
Taupo, New Zealand

'OK, chaps, we have a ferry to catch. Shall we hit the road?' I clapped my hands.

Jonathan, now 15, Charles, now 12, my friend Alexander and I piled into the 1983 Series III Land Rover. Hands down, it was the coolest vehicle I'd ever owned and I loved it. It was ex-Army, matte green, with a canvas roof and large, long-range fuel tanks. It was also a beast to drive. Usually, there would be Alexander and me in the front, and Jonathan and Charles in the back, on top of the sleeping platform we'd built, where there were no seatbelts — a fact that caused Mum no end of anxiety.

I started the Land Rover up. There was quite a trick to it — you had to pump the accelerator with just the right frequency and use just the right amount of choke. The sound of the engine roaring into life was thrilling, all eight cylinders brimming with power as they screamed in the sports-car-inspired aluminium engine.

We were heading down to the South Island for a month of exploration. Mum and Dad had decided to go overseas for Dad's fiftieth birthday and were renting out the house in Taupo to help pay for the trip. This meant that we boys would be homeless for four weeks around Christmas. I was desperate to get out and explore, to

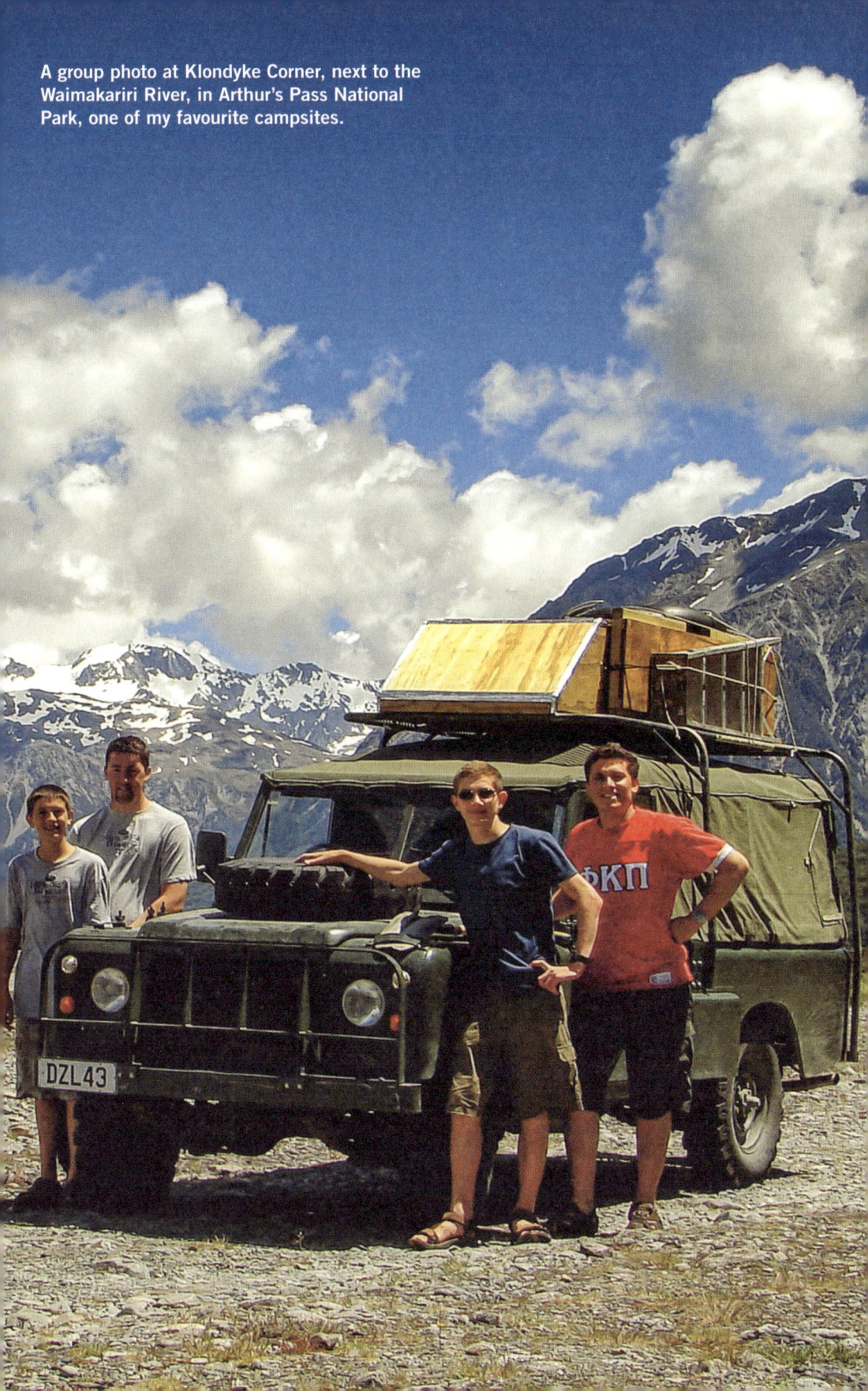

A group photo at Klondyke Corner, next to the Waimakariri River, in Arthur's Pass National Park, one of my favourite campsites.

enjoy the New Zealand landscape again, and had suggested a road trip to Jonathan and Charles. Our plan was to free-camp all the way around the South Island for the entire period Mum and Dad were away. Using our savings and a small amount of housekeeping from Mum, we figured we could get by on a total of $80 a day: plenty of money, we thought, for the trip of a lifetime.

Moving back to New Zealand had been hard. The uncertainty and unpredictability of my health made it hard to settle into the security of a routine and a steady job. Some days I would be OK; on others I would be entirely incapacitated, seemingly without reason. Months of consultations with doctors, neurologists and other specialists had failed to result in a definitive diagnosis, leading me to wonder if I was crazy, if all this was the product of a sick mind. The one thing the doctors did establish was that I should avoid anything stressful or I could regress. It was likely that I had chronic fatigue, they said, so I should take it easy and I might get better again.

Avoiding anything stressful meant I was unable to participate in many outdoor activities. But I was desperate to get out and I tried a few easy day walks, although they always left me bedridden for the next week or two. I found the subsequent sense of alienation from the outdoors incredibly difficult. One consolation was that my parents had a 4WD, and around Taupo are a good number of wilderness areas where I could take it. The 4WD provided a great way to get into places that scratched my itch for the outdoors. Nevertheless, working irregularly combined with the doctors' instructions to avoid anything stressful meant that I also struggled with a lack of purpose. I needed a goal to work towards, something to look forward to, something to keep me moving through the bad times. That's the reason I'd been keen to buy the Land Rover in the first place.

The Landie and the prospect of the trip south brought a tremendous amount of focus and purpose — which is probably why I loved the Land Rover so much. I had spent several months tinkering on it, fitting it out for our trip with help from Jonathan and Charles. I stripped out some of the old army gear, upgraded various parts, fixed a number of problems, and then built cabinets and beds into the back, enough so that we could live out of it. Then there was all the planning for the trip. I researched it extensively, finding places to stay and tracks to drive on. I took into account everything from hours driven per day (I could only handle so much) and how to make basic repairs to the location of petrol pumps and how much spare fuel we might need to carry at any given time. Having this focus was a massive help on those down days, giving my mind something to focus on other than how miserable I was feeling. The trip also helped me to focus on the physical care of my body. I was trying to learn how to read and manage my symptoms; I knew that would be key to the success of the trip.

The only problem was that the Land Rover was physically demanding to drive. Between the massively long gearstick, which almost needed two hands to manipulate, an industrial-weight clutch, the lack of power steering and ineffective drum brakes that required you to stand up out of your seat if you needed to stop fast, you felt as if you really were driving a machine. I could only manage it for an hour or two at a time. Jonathan had his learner's licence, but because the Land Rover had the aerodynamics of a brick it was difficult for him to drive as well. That's why I had invited Alexander, one of my close friends, to join us as the designated driver.

I felt a strange mixture of excitement and fear as I backed out into the driveway. I was excited to be finally hitting the road, but nervous about making the ferry on time, and of the possibility of the Land Rover breaking down — something that was a distinct possibility if you believe what everyone says about their reliability.

'Have you got sunhats? And what about sunblock?' Mum shouted.

'Yes, Mum,' I replied, leaning out of the window.

We gave a final wave, bumped down the driveway and, with a throaty roar, turned south, towards Wellington and the ferry.

It was during the third day, a couple of hours out of Westport, when the throaty roar of the engine began to cause concern. Loaded up with a month's worth of food and gear, we'd had to push the Land Rover a bit harder than I had expected and, as a consequence, were using more fuel than I had calculated. But then, we were making our way through the Buller Gorge, a serpentine stretch of road that would use more fuel in any car, I thought.

We'd spent the morning exploring the remains of Lyell, a ghost town deep in the Buller Gorge. The day was overcast, wisps of cloud hung around the valleys, and Lyell, now just a mown patch of grass, was surrounded by dense beech forest darkened by the morning's rain. A track runs up Lyell Creek to the Croesus Battery, both remnants of the gold rush that gave rise to the once-booming town. We decided to walk out to the battery, a route that took us past the old Catholic graveyard, now an eerie cluster of tombstones in the bush, and across an arched bridge to the tunnel the miners used to divert the water around Maori Bar, where gold was first struck. Continuing along the old dray road through the bush, we finally arrived at the old battery, marked only by a few foundation stones, sheets of corrugated iron, and the rusted steel hulk that was the stamping battery. Mist hung about the bush, adding to the atmosphere of mystery and intrigue.

By midday our stomachs had developed appetites worthy of explorers, so we made our way back to the Landie for lunch before continuing on to Westport. We had filled the tanks at St Arnaud, and that had cost a lot more than I'd anticipated. Now it was early evening, about an hour and a half out of Westport, and there was an unusual silence in the vehicle.

'Why are you guys so quiet?' I shouted, trying to make myself heard over the drone of the engine and the hum of the old mud tyres.

No one replied.

'Guys? Are you all right?' I asked again, turning round in my seat to look at the boys.

Charles, the most vocal of us all, shouted back, 'Nick, I'm hungry! Like, soooo hungry! We didn't have enough lunch and I really need something to eat. Can you please pull over at the next dairy and get some biscuits?'

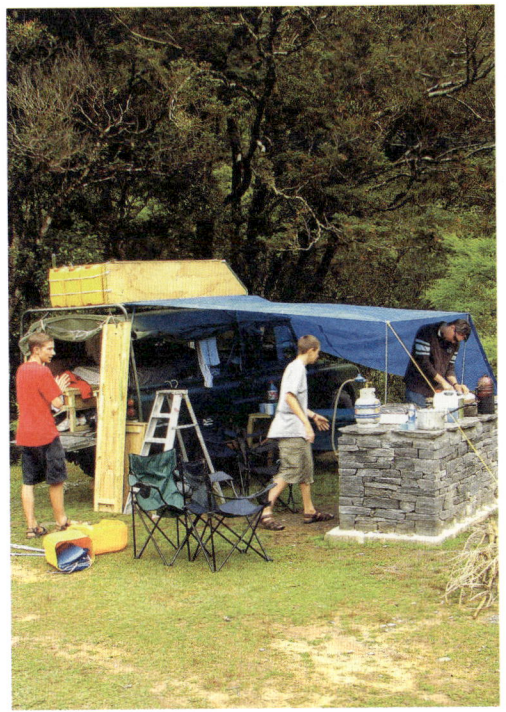
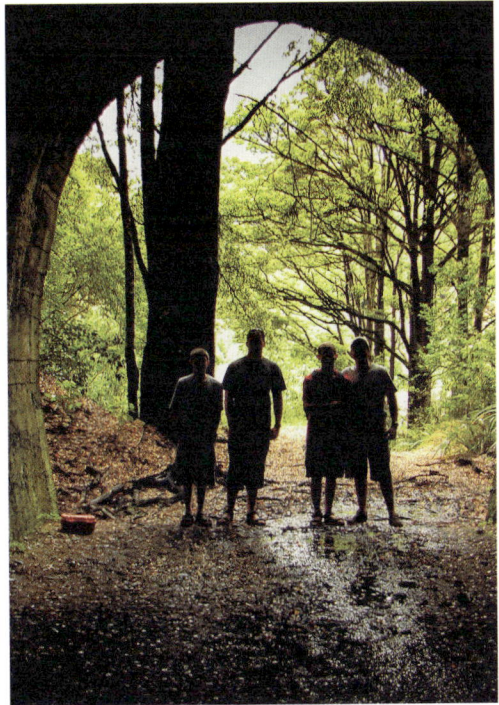
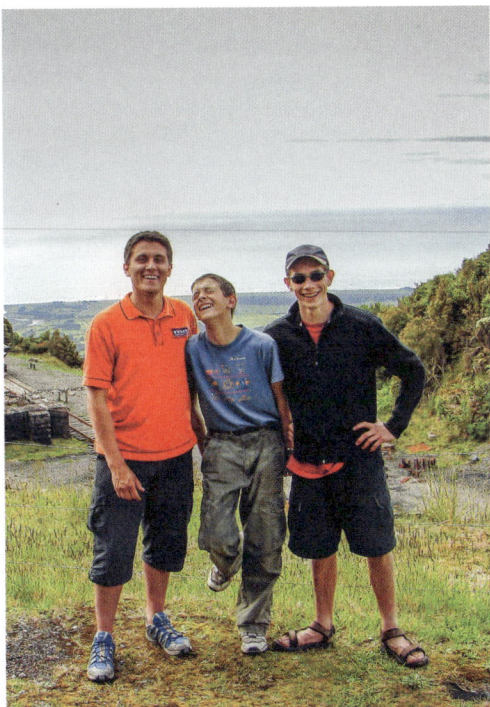
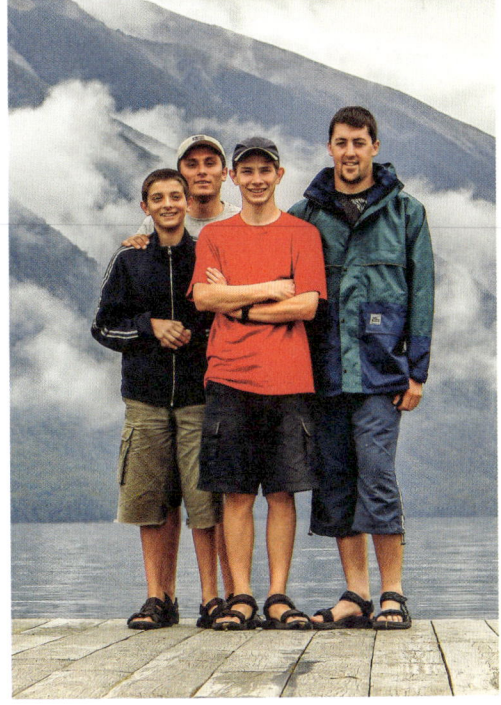

Clockwise from top left: Camped at Lyell; Kawatiri Tunnel; Lake Rotoiti, Nelson Lakes; At the top of the Denniston Plateau.

'Yeah, I'm pretty hungry too,' added Alexander, who was driving, with a subtle nod.

I looked over at the fuel gauge — it was already sitting on the three-quarter mark. We were consuming fuel at an alarming rate.

'Yeah, I know, I'm starving too,' I replied, scratching my head.

'I don't think one loaf of bread is enough for lunch, Nick,' Jonathan said.

'I know,' I replied. 'The problem is that it cost us just under a hundred to top up at St Arnaud, which is more than our daily budget. And then the bread was so expensive there, too, which means that we have already eaten into nearly a third of tomorrow's budget.'

I was silent for a moment, thinking. It was rather annoying, all this. I had done all my calculations and planning so carefully, I thought, but I hadn't considered the possibility that the cost of fuel and bread would be higher in remote West Coast towns.

'Nick, can't we stop at the next dairy and get something to eat?'

'Charlie, if we do, we'll be using up tomorrow's money, which means we'll be hungry tomorrow as well.'

'But, Nick, I'm so hungry. And a packet of biscuits won't cost much! Come on! Don't be a meanie.'

'Charles,' Jonathan grumped, 'if we buy the biscuits today we won't have enough money to buy biscuits tomorrow. End of story.'

'Joni's right, Charlie. Sorry,' I said, as understandingly as I could.

Alexander didn't say anything.

Charles sank his head in his hands and a lethargic silence reigned once more. The engine continued its thirsty drone. It had been a long afternoon.

That night we parked just south of Westport, on the edge of Constant Bay, near the town of Charleston. I jumped out of the Landie with my camera, wanting to take some photos before it got too dark. I took a few shots and then stood on the edge of the beach, not far from the carpark, just admiring the scene. The evening was slightly overcast and way out to sea sheets of rain shrouded the setting sun. The water in the sheltered cove was calm, but a slow swell was rolling through, making a steady run up the pebbly shore. I could see a seal edging its way along the rocks at the mouth of the cove beneath the thick flax. A very slight breeze came off the sea. I took a deep breath.

'Nick! Can we hurry up with dinner? I'm starving!' Charles shouted.

'Sorry! I'll get on to it now,' I shouted back, walking over to the Land Rover. Poor chap, growing and interminably hungry, I thought.

I suggested that the boys light a small fire while I got everything set up in preparation for dinner, something to keep them occupied. They'd gathered driftwood, but most of it was wet. I pulled out a portion of dehydrated mince — it looked like two or three tablespoons of instant coffee sitting in the bottom of a small zip-lock bag. Before we had left I had dehydrated 10 kilograms of beef mince stolen from Mum's freezer, and this was our first night of it.

'Is that all we're getting for dinner?' Charles whined, slightly disgusted.

'It'll expand, Charlie, I promise. And we'll have it with a sauce.' I pulled out a handful of Maggi sachet sauces. 'Do you want Beef Bourguignon, Lamb Goulash or Mexican Mince?'

'I don't care, just give me food!' Charles said in exasperation, collapsing into his camping chair. He rubbed his eyes, sore from the smoke billowing from the smouldering wood.

My map, which was probably 20 years old, told me there was a petrol station at Punakaiki. We considered heading back up to Westport from Constant Bay to fill up with petrol, but we were keen to continue south so we decided to do it at Punakaiki. I really should have filled up at Westport the previous night, as we passed through, but we were all too tired and hungry.

First on the list was a stop at the Mitchell's Gully gold mine, where gold had been sought in the soft sandstone of the ancient seabed formed from the silts washed down from the mountains. A somewhat short, scrawny gentleman, with a long white beard, stood behind the counter in the office, which was crammed with dusty mining paraphernalia, old glass bottles and sepia photographs.

He told us how the mine had opened in the late 1800s, and how his great-grandfather had worked there. 'But did you know,' he continued in his raspy voice, enunciating delicately in a tone of pure wonder, 'the whole universe is magnetic, flowing with energy and life-force — which is magnetism, of course. And not just that —' he leant forward slightly, his eyes big — 'we're magnetic. Yes! The very blood pumpin' through your veins is magnetic!'

He flung his arms into the air.

'You see, all the problems of humanity — all our sicknesses and ailments — are because we have become disconnected from the life-force. But magnets concentrate the life-force, allowing us to connect with it again. That's why I have these.'

He pulled out a couple of large rare-earth magnets from beneath the glass-topped counter and ran them up and down his forearm, across his well-defined veins.

'Oh, wow,' I exclaimed, surprised and bemused.

The old man explained the healing benefits of magnetism with enthusiasm and at length. About 15 minutes passed. 'So when I heard that the kids were playing up in the car, all agitated and what not, I told the parents about the magnets and ran the magnet over the little boy's arm. They popped in on their way back and told me that the boy had slept like a baby for the rest of the trip — all because of the magnets!'

By now Alexander was examining the photos on the wall of the office for the third or fourth time. Charles looked longingly out of the door, then back at me, as if he was almost ready to die.

'That's amazing! Thanks so much for telling us about all that . . . Hey, how much does it cost to get in to see the mine?' I interrupted as soon as there was a slight pause.

'Where are you guys from?' the old guy asked, raising a bushy eyebrow.

'We're from Taupo,' I said, pointing to myself, Jonathan and Charles.

'I'm from Auckland,' Alexander added.

'Auckland, eh?' He didn't seem too impressed at that, and looked

Alexander up and down. 'I'll just pretend you said Taupo, my boy. That will be five bucks each.'

It was possibly the best $5 I'd ever spent. We took a good hour exploring the warren of cold, damp tunnels and shafts that riddled the area. After a while the old gentleman found us and gave us a guided tour, explaining how the mine worked and showing us some of the local fauna: trapdoor spiders and wetas in particular. He was a real character and we enjoyed lots of laughs.

When we walked back to the office with him there were a couple of tourists waiting.

'Hello!' the old gent said cheerfully.

'Hi,' the couple responded timidly. 'Um, how much is it to visit the mine?'

'Where are you from?'

'The UK.'

'That'll be twenty dollars each, thanks.'

The couple handed over the money.

'Thank you,' said the old man, quickly counting the cash. 'Before you walk in, let me tell you about these.' He picked up the magnets, which were still lying on the counter. 'Did you know that the whole universe is magnetic, flowing with energy and life-force?'

We gave him a wave as we quickly exited, but he was too engrossed in his story to notice.

It's a stunning drive as you head south towards Punakaiki. We pulled over just after a hairpin corner high above the sea cliffs of Meybille Bay, and walked the few metres to the lookout. The wind was gusting strongly enough to make our eyes water, and the view was inspiring. A big swell rolled in, erupted on to the rocks then washed back out to sea. The hills, rising steeply out of the sea, disappeared into the mist. The coast felt rugged and remote, and I soaked it in, amazed to be able to enjoy an environment like this again and yet be only a few metres from the road.

I let out a loud 'Woohoo!'

'What do you think of this, guys? Isn't this awesome?'

'Real good view,' Alexander replied, understated as usual.

'Inter-westing. Weal inter-westing,' Charles said with a cheeky grin, as he tried to get his face in the shot I was attempting to frame.

The empty light on the fuel gauge began flashing on both tanks as we rolled into Punakaiki. We all kept a lookout for the petrol station, but when we reached the famous Pancake Rocks on the southern tip of town there was still nowhere to fill up. We pulled into the Pancake Rocks cafe, and I ran inside and approached the guy behind the counter.

'Gidday. Where's the petrol station?'

'Petrol station?'

'Yeah, the petrol station.'

'There hasn't been a petrol station here for years, mate.'

'Damn.' I was a bit shocked. My mind raced as I tried to think of a solution. 'Well, look, here's my situation: I'm on empty and I need some gas. There's no way I'm gonna make it to Greymouth. Do you know of anyone in town who has a supply of fuel, anyone who would be willing to sell me some?'

'Yip. The DOC office has some. Try them. Head back up the road and they'll be on your left.'

'Thanks, mate,' I said, and headed back out to the Landie.

Alexander drove us to the DOC (Department of Conservation) office. There was no one on duty inside so I went around the back.

'Kia ora, bro. Can I help you?' I heard a voice behind me.

I turned round. 'Oh, hi! Hey, do you sell petrol here?'

'Youse driving the Landie?' the guy asked, nodding at the Land Rover. He didn't sound like your typical DOC ranger, but he was covered in grass and walking around with a weed-eater, so I assumed he sort of belonged.

'Yeah, that's right.'

The man burst out laughing. 'You're buggered, mate! Youse couldn'a chosen a worser vehicle! Those bloody Landies'll suck youse out of house and home. Your dad had better be a bloody Arab prince or something too, eh, 'cause youse'll need one to feed that beast!' He roared with laughter again.

I laughed too. After all, my naivety at thinking that $80 per day for fuel, food and accommodation would suffice to get by on *was* pretty laughable. At least, I thought it was laughable; I don't think Charles and Alexander thought there was anything funny about it.

'I know! She's proving to be a bit thirstier than I expected. But it's good for losing this,' I said, patting my puku. 'So how much do you want for the fuel?'

'We get tourists runnin' outta fuel all the time, so we've got the big tank out back just for fullas like you.' He laughed again.

'Oh yeah? And how much do you charge?'

'Five bucks a litre, eh. How much do ya need?'

I let out a low whistle. Loaded up with all our gear, we were getting about 4 kilometres per litre of fuel. It was about 50 kilometres to Greymouth. 'Thirteen litres should do it.'

As I hopped into the Land Rover Joni asked, 'How much was it?'

'Sixty-five dollars.'

'Agh! Another day's food gone,' Charles groaned.

By the time we reached Franz Josef the situation had not improved much, except that we had all got used to eating less food. The best days were those when we had enough money to buy a loaf of bread and a packet of potato chips. Alexander and Jonathan were always given the responsibility of divvying our daily rations into neat piles. As naturally precise people, they excelled at ensuring we all got an equal number of big, medium and small chips, as well as an equal portion of crumbs. It was a serious business.

By now it was just a couple of days before Christmas. We had driven from Franz Josef down to Fox Glacier so Alexander could do a guided walk up on the glacier. Originally, I had planned to go as well, but by this point, not only did we need the money for food, but I also knew I would not handle the requisite five or six hours of walking. The short 30-minute walks we had been doing on the way down to the glaciers were leaving me feeling tired and in need of a rest.

Jonathan, Charles and I sat eating lunch at a lookout with a view of

Fox Glacier framed by ponga fronds. I didn't say much that day. I felt pretty flat about not being able to go on the glacier walk, something I'd always wanted to do, something I'd hoped I might be able to do if I managed my sleep and rested appropriately. But the periods of rest and sleep offered by the trip were not enough and I was beginning to feel worn out.

Suddenly a thunderous roar echoed up the valley and our eyes shot up towards the glacier. A massive block of ice had carved off the terminus, but we caught only the explosive spray of ice that showered down on the tourists as they ducked and ran away from the 'Come no closer' sign.

As I looked at the crevassed icefall above the terminus I imagined the glacier groaning under the weight of the magnificent snowfields above. The poet Stephanie de Montalk puts it so well in her poem 'Violinist at the Edge of an Ice Field':

> *At first only silence,*
> *and then slowly a dull roar*
> *. . .*
> *a crevasse stretching,*
> *or a solidified stream adjusting*
> *to shear stress*
> *and the immediate prospect*
> *of decoupling*

There was more splendour than I could handle and I felt a twinge of grief, just as I had when we'd been at Arthur's Pass days earlier. On the one hand, I had just loved it; it's a supremely beautiful part of the country. We'd camped for a night at Klondyke Corner, where the Waimakariri meets State Highway 73 and the Bealey River, just before the township. It was a magic spot, looking up the valley and into the Alps, the Jellicoe, Shaler and Black ranges still crowned in white, while the river ran deep and cool beside us. In a setting like that I always find my eyes being drawn upwards, along the ridges and across the glaciers, up to the peaks. I felt an overwhelming desire to

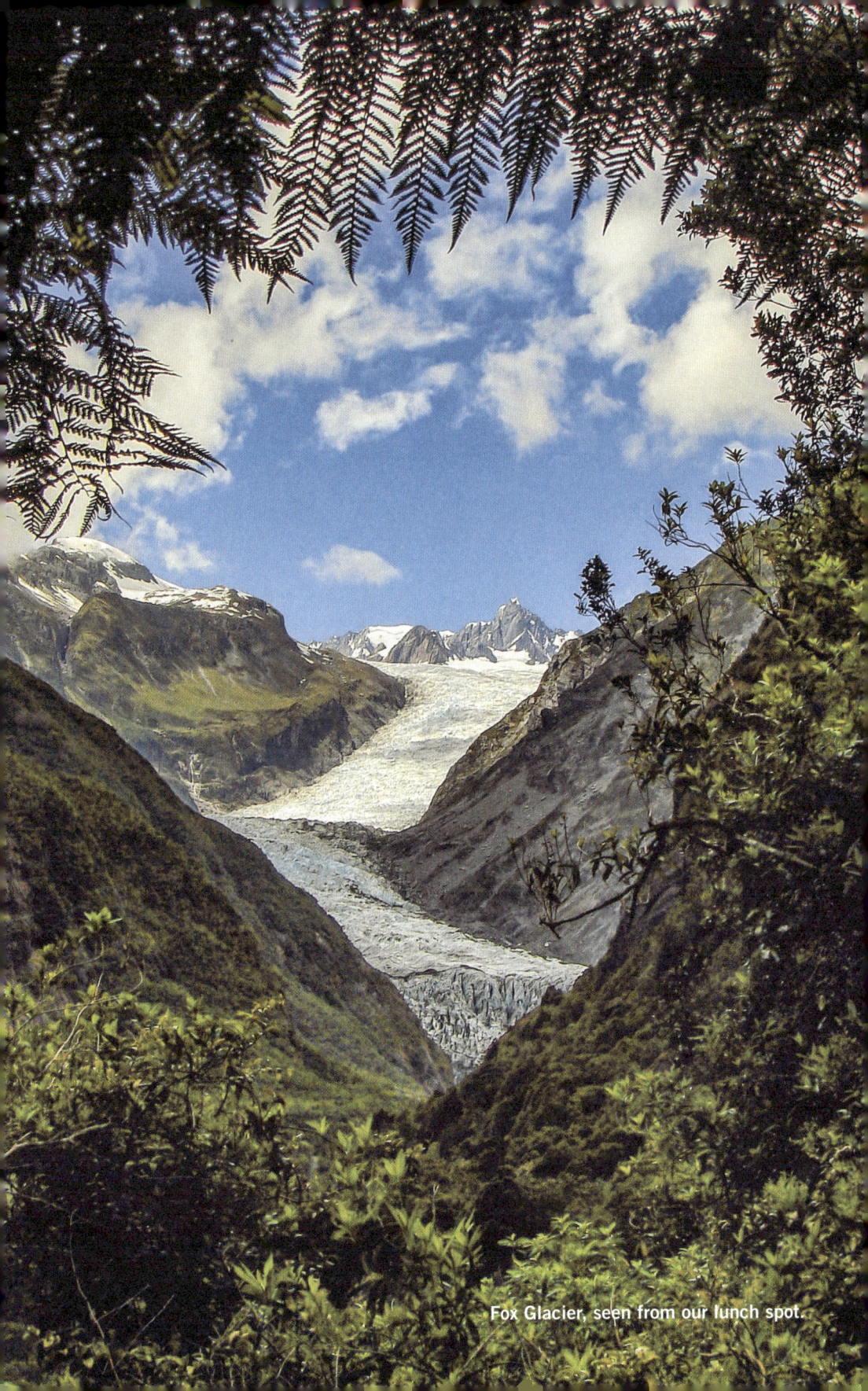

Fox Glacier, seen from our lunch spot.

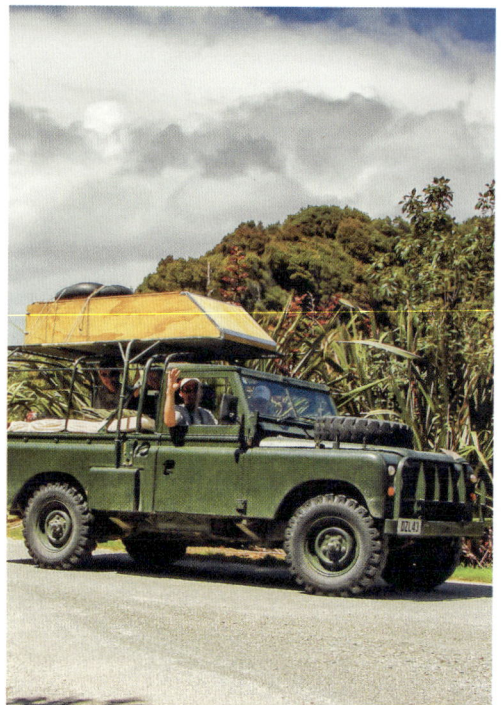
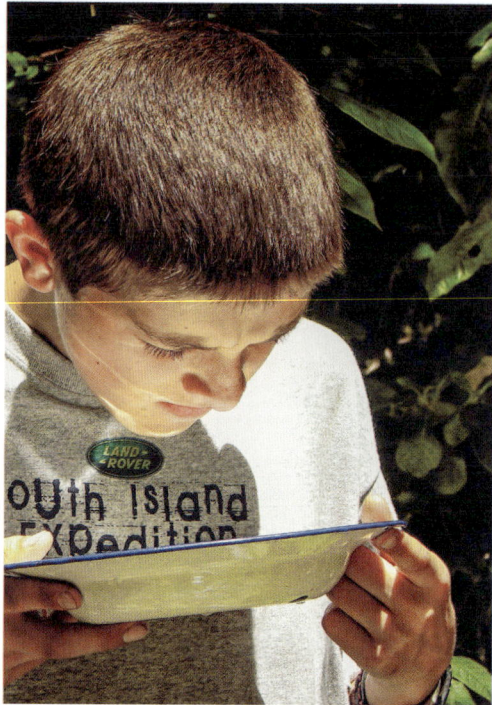

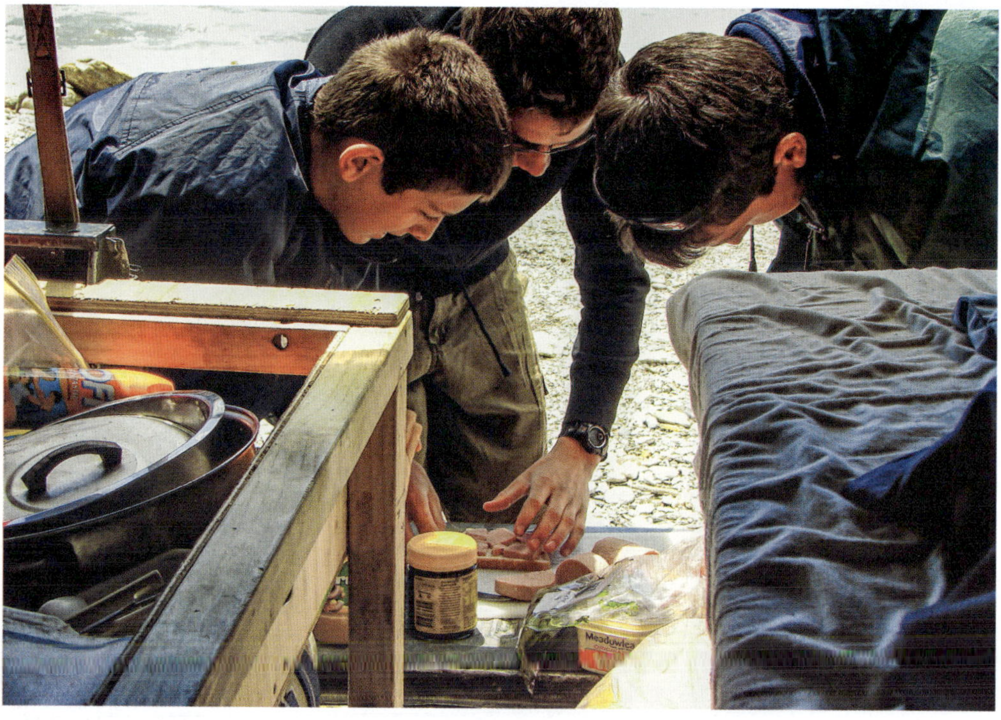

Clockwise from top left: Driving with the roof off; Charles panning for gold near Ross; Dividing up the daily rations.

be up there, among the rock and ice. Yet I knew that there was no way I could be. It felt as if the peaks were taunting me, flaunting their beauty and mocking my weakness. The sense of impossibility and limitation was crushing.

The Land Rover was great and I loved the fact that it enabled me to get out into the wilderness. I also loved the way it helped me to overcome certain social barriers. Many people my age had moved out of Taupo for work, and those who remained tended to be super-outdoorsy types — at least, the people I liked to hang out with were. This was a source of conflict for me as I wanted to be part of this group but I was constantly confronted by all the things I couldn't do anymore. My inability to participate had become a barrier to enjoying community.

With the Landie, it was a different story. It gave me access to a welcoming community. Through the process of upgrading and outfitting the Land Rover I was constantly in conversation with the New Zealand Land Rover Owners Club internet forum. I had only very basic mechanical experience and I needed the advice of these veteran Land Rover owners. I felt as if these guys were my mates, particularly as I asked them questions, gave them updates, and enjoyed a bit of banter. Also, because the Land Rover was a classic vehicle, all kinds of people would come to have a look, telling me stories of the Land Rovers they'd owned back in the day. It was a lot of fun and I enjoyed being part of a community where my illness did not really matter.

Nevertheless, the Land Rover could not get me up there, into the mountains, or on to a glacier. I still felt isolated from the fullest expression of my love of the outdoors. And, while I loved being part of the Land Rover community, that involvement could only be sustained for as long as I was able to drive the vehicle, something I was now struggling to do. Apart from short stretches, I'd given the responsibility of driving entirely over to Alexander. I found this hard, both because it felt as if I was abdicating my responsibility as the trip organiser, and because it was one step closer to losing access altogether.

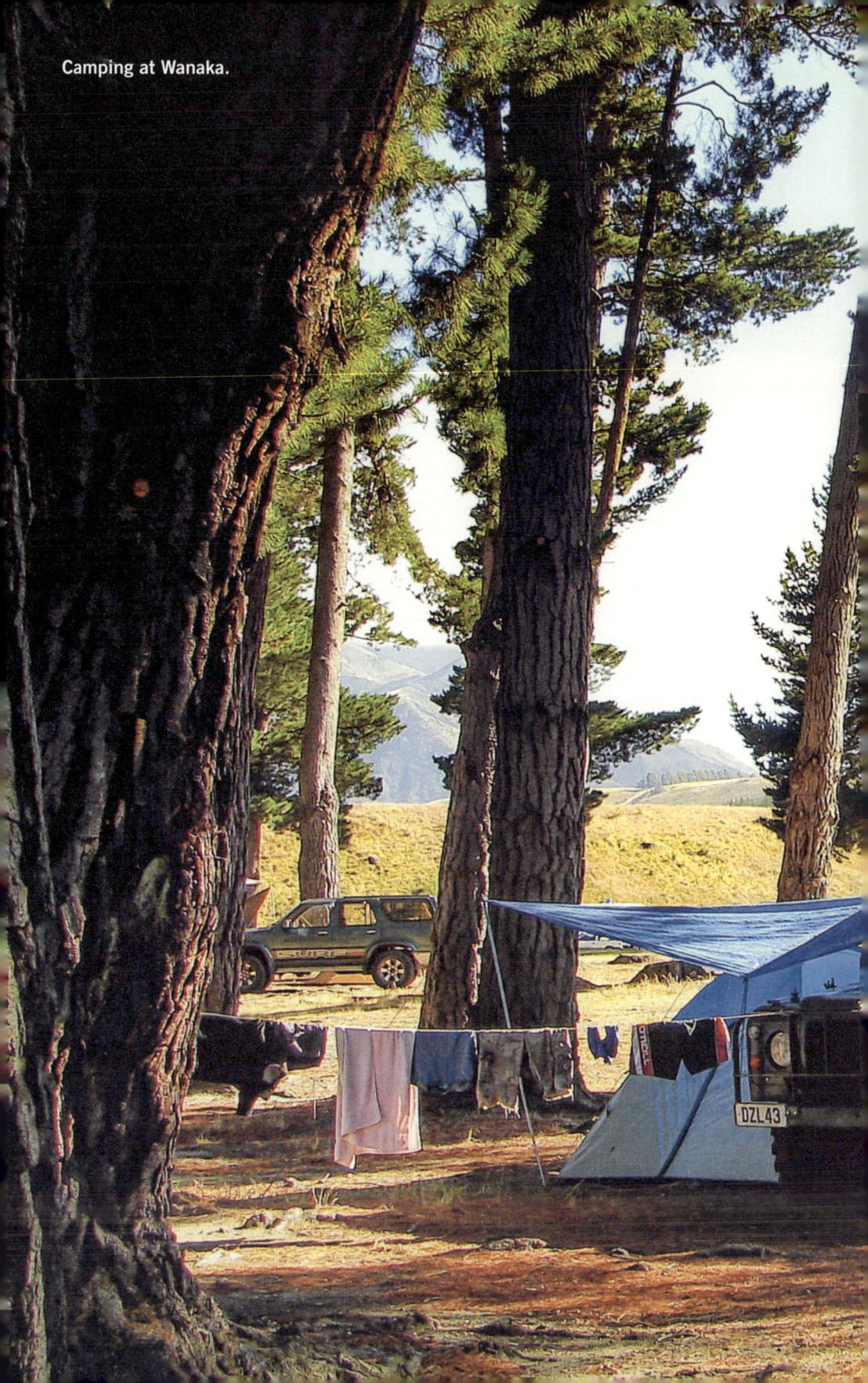

Camping at Wanaka.

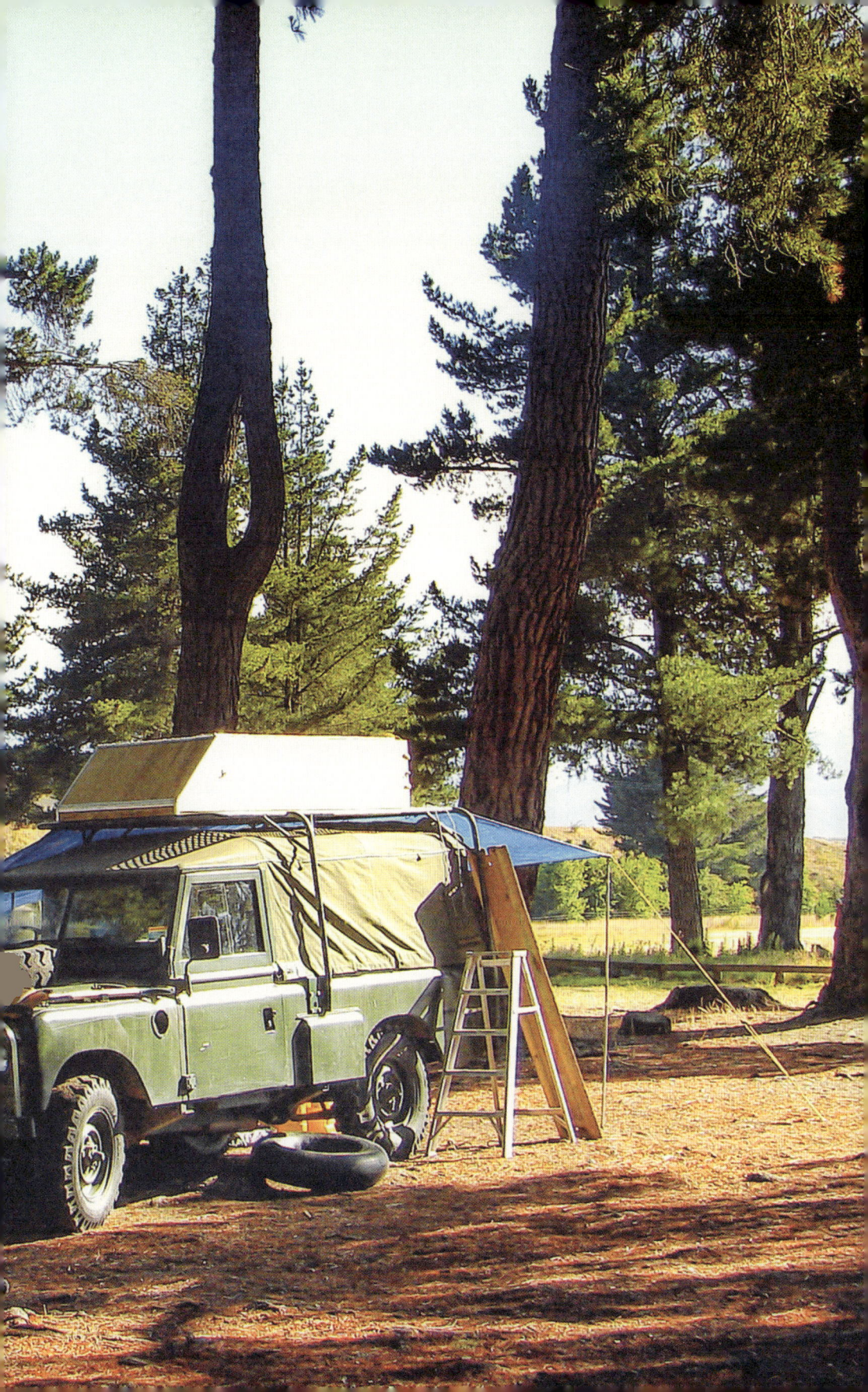

Then came our greatest moment of desperation. Wanaka. We were wretchedly hungry. It was a beautiful sunny afternoon and we were walking past the cafes that line the waterfront. Now in our third week of travel, we had managed to spend a total of $1400 on fuel, leaving each person $3.25 a day for food. We still had enough dehydrated mince for dinner and the porridge for breakfast went on Mum's emergency credit card — it was a pretty dire situation, after all — but that still left lunch. With our budget, we could barely afford a coffee, much less lunch.

'These smells make me so hungry,' Charles said.

'Me too,' Alexander agreed.

'Oh, look!' whispered Charles, pointing. 'Look at those people.'

A couple had just walked away from their table, leaving behind a big bowl of fries evidently untouched. Never in my life had a bowl of fries looked so tempting. My stomach growled.

'We should get them!' Charles said, wide-eyed with excitement.

Jonathan stood a short distance away, ogling the fries.

'Quick, let's go! They'll be wasted otherwise,' Charles urged.

It was very tempting. The chips were sitting there, waiting to be cleared, and it seemed wrong for them to be wasted. Nevertheless, I felt stuck in an ethical dilemma: would we be stealing these fries if we ate them?

'What do you reckon?' I asked Alexander.

'Dunno,' he replied, glancing around nervously.

'Would it be stealing, do you think?' I asked.

Alexander didn't say anything, and stared down the street.

Jonathan turned to me and said, 'I think it would be. We should just go.' He started to walk away.

'I agree,' Alexander added, taking a step away.

I grunted. I knew they were right, but I was desperately hungry.

'Come on!' Charles whined. 'Why can't we just do it?'

'OK, let's go, quick,' I said to him, and I started to walk towards the table.

Just before we reached it a fat seagull landed on the fries, jumped down on to the table, and started eating them. Fighting a seagull for food seemed to be a stoop too low, so we walked on.

We sat down by the edge of the lake and discussed the situation. I was not in good shape physically and we had run out of money. Starvation, we decided, was not that much fun. It was time to head back north.

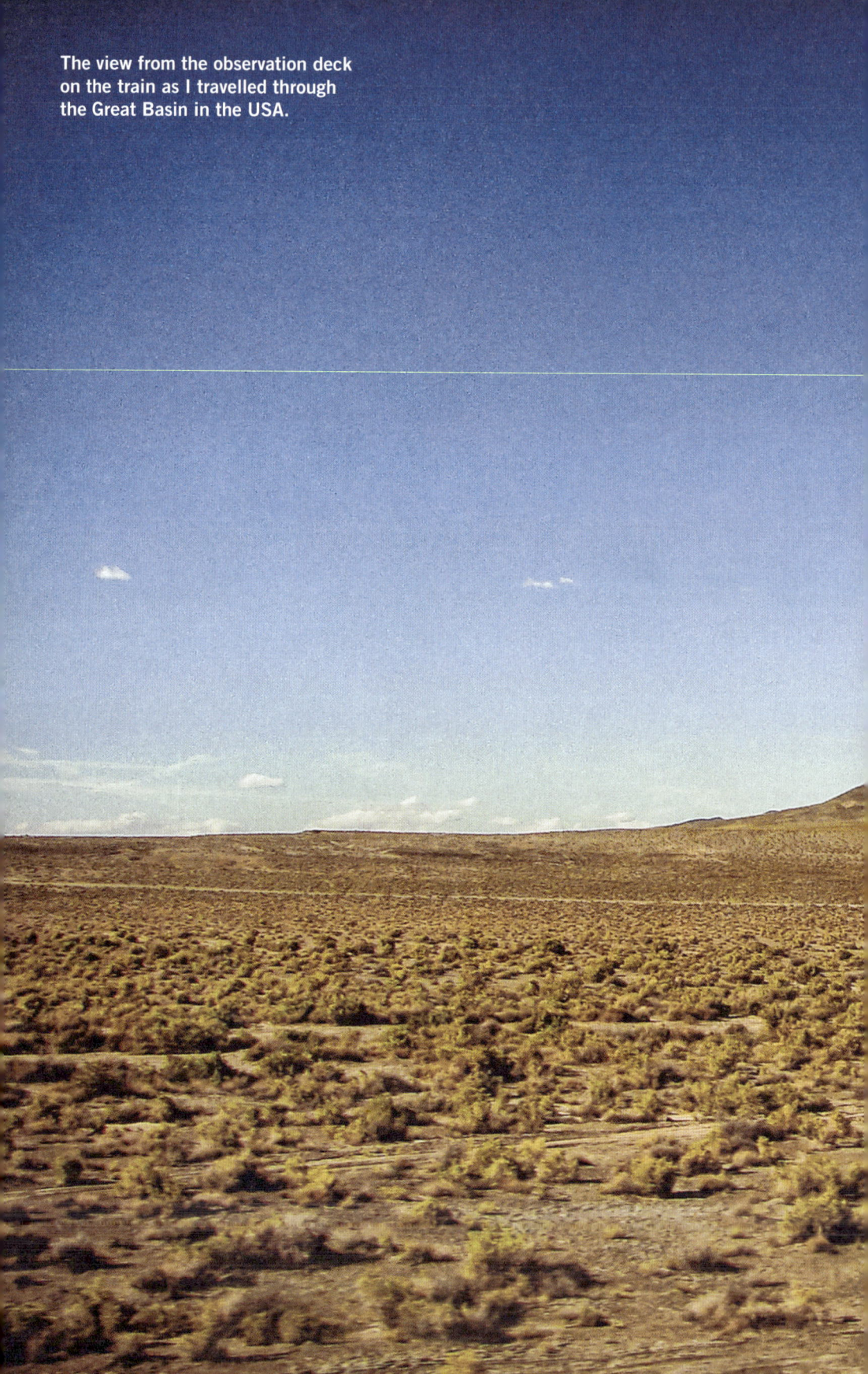

The view from the observation deck on the train as I travelled through the Great Basin in the USA.

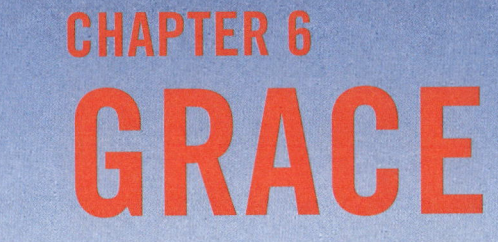

CHAPTER 6
GRACE

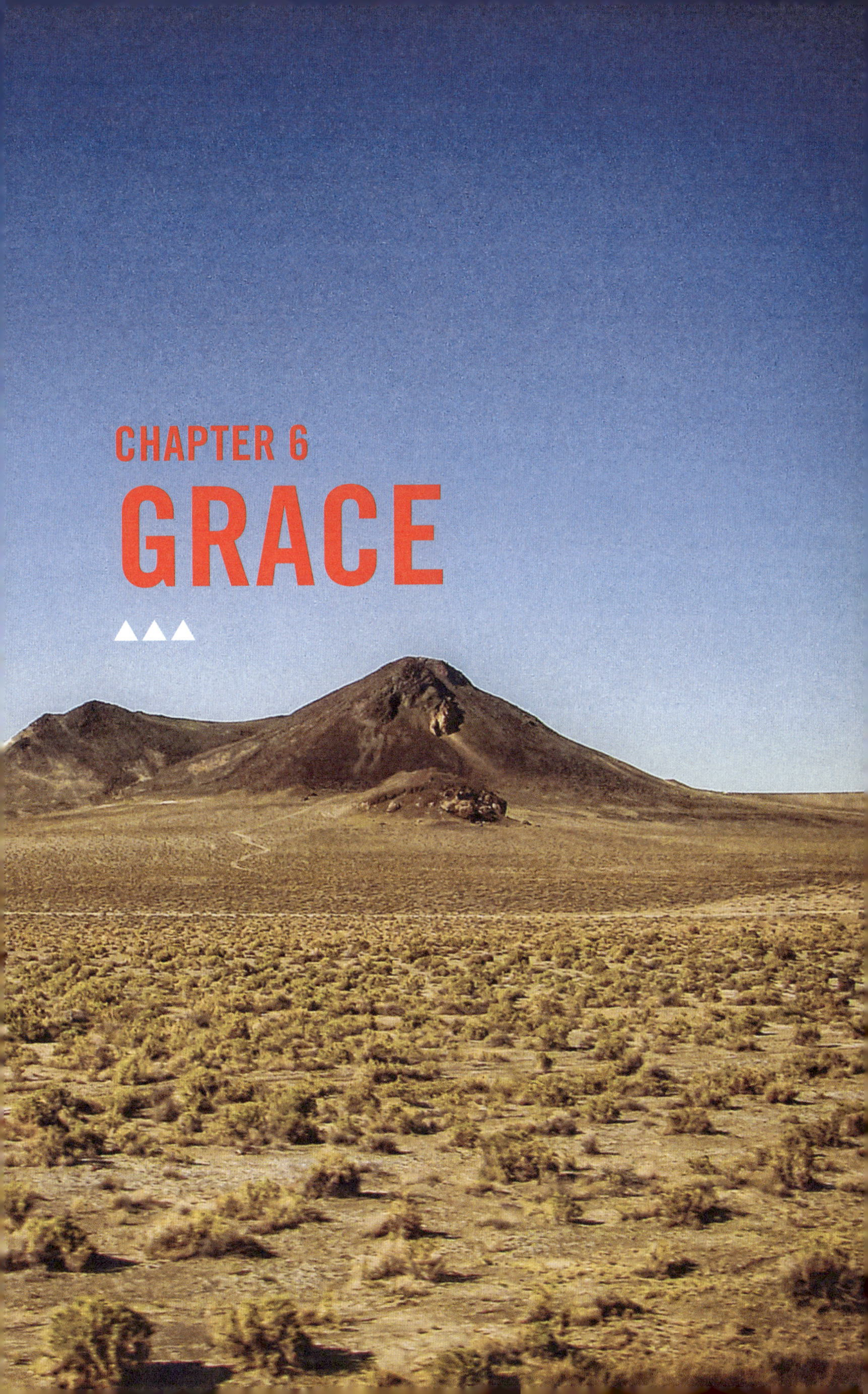

▲▲▲

August 2009
Nebraska, United States of America

Endless cornfields raced past my window, punctuated by power poles and the odd shrub. I had never seen land so flat. Nothing broke the horizon but the occasional barn. I felt uncomfortable without the view of a mountain or hill on the horizon.

I returned my focus to my computer and pressed 'Send' on the email. I felt an intense sense of heaviness. I knew I had just dropped a bombshell, but I didn't want to go back — I knew it would never work. I looked back out through the dusty window, watching the power lines plot hyperbolic curves as they raced up and down in the frame.

I was taking the train from San Francisco to Chicago, on my way back to university in South Carolina. The trip had begun at my aunt's place south of San Francisco, in Redwood City, on the hill that looks across San Francisco Bay. I'd had a great few days resting after my flight from Auckland and I felt quite at home there. Perhaps it was the many references to New Zealand in the design and decor of my aunt's home that made me feel that way. I also enjoyed the openness and liberality of the few Californians I had met, and I loved the smell of salt carried by the air — a smell redolent of my childhood in Auckland.

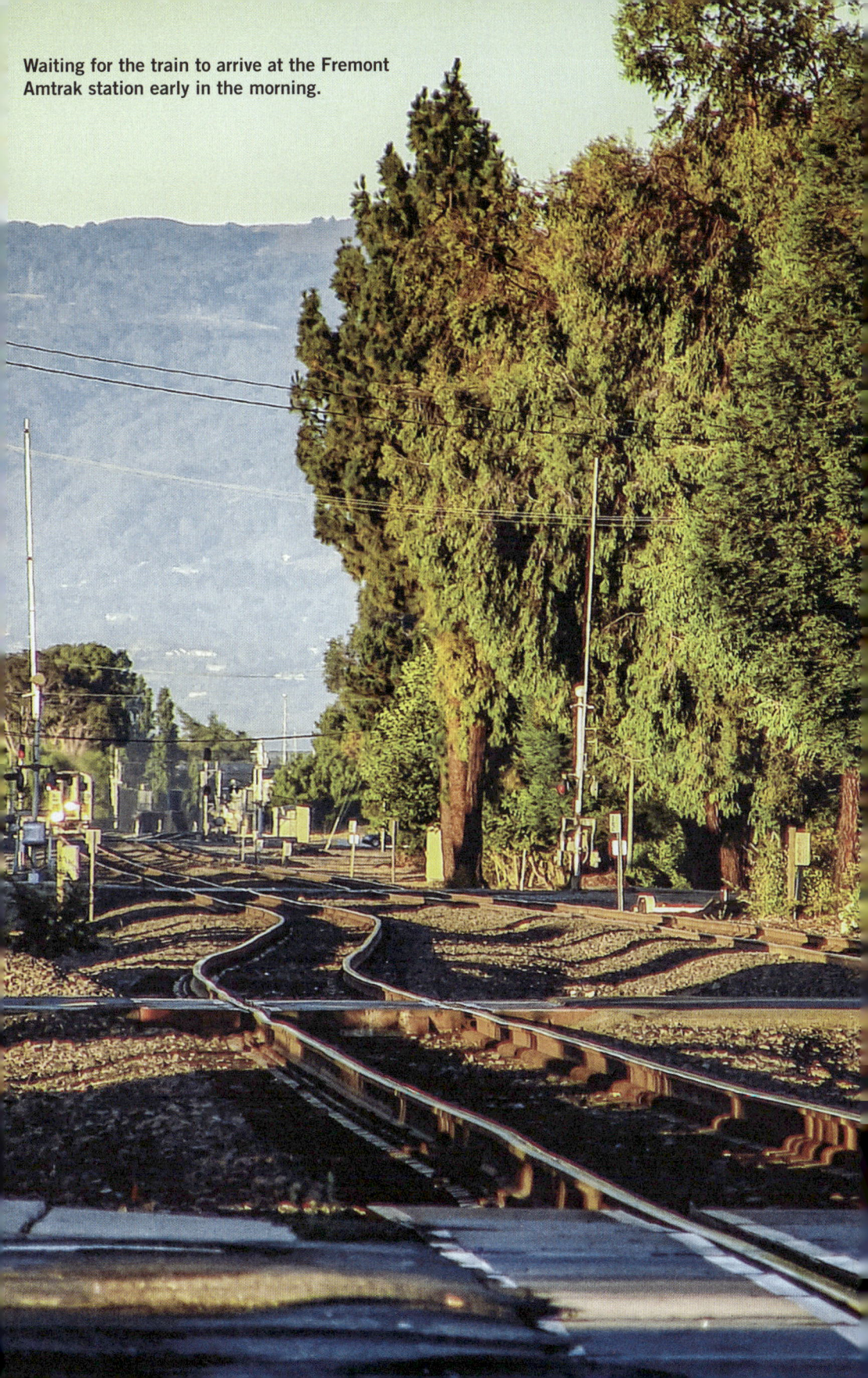
Waiting for the train to arrive at the Fremont Amtrak station early in the morning.

The morning I left California had started at around 5.45, when a taxi had picked me up from my aunt's house. I had been surprised to find that the taxi was actually a small limousine. We had cruised along the highway in style, crossing the Bay on Highway 84, as we headed for the Amtrak station at Fremont. I felt tired from the early start and the seats were supremely comfortable, so I was slightly disappointed when we arrived at the station and I had to rouse myself. I hoisted my pack on to my back and staggered the short distance into the station, grabbed a very quick selfie looking strong and adventurous, then dumped the pack and sat down. It was a good picture, I thought; one for Facebook.

It was as I wound my way along on the Amtrak, heading towards Sacramento, that I first began to feel a sense of unease, even dread. We were rolling past the mothballed Suisun Bay Reserve Fleet, a collection of about eighty ships sitting rusting in the muddy waters of the Bay, a sight made quaintly beautiful by the delicate morning light. As I watched the chop lap against the Second World War battleship the USS *Iowa*, a massive hulk, I felt a sinking feeling.

I felt as if a good thing had just ended — the kind of feeling you experience at the end of a great holiday, when you arrive home to an overgrown lawn and an inbox full of emails, when the dreary reality of life kicks in and pushes the memory of holidays into the realm of dreams. Or perhaps I was feeling the weight of a suspicion that something unpleasant was about to start. I couldn't decide which it was, but I found it troubling nonetheless. Why would I feel this way at the beginning of a great adventure?

It was not the fact of being in the USA per se that made me feel unhappy — the US is a stunning country. I loved the scenery I saw through the train window. I'd decided to travel by train because flying over mountains always seems like a waste to me, the convenience of speed coming at the cost of enjoyment of the physical landscape.

The train climbed out of Sacramento, through the granite hills of Tahoe National Forest and into the Sierra Nevada mountains. Small patches of snow clung to the tops of some peaks, feeding the pines and firs that sit as steepled woods in the dips and valleys. The gnarly granite knobs and ridges drew the eye down to the sapphire-blue alpine lakes. We made a stop in the small town of Truckee, where the old Western-style shops had weatherboard facades and the taverns were rough-plastered, Spanish style; they seemed cradled by the gentle boughs of fir and pine that surrounded them. Occasionally we'd pass an old water race or viaduct. I wondered if they were remnants of the gold-rush days — they certainly looked like it.

Coming off the Sierra Nevada we entered the Great Basin, a desert area of massive basins and ranges that have no draining point other than the saline lakes that lead to Death Valley. The reds, browns, greys and greens of the eroded mountains, now smooth mounds, were hauntingly beautiful in the late-afternoon sun. The landscape was barren, supporting only a smattering of woody shrubs and tumbleweed. Occasionally we'd cross large areas of mud-cracked earth, low points that became shallow seasonal lakes. Precipitation, which mostly falls as snow, melts and evaporates beneath the harsh desert sun. I sat in the train's glass-roofed observation car, enthusiastically photographing the landscape and soaking in the glory of the desert sunset.

The next morning we were winding our way into the breathtaking Rocky Mountains. Still in the desert, we moved through great mesa-ridged landscapes. At times it felt as if we were on the set of a Western movie, and I half expected to see John Wayne appear round the corner. When the train stopped at the little towns along the way I felt I was being given a distant glimpse of the lives of people whose everyday experiences were a world away from mine. We passed plenty of ruins, too, brick-walled buildings with roofs that had collapsed. It amazed me that anyone could live in such a barren environment, it was so dusty and dry. The textures of the earth flashed by my window, the coloured lines and layers of the ridges and mountains, the water-scoured faces that looked like elephant skin.

As the train moved into the Rockies the mountains grew larger and steeper, and the valleys deeper. The train was moving slowly now, hugging the sides of ravines, torrents raging below. From time to time we'd see people rafting beneath, throwing quick glances up at

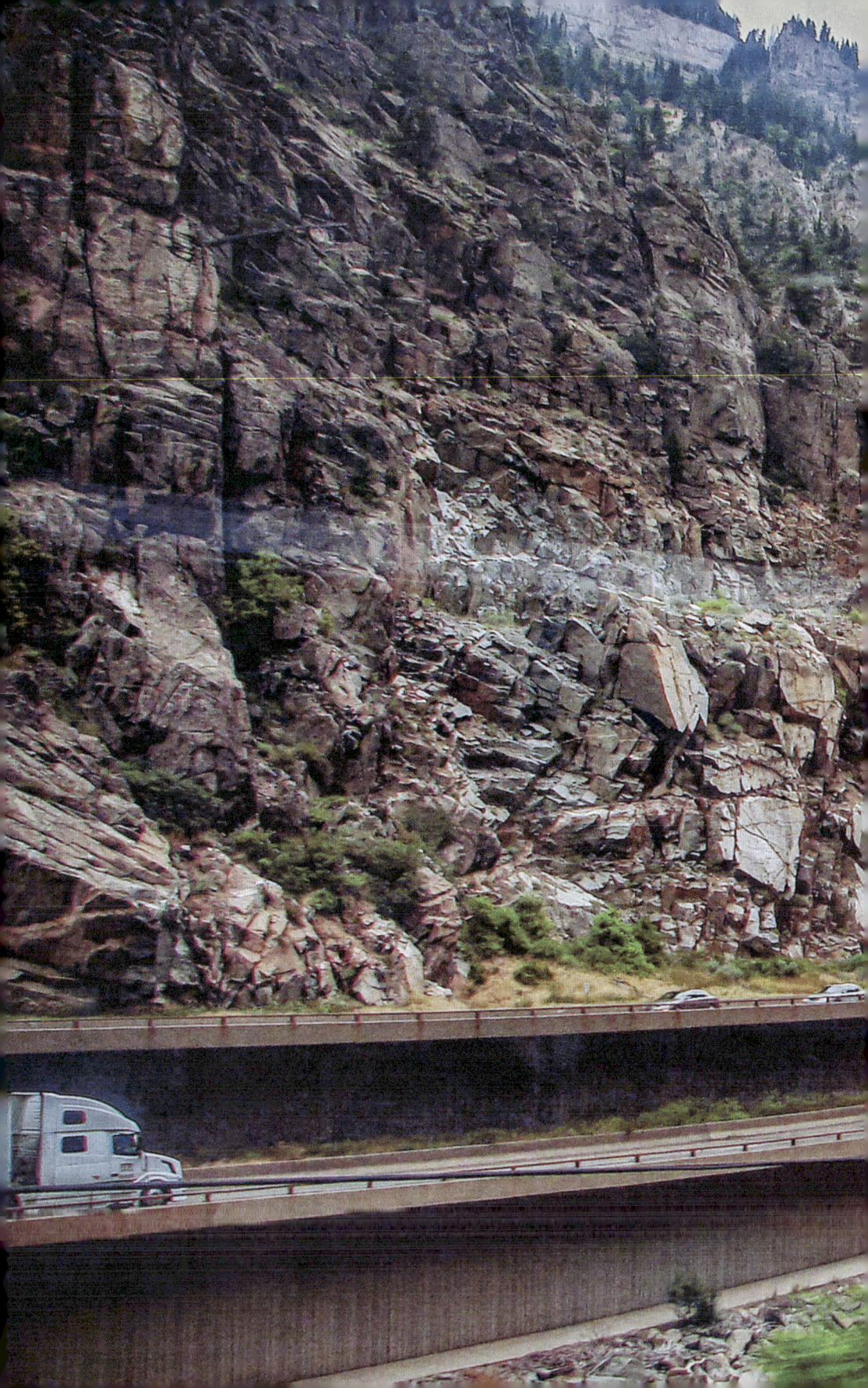

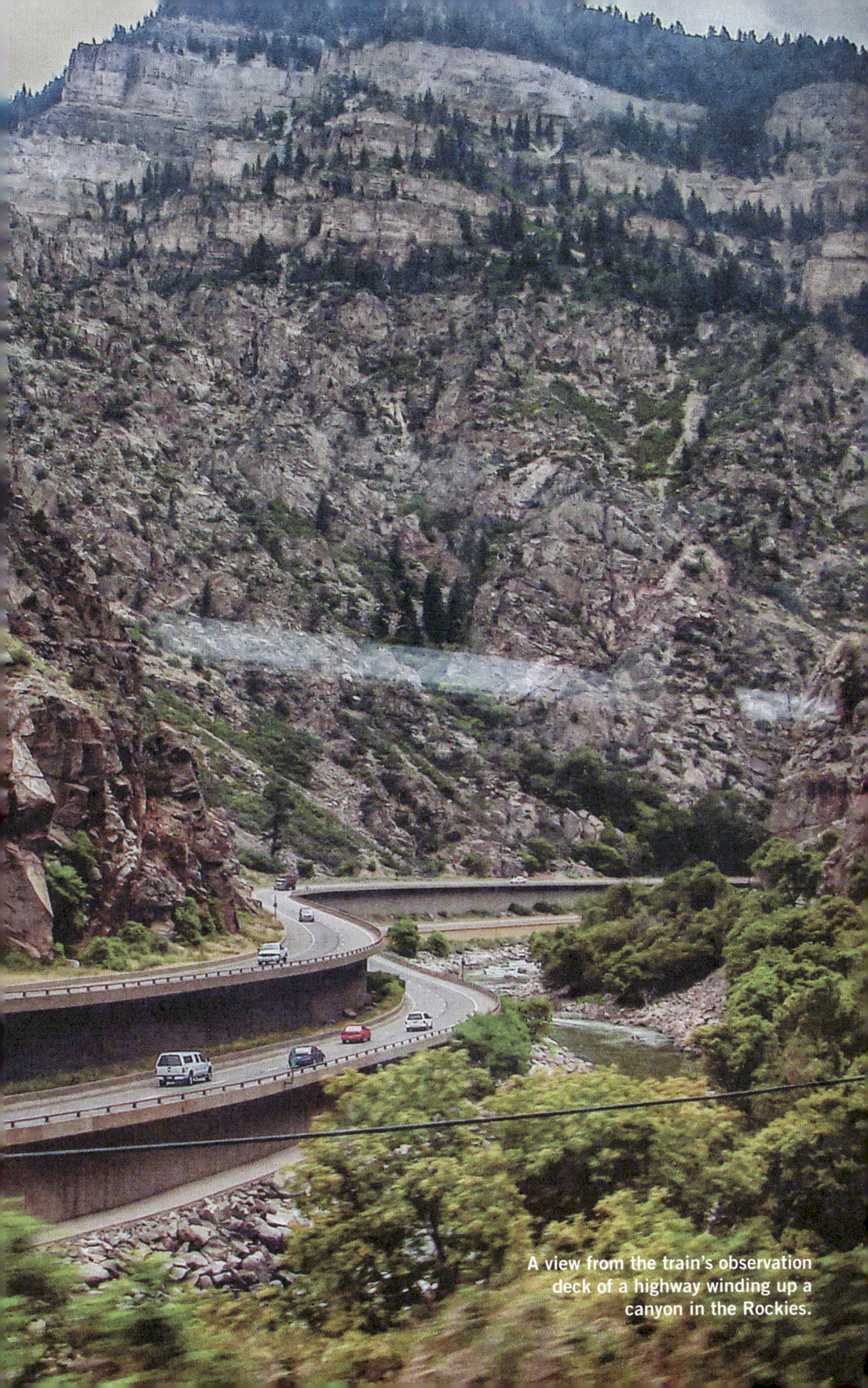
A view from the train's observation deck of a highway winding up a canyon in the Rockies.

us as they crashed through the rapids. Around Glenwood Springs, a resort town nestled high up in the heart of the Rockies, there were even more people swimming and fishing in the river. Every now and then someone would pull down their pants and expose themselves to the full and bemused view of the train's passengers. The steward announced that this 'mooning' was a tradition among the people who lived in the area, and suggested that if passengers were offended by it they should move to the other side of the train.

I got talking to a young Mormon woman who was a postgraduate student at a university in Utah. When I told her where I was going she looked surprised and slightly amused. 'You're studying there, at that university?'

'Yeah.' I tried to laugh, cringing slightly inside.

'You know that's a crazy-strict, super-conservative university, right?'

'Yeah, I know.' I looked at the floor, surprised at how embarrassed I felt. 'I've been there before.'

'Wow! And you're going back.' She looked at me sideways. 'I've heard about it, but I've never met anyone from there before.' She paused. 'So are you one of those super-conservative types? You don't look it.'

I thought about this for a moment. I felt as if I had suddenly happened upon the core of the issue: What was I? What did I want to be?

'Um, no. No, not really,' I said, scratching my head.

'Jeeze. Then why the hell are you going back?' She looked at me, completely mystified.

'Yes, it's crazy, I know.'

'I'll say it's crazy.' She sat back in her seat and looked out the window. 'Gosh. I don't know why anyone would go there.'

I couldn't think of a reply to this so I decided instead to change the subject. 'So, tell me about your thesis,' I said.

As we began the descent from the Rockies, towards the foothills of Colorado and beyond, I thought about our conversation. Why was I going back? Did I really want to be subject to the rule of the bell and the threat of the student discipline committee? Even more troubling was a brooding dread of theological conflict. I was a Presbyterian entering a predominantly Baptist university with a reputation for an unflinching commitment to a particular set of very conservative American beliefs. The potential for conflict was very real.

I had made my beliefs clear when the university offered me the scholarship, and I was aware that I was likely to be pressured to change. It wasn't that I intended to be inflexible or closed-minded, but at the crux of my faith was a belief in the importance of grace — the free and unearned favour of God, uninfluenced by how well I perform. Much larger than denominational affiliations, I knew this would be at odds with the university's conservative values, which encompassed a meritocratic, performance-based relationship with God.

I knew that returning was not going to work. Deep down I'd known this when I accepted the scholarship — I'd just explained away my dread of going back by conflating it with the fear of becoming unwell again.

When I finally arrived at Denver's Union Station I was met by David, a good friend who I'd known growing up and hadn't seen in years. He lived a little way south of Denver, in Roxborough. It was fantastic seeing him, and as we passed through the outskirts of Denver the conversation naturally drifted to the reason I had come back to the US. I explained that I'd been awarded a scholarship to study in Greenville.

'That's cool, man! How did you manage that?' David asked.

'Well, it was funny actually,' I told him. 'When I was there this time three years ago, I made friends with the guy who's in charge of international admissions. After I'd left in a bit of a rush, he put my name forward for the scholarship, without even telling me. I guess he felt sorry for me, after I'd had to drop out and return home. At the beginning of this year I just got an email one morning offering me the scholarship — that was the first I'd heard of it.'

David laughed. 'That's awesome. What are you studying?'

'Divinity. The scholarship is for me to study divinity.'

'Sweet, man — so you want to enter the clergy and become a minister then?'

'Yeah, I think so. I got pretty involved in my church back home, and I think it would be an interesting job. I love working with people and helping them. I think it could be really great in that regard.'

'Isn't that a bit of a change? I mean, weren't you studying engineering or something?'

'Yeah, I was, and I worked as a design engineer for a bit too.'

'Why the change?' David asked.

'Well, I guess I just never found it as satisfying as I'd hoped. I enjoyed the design work and I had a cool boss, but I suppose I realised I was not really into working on machines and circuits and stuff.'

I paused for a moment.

'But, to be honest, part of the reason is that I want a qualification, and I'm not sure I could get one in engineering. Since I got sick last time I was here, my mind has been thick with this intense brain fog. It's crazy, and I find it really hard to think analytically. I just can't handle calculus and hard-core maths anymore — at least, not enough to complete an engineering degree. And then I got offered this scholarship. It provided a goal, and no other options presented themselves, so I went with it. And, hey, it's an all-expenses-paid scholarship — worth over a hundred thousand New Zealand dollars. I mean, how often do you get offered one of those?'

We both laughed.

'Yeah, that sounds like a pretty good deal, all right.'

I paused, trying to psych myself up, trying to overcome the knot that was growing in my stomach. 'Yeah. It should be good.'

David smiled. I could tell he was unconvinced. 'How are you feeling about Greenville?' he asked.

'Oh, OK, I suppose. You know what it's like, eh?' I said.

'Yes. Yes, I do.' He looked at me, squinting slightly. He seemed to be asking, And you really feel OK about it?

I grunted and looked out of the window, wondering whether or not

I should tell him the truth. After a moment I took a breath and said, 'To be honest, I'm dreading it. Theologically and ideologically, the university and I are on different boats. I just don't know how I'll handle that difference without being either assimilated or flogged for it.'

I drew another breath and went on, 'And then, with the scholarship comes the expectation that I'll take over a church in Taupo, and I'm really not sure that's what I want to do. The church is broadly Baptist and roughly on the same page as the university when it comes to grace, so the expectation that I'll change is enormous. I mean, it's a great little church and Taupo is a cool place to live, for a while at least, but the prospect of living there for years . . .' I trailed off, trying to think of the right words. 'I don't know. It leaves me feeling listless . . . and compromised.

'And then,' I added, 'the last time I was at Greenville it wasn't a great experience. I've nearly pulled out a couple of times — perhaps I should have — but the sense of being aimless, powerless, for the last couple of years has been crushing. The scholarship is a way to get going again, to regain purpose. And the university has been really keen to work with me to overcome the obstacles created by my illness. I need a mobility scooter to get around campus, and they've even given me my own wheelchair-accessible room on campus.'

'That all kind of makes sense, I suppose.' I could tell David still wasn't totally convinced.

Our conversation continued over the next few days. David was a great listener and asked probing questions that really got me thinking; I valued his perspective and insight. The process of verbalising my feelings and reflecting on them led me to seriously question my reasons for accepting the scholarship, and to explore the fears that I'd tried to sublimate. By the time I rejoined the Amtrak to continue to Chicago, several days later, I knew I did not want to return to university in South Carolina.

'Well, that's that. The email's sent,' I told Robert, the guy sitting across the table from me in the dining carriage. We were sharing one of the train's few power sockets — I was charging my laptop and he was charging his phone.

'All three pages of it?' Robert asked. It had taken me quite a few hours to write the email, and Robert and I had chatted off and on throughout that time. He was a gentle, empathetic type of guy, on his way back from Reno. And you do talk when you share a booth with someone for the better part of a day. I'd told him everything — it was hard not to, when it was weighing so heavily on my mind.

'Yes, all three pages.' I grimaced. 'I hope it won't be too much of a bombshell for my parents that I've decided to return home.'

'I'm sure it will be fine.' He smiled. 'You know, I had to write an email like that once, when I told my parents I was homosexual. I'm not gonna lie, it was pretty hard at the beginning, with people freaking out and all — but, you know, it's better to be honest and upfront than to keep it all caged up and be unhappy. I'm sure you'll be fine.'

I appreciated Robert's non-judgemental demeanour and his calm reassurance — a gracious acceptance you can only experience through vulnerability.

I looked outside again, into the endless Nebraskan cornfields. I felt relieved that I'd been able to express my thoughts, but I knew that a storm was coming — it wouldn't be easy to shake my connection to the university. There were too many interests and expectations involved.

'Here it is, y'all!' Tom said enthusiastically as he brought my mobility scooter, a new Victory 10, into the showroom where my friend Kyle and I were waiting.

Tom's snowy-white hair and moustache gave him a friendly air. He was gently spoken, kind and eager to help. 'Oh . . . it looks good,' I said, wanting to appear enthusiastic.

I had bought the scooter online a few months earlier. Now that it was standing in front of me, I tried to think of something positive to say. 'The blue looks really good. Oh, and it's got a metallic finish. That's nice.' I tried to feel grateful and not full of disdain as I ran my hand over the smooth paintwork. It looked good, as far as mobility scooters go, I told myself.

'Sure is,' Tom replied. 'And the wheels — what did you call them in the email? Mags? Well, they make it look real sporty. At least, that's what I think, I don't know 'bout y'all.'

I agreed with him. It didn't look like an older person's scooter, which was something of a relief. But it was hard to feel too pleased about the scooter; after all, I was about to forfeit my legs for some wheels.

I thought back to the first time I'd tried out a mobility scooter, just a few months earlier. I was with Dad in Penrose, Auckland, and he was so excited about the scooter and its potential to get me mobile again. By that stage any physical activity left me feeling so fatigued that walking any significant distance without extended periods of rest was not feasible, especially when it was hot. Hurriedly traversing a large campus every day would not be sustainable without the aid of something like a mobility scooter. My doctor had suggested it as something to help me to cope with university in the US.

Dad had driven me to the scooter shop — I could not handle driving in heavy Auckland traffic anymore; my mind was too encumbered by a deep feeling of fogginess. As we pulled into the carpark I felt sick to my stomach. I did not even want to enter the shop, or to be associated with something as defining as a mobility scooter. The idea was to figure out what type and size of scooter would suit me, but as the salesman started explaining the features of the different models I didn't want to listen. I didn't even try. I knew there would be more information than my mind could process. Dad was taking it all in, though, so I left it to him. I just stared out of the window.

'OK, Nick, what do you reckon?' Dad asked after a while. 'I think something like this would be the way to go. How about you?'

The question forced me out of my daze. 'Um, yeah. Sure,' I replied unenthusiastically.

'Cool! Do you want to try it?' Dad asked.

I looked at the salesman, who nodded and smiled, and then back at the scooter. I despised it and I did not want to touch it, let alone sit in it. I would rather die than sit in it.

'Nah, it's OK.' I kept my hands in my pockets.

'Please, feel free to give it a go if you want,' the salesman said. 'We find it's helpful for people to get a feel for a scooter, just to make sure it's the right size and stuff.'

I looked at Dad.

'It makes sense, Nick, to check it out for size.'

I sighed and shrugged my shoulders. 'Fine.'

I don't think I will ever forget that first step on to the scooter, the moment my shoe touched the black non-slip surface. I felt utterly defeated. It felt like an act of surrender, that I'd relinquished every last hope of climbing or tramping ever again. I had already sold the Land Rover by this point, as it was both too expensive and too demanding to maintain. I plonked myself down in the seat.

'Awesome.' The salesman smiled. 'Right, so, let me turn it on and you can take it for a quick spin outside.'

'Oh, it's all right. This is fine. It feels about right,' I said curtly as I turned to get out of the chair.

Dad crouched down beside me and put his hand on my shoulder. 'It's OK, Nick. This will be great. Why not give it a quick go?'

A part of me knew that I needed to give it a go, particularly as I was looking at buying Tom's scooter online, and a part of me knew that this was the only thing that would realistically allow me to get outside. Nevertheless, the rest of me hated everything about this moment.

The salesman opened the door and I drove out on to the footpath beside Great South Road. It was late on a busy afternoon. I wanted to cry. I felt incredibly self-conscious, as if every person in every car driving by was staring at me, despising me. I felt as if I might as well be holding up a sign screaming 'Look at this Failure!' or 'This Guy is a Worthless Weakling!'

Objectively, I knew that none of this was true. I looked at the passing cars and saw that nobody was taking any notice of me, and it's not as if *I* think those things about people I see in wheelchairs or mobility scooters. Clearly I had a double standard, judging myself differently from others. Nevertheless, at that moment I felt a total loss of worth. I'd believed that people would like me if I was masculine: cool, athletic and strong. I felt that the scooter robbed me of these things, casting me out of the mainstream narrative of what life should look like for a 24-year-old Kiwi male and into an emasculated netherworld of meaninglessness and marginalisation. Nevertheless, I was determined to maintain some level of masculine respectability, and I refused to let my emotions get the better of me. I would show that I could at least control my emotions.

Now, standing in Tom's showroom in South Carolina, I experienced similar feelings. I had to work hard to appear excited about my new scooter, to remain focused as Tom explained details of its care and use. As he helped us to load it into the boot of Kyle's car Tom said gently, 'And please feel free to give me a call if y'all have any questions or problems.'

'Thanks heaps, Tom — I tend to forget stuff all the time, so I'll definitely give you a call if I have any questions. Hey, and I really appreciate your help with all this, you know. Thank you,' I said, shaking his hand. Despite my feelings about the scooter I felt deeply grateful for Tom's help and humbled by his compassionate and graceful attitude. He hadn't treated me as an emasculated young man, but with simple dignity, as a human.

Kyle closed the boot and I gave Tom a final wave as I lowered myself into my seat. We drove the short distance back to campus. Not much had changed since I'd left three years earlier — some paint here, a facelift there, but otherwise the same, a fact that made me nervous. I had a growing feeling of oppression as we drove beneath the avenues of trees, around the yellow-brick buildings, and past the meticulously manicured gardens. Memories of the last time I was here and the enormity of the difficulties I would face came flooding over me.

I was still living under the cloud of the email I had sent from the train somewhere in Nebraska. The email had sparked a storm of messages and phone calls from the various parties involved, some of them angry and condemning, some gracious but firm, and almost all of them adamant that I should continue with my studies in the US. I felt as if I was being steamrollered by the agendas of one or two powerful people, that I had lost my voice, and that no one back home could see it. I seemed to have been presented with an impossible choice: disappoint my friends and family by pulling out, or become a spineless coward by staying in.

Stress, I had learned, was one of the main triggers of physical decline, and this situation was intensely stressful — something my body was quick to let me know. In fact, it was more than I could cope with. I found the emotions and pressure of the situation overwhelming. After a week, I caved under the pressure; I decided to stay. The decision made me feel like a coward and reinforced my sense of powerlessness; I felt as if the sickness, by causing me to crumble, had robbed me of both my agency and my ability to independently pursue what I thought was right. Nevertheless, I managed to negotiate a compromise, promising to try the university for one year, at which point I would reassess the situation.

'Here we are!' Kyle announced as we pulled into the dormitory carpark. 'I'll give you a hand unloading the scooter and getting you moved in.'

'Thanks, man.' I smiled.

We hopped out of the car, pulled out my gear, and reassembled the scooter. I could not bear to ride it — I still felt far too self-conscious, so I opted to push it from the car to the dormitory. It was a heavy machine and I struggled, especially when it came to getting it through the front door of the dorm. Kyle, loaded with my bags, held open the door for me. The scooter was just slightly narrower than a standard door frame and there was no way of getting both me and it through the door at the same time. I tried pushing the scooter from behind, without holding the handlebars, but that only resulted in the front wheels taking a hard left or right, smashing the scooter into the door or the frame. It made quite a racket — so much for being inconspicuous.

After several attempts I realised that the only way to get through the door was to drive the scooter through it. Kyle helped me to pull it back out from the doorway and continued to hold the door as I

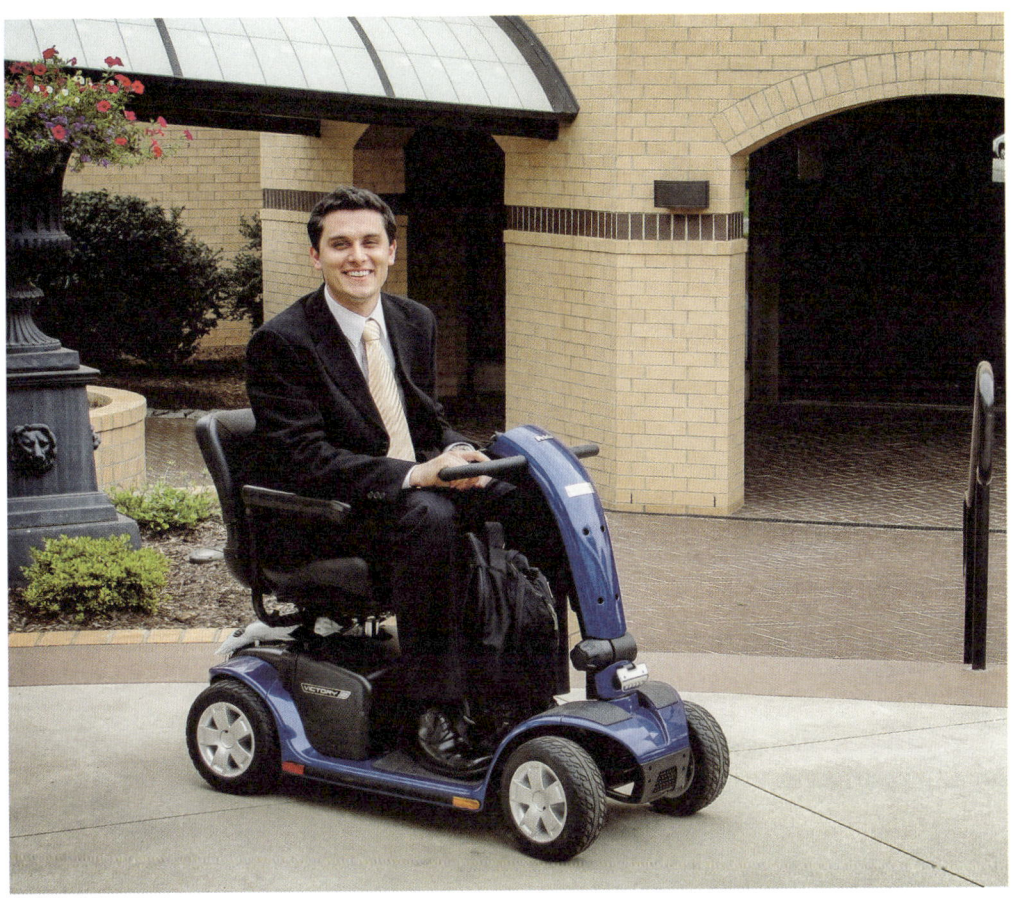

Me on my mobility scooter, the Mighty Blue Beast. I did think about attaching blue LED lights underneath it, to bling it out, for a laugh.

hopped on the scooter and turned the key. I was acutely aware of people watching and I wanted to get through the door as fast as I could. I opened the accelerator right up, but found myself travelling at a snail's pace. Annoyed, I looked down at my little instrument panel and realised that the speed-governor was at its lowest setting. I quickly turned the dial, putting it on the highest speed setting, and once again pulled on the accelerator.

This time, the scooter launched through the door, throwing me back in my chair — the motor put out serious torque, I discovered. Alarmed and barely in control, I let go of the accelerator, which brought me to an abrupt stop, throwing me into the handlebars. A guy manning the info desk in the lobby looked at me with wide eyes. I was mortified.

The accelerator was pretty touchy, so I turned the dial right back down again and drove slowly down the hall towards my room, parking the scooter beside the door. Kyle opened the door and turned on the light.

'A room to yourself, eh? You lucky man.'

'I know, right!' We both laughed.

Kyle put my bags down. 'Right, well, it's been so good visiting with you, Nick.'

'It's been awesome to see you, too,' I told him. I was enormously grateful to Kyle for picking up my scooter and helping me to move in. 'I couldn't have done it without you,' I told him.

'My pleasure, man.' Kyle smiled and turned to leave. 'Anyway, bro, I'll leave you to it. I have to get home — Sarah and I are going out tonight.'

'OK, sounds good,' I said, walking him to the door of my room.

I waved Kyle off and closed the door behind me. I felt profoundly depressed. The smells, the feel and the look of the place brought back all kinds of memories. Why was I doing this? Why would I put myself through this again? Because you're a bloody coward, a weakling!

At that moment I felt profoundly alone: physically, emotionally, relationally and philosophically alone in an ideological enclave that threatened to steamroller me, to make me into its own image.

▲▲▲

Several days later I still did not want to be seen on my scooter, much less take it to meet a stranger in the foyer of a girls' dorm. However, it was a scorching day and I would be late if I walked, so I drove.

It was the first time I had driven to the girls' side of campus, and the first time I had used the scooter with a lot of other people around. My aim was to be as inconspicuous as possible, but I was surprised at how difficult this was. For starters, I was riding in a shiny, bright blue mobility scooter on a sunny day. Then, because I was in a mobility scooter, I couldn't cross the campus with the general flow of traffic, something that would have allowed me at least a chance to blend in with the crowd. Curbs, grass and stairs provide obstacles to wheelchair users, so I was forced to break out of the flow and take routes that fringed the main thoroughfares. I felt as if the mobility scooter impeded my ability to fit in, and I felt stupid, my inabilities on full display.

Often, when faced with a particularly dense area of foot traffic on the narrower footpaths, I was forced to stop while people passed, or I was pushed dangerously close to the edge of the curb if I wanted to keep going. It was not just the inflexibility of people as they streamed past but the campus itself that gave rise to this sense of my body being a problem to others. It appeared that wheelchair accessibility on campus was an afterthought, an issue of compliance not of compassion. Spots in the curb had been ground down at sharp angles to grant a form of access to wheelchair users. Difference was tolerated but not really accommodated — at least, that's how it felt.

This was the frame of mind I was in when I pulled up in front of one of the girls' dorms. People were streaming past as students moved in, ready for the start of the new school year. I struggled to park in a place that was not in the way and entered the dorm feeling both unaccepted and unacceptable, a sense that was reinforced as pretty American girls streamed past, each one seemingly out of my reach. Who would want to go out with me? I thought.

The stranger I was there to meet was Dr Chetta, a friend of a friend.

He was one of the many fathers moving their daughters in, and he had agreed to talk about my medical situation and to offer ongoing support, free of charge. This was a huge help to me, for which I was very grateful, given that accessing medical help through a doctor's surgery was incredibly expensive.

I recognised Dr Chetta from a photo I'd seen, and somewhat warily approached him. 'Doctor Chetta?' I asked hesitantly.

'Hey, you must be Nick,' he said, giving me a hug. 'It's so nice to meet you.'

I was slightly taken aback by his warmth and his embrace.

'Yes! Nice to meet you, too.' I laughed nervously. 'How are you?'

'I'm good thanks, Nick,' he said. 'Hey, I need to quickly finish up something for the girls. Why don't you find a seat and I'll be right back.'

I sat down and waited, feeling awkward, until Dr Chetta hurried back a few minutes later. 'OK, Nick. I'm sorry about that. Let's find somewhere quiet.'

We moved over to a quiet part of the room and chatted for a few minutes, getting to know each other a bit. I could tell that he was a big-hearted man and genuinely eager to help.

'So,' he said as he leant forward slightly, 'tell me about you.'

My stomach churned, as it always does at this question. I felt as if I had already been exposed enough for one day, and I was not eager to immediately divulge all my weaknesses and problems to him. On the other hand, I needed his help.

'Oh, well, where to start?' I said nervously.

I went right back to the beginning, telling him about everything from weak legs and leaking bladder to the tingling and vision problems I'd been having. He asked me lots of questions and conducted a basic physical examination, testing my reflexes and sense of touch, and then he asked more questions.

'So, that's me,' I said as his questions came to an end. 'My doctor back home said the picture is looking increasingly neurological. What do you think?'

Dr Chetta looked at me for a moment then he nodded. 'Yes, I would agree.'

He then began to summarise what I had told him, linking the symptoms and signs with neurological dysfunction.

'You know, Nick,' he said in conclusion, 'considering everything you have told me, and based on these quick tests, I think we can confidently say that you have multiple sclerosis, and that you are currently in remission.'

His words were spoken softly, but they pounded in my head. Multiple sclerosis had been mentioned before, but never after the words 'you have'. It seemed that Dr Chetta was used to delivering diagnoses like this, as if it was no big deal. I, on the other hand, was shaken to my core and crushed. I thought something was wrong with me that my emotions should be so affected by it, so I tried to appear calm and strong, as if I was taking it all in my stride. Nevertheless, I found myself fighting a sense of ground-rush as my focus narrowed and the whole room seemed to close in around me. I felt dizzy, my head throbbed.

Dr Chetta stood up. 'OK, Nick, well, I probably need to keep going, but please keep in touch and let me know if there is any way I can help you,' he said.

I thanked him and he gave me another big hug that lingered for a moment. I appreciated this sense of being valued beyond my illness. He would be a good friend and helper in the months ahead.

I walked outside to the scooter and navigated my way back to my own dorm, trying not to burst into tears. The weight of Dr Chetta's diagnosis was devastating, even though it was not entirely unexpected. In a way it was a relief to finally have my neurological symptoms recognised and to have a peg in the ground, a point from which I could start working to regain control. But it was the permanence of the diagnosis that really got to me, the prospect of a future in which I was relegated to the fringes, tolerated but never fully accepted.

When MS had previously been suggested as a possible diagnosis, I had done my research. I'd discovered that multiple sclerosis is a disease of the central nervous system, causing damage to the myelin sheaths — the insulation surrounding each nerve — in the brain and spinal cord. A nerve's ability to conduct signals is disrupted, resulting in the neurological symptoms I was experiencing. One in every thousand New Zealanders gets MS. Having read about the debilitating effects of the disease, I felt as if I had been handed a death sentence.

I got back to my room and called home.

'Mum, I saw that doctor guy. He said that it's MS.'

'Oh, darling.'

A single hot tear rolled quietly down my cheek.

'Sweet! Where did you get this from?' I was ecstatic, my mind racing with possibilities as I examined the shopping trolley that had been hidden in an empty dorm room down the hall from mine.

'Perhaps it's best you don't ask,' Luke said, winking.

'OK.' I laughed. 'Do you reckon the others will be up for it tonight, after the work meeting?'

'Yeah, buddy,' Luke replied, nodding with the decisiveness you would expect from a hard-core US Marine with a buzzcut.

I giggled with excitement. 'Can you source some rope?'

'Sure can. I think Andrew or I have some rope in the car — I'll get it before the meeting.'

As part of my scholarship agreement I had to work between 16 and 20 hours a week, one of a team of guys who manned the info desk for all the guys' dorms — it was regarded as one of the more responsible jobs on campus. Our work meetings were always late at night, the only time when everyone was on campus and not doing anything else. This particular night the meeting had finished well after midnight, and a few of us were gathered in the dimly lit, otherwise empty dorm foyer. It was my job to supply the mobility scooter.

'OK, so how we gonna do this?' Victor asked, in his heavy Ukrainian accent.

'Well, I think it would be best if we tied the rope to the seat post on the chair,' I replied. 'How about someone ties an end to the trolley?'

'What length shall I tie the rope?' Greg asked.

'Oh, I don't know. Perhaps two or three metres — six to nine feet?'

I checked the knots as Micah jumped on the scooter, nominating himself as driver. I enjoyed seeing people having fun on the scooter and was happy for him to drive.

'Are you guys ready?' Greg asked as he opened the door.

'Ready for some fun!' Victor laughed.

We pushed the scooter and trolley out through the door. It was now around 1 a.m. and we spoke quietly, trying not to disturb anyone as we left the building.

Victor and Tyler jumped on the side of the cart, wanting to ride it in the way your mother never let you at the supermarket.

'Guys!' said Jeremy, momentarily forgetting to whisper. 'Oops! Guys, you can't ride it like that — it'll be too unstable. We need to get in.'

Victor and Jeremy both climbed in. It was a bit of a squash but it worked.

Micah drove forward slowly, taking up the slack in the rope. I turned my camera on, to try to capture some of the action.

'Ready,' Micah said in a loud whisper.

'OK!' shouted Victor, laughing in his high voice.

Micah pulled back the throttle and launched the trolley into a high-velocity rampage down the footpath past the dorms. It had a rather rough surface and the shopping trolley made an almighty racket as it rattled and clattered along.

It was on our second or third pass of the dorms that we saw the headlights of a security car round the corner, heading down the road towards us. This was not good. We needed to hide.

'Guys! Security!' I whisper-shouted.

'Shoot! Wadda we do?' Micah asked as he flew past, still at the helm.

'Quick, down there between the dorms!' I said, pointing to the hedged path that led between the dorms, giving us access to one of the back doors.

Micah pulled a hard right, shooting down the path as fast as he could. The only problem was that the trolley could not change trajectory as easily. It ploughed straight into the hedge, throwing Jeremy into the garden and spilling Victor on to the pavement. We all erupted into laughter.

The scene was too funny not to photograph and I took a quick shot. We hurriedly helped Jeremy and Victor to their feet, then dragged the scooter and trolley inside the dorm and hid in the stairwell, hoping security would not find us. We sat there for a few minutes, all trying desperately not to laugh. No one came.

'Maybe he didn't see us,' Tyler said quietly.

'Yes, we got away with it!' Victor laughed.

There was a combined sigh of relief, followed by a round of high-fives.

We came out of the stairwell and were walking down the hall, enthusiastically reliving the spill, when a security guy appeared at the other end and started walking towards us. We immediately fell silent. As the owner of the scooter I knew that I would be the one held responsible.

'Hey, man, how's it going?' I asked. I recognised the guard from one of my classes — he was also a student — and I had talked to him before.

'I've had calls from people complaining about the noise. What were y'all up to?' the guard asked sternly, skipping any pleasantries, as he walked down the hall with his hand on his firearm.

'Noise complaints? Oops. We were just messing around outside, that's all.' I tried to sound upbeat and cheerful, but I could see that he was not buying it, particularly since the scooter and trolley were behind me.

'What's this?' he asked, pointing to our rig.

'Oh, this is just the stuff we were messing around with.'

He stared at me sharply for a few moments. 'You know what, I don't even want to know what y'all were doing. But I saw the flash of your camera —' he pointed incriminatingly at me — 'and I seen what y'all did to the hedge out there. You de-stroyed it.'

'Oh,' I replied. I had been in too much of a hurry to think about the

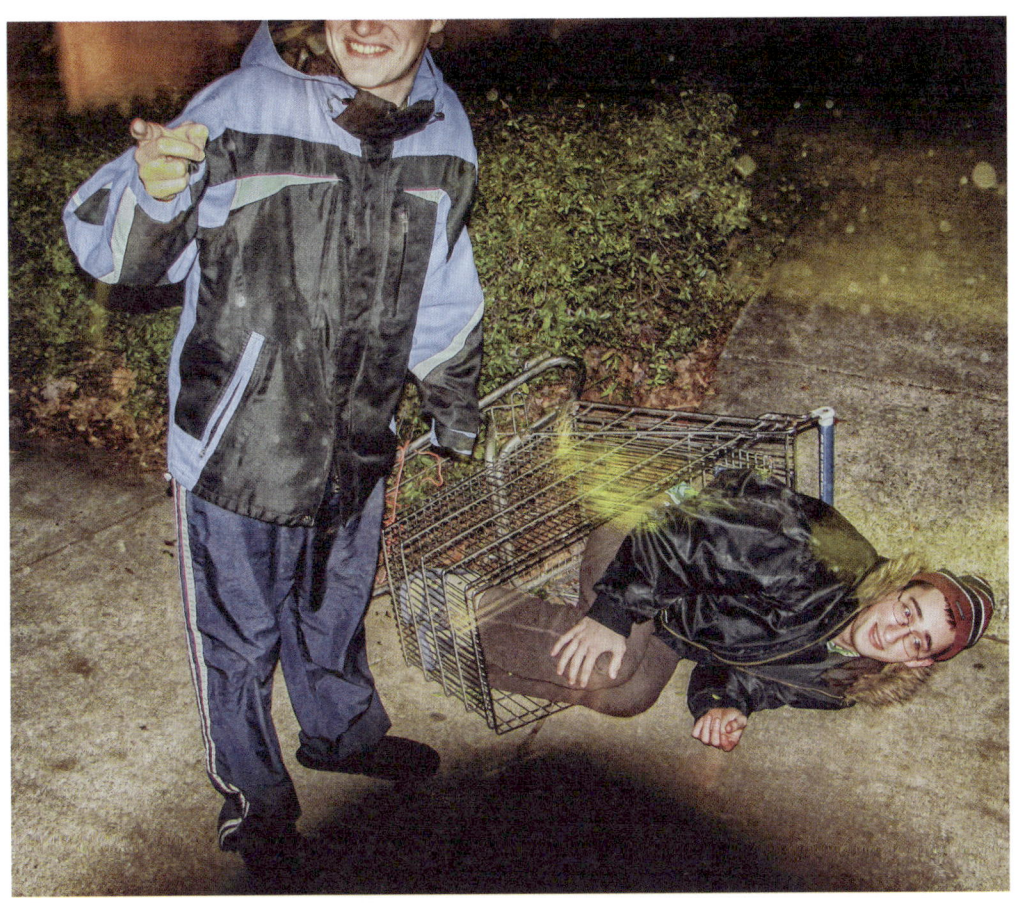

Victor on the ground and Jeremy pointing at the approaching security car immediately after the crash.

hedge. Neither had I thought about the camera flash when I took the photo.

The guard paused again, thinking, looking severe.

'Y'all know I could get y'all hit with major demerits for an offence like this. And the DC would not look kindly on it. No one is allowed to leave their dorm after midnight, and y'all have caused significant damage to university property. You know you could lose your campus jobs for that,' he said with a gruffness that was surprising — out of uniform, this guy was friendly and chatty.

'Really?' I exclaimed, trying to play dumb. 'Oh, man, thanks heaps for letting us know. We'll all be sure this doesn't happen again.'

He shook his head. 'OK. If it does happen again, I will throw the book at y'all — understand?' he said, jabbing his finger at us.

'Yes, absolutely,' I replied. I stepped towards him, gave him a pat on the shoulder, then thanked him again.

While threats of being hauled up before the DC were moderately stressful, it was the chasm between my theological beliefs and those of the university authorities that eventually brought me to breaking point. Although I had disclosed my theological background and perspective at the beginning, and although I had been aware that I might come under pressure to change my thinking, what I hadn't expected was that the authorities would threaten to withdraw the scholarship unless I changed my beliefs and conformed.

I had managed to fly under the radar for the first few months and had begun to think that I might just make it through. That's until I was unexpectedly called to a meeting in which I was informed that I had until the beginning of February — two and a half months — to decide whether I would agree to change my beliefs. If not, the scholarship would be withdrawn, and I would have to repay all the costs the university had covered under the scholarship.

I was shocked; I was being asked to give up the freedom to think independently. In particular, I felt as if I was being asked to abandon my belief in grace as the overarching framework of my Christian faith. Adopting a graceless religiosity was a horrifying thought.

For me, grace represents an overflow of Divine goodness that provides unconditional acceptance, the power to change, peace in hardship, and strength under trial. For some at the university, however, grace appeared to represent a modality that was enjoyed only if you performed, and came with the suspicion that too much of it brings a licence to sin.

The university's Chancellor chaired a weekly seminar that all theology students had to attend, and he often spoke out against those who held a similar theological position to mine. Although these students, who were few in number, held similar beliefs to me, they weren't on scholarships under the Chancellor's patronage, and I often felt as if I was personally under attack. As a group who believed in the importance of grace, we felt a growing intolerance of our position among a number of the university's staff and faculty, and felt there was an increasingly hostile atmosphere within the student body.

Once again, I felt deeply isolated. Friends and family back home wanted to be helpful but they could not fully grasp the situation, which had grown out of a set of distinctly American cultural values.

Adding to the pressure was the suspicion that my response to the university's ultimatum would dictate the direction of my life. My conversation with the Mormon student on the train often played through my head. What was I? And what did I want to be? Was I going to define my life by religious conservatism, or by something unstinting, more gracious, more open-minded? Added to this was the continued, plaguing sense of cowardice that had come with my decision to remain in the US. I did not want to make this mistake again, nor did I want to continue in a situation where I could not express my beliefs openly.

The pressure of the university's ultimatum provoked a significant physical decline over the next couple of months and had a massive impact on my health. Combined with the already considerable stress of full-time study and part-time work, and despite my best efforts to

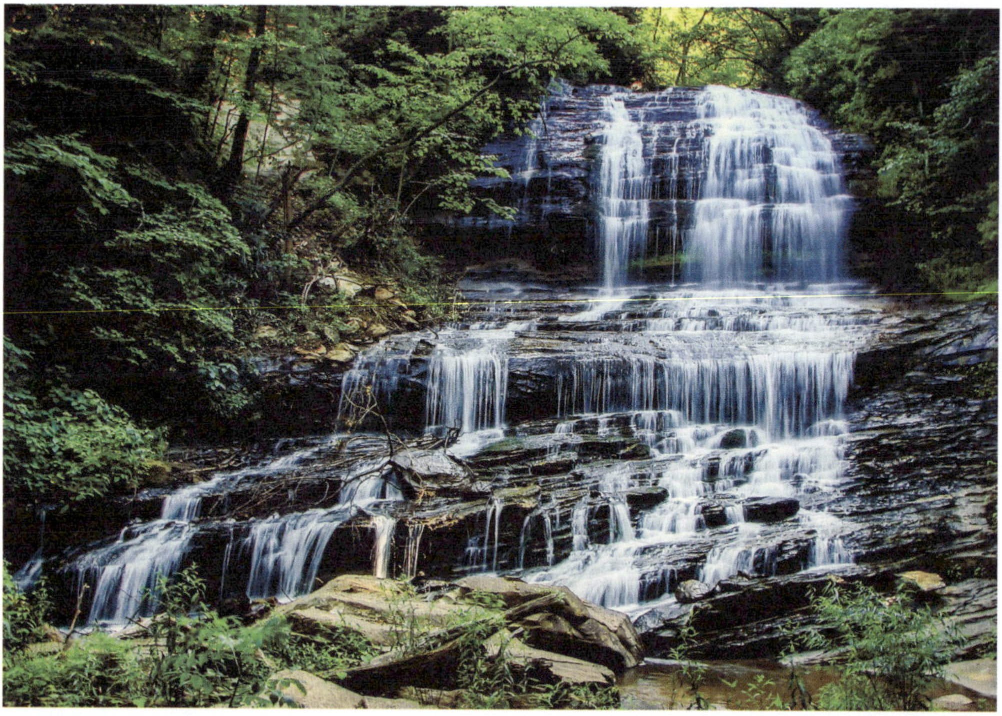

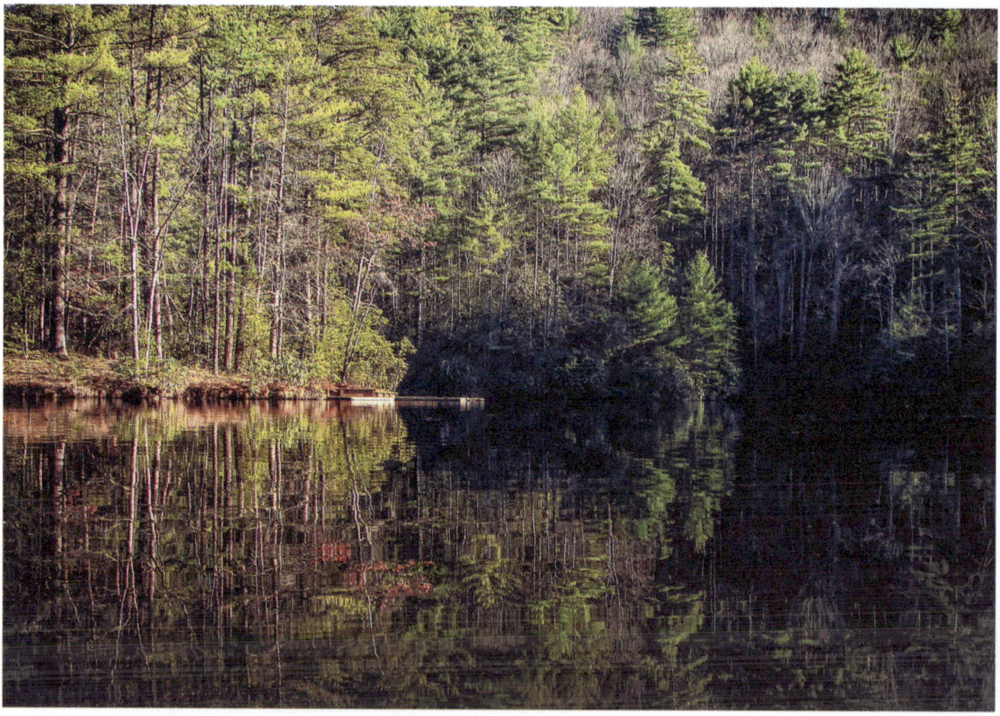

Top to bottom: Pearson Falls; Lake Placid at Paris Mountain State Park.

mitigate the physical pressures of university life through the use of the scooter, it all proved to be too much.

Bladder control was among the first things to go. I saw Dr Chetta regularly, and he and another friend, Dr Walker, supplied me with medication that reduced the dribbling that always threatened to wet through my pants. But then I began to have major problems with urgency, feeling as if I was busting to go to the toilet every 15 or 20 minutes. Rushing to the toilet, I would then find that I could only pass a few millilitres of urine, which was very frustrating.

My ability to walk also began to be compromised. This was most clearly illustrated when, on a trip with a friend to Paris Mountain State Park, I felt incapable of walking 10 minutes along a well-formed forest path to see the reportedly picturesque Mountain Lake and waterfall.

It became clear that my reliance on the scooter to get me around campus, combined with an unrelenting sense of profound fatigue, was quickly diminishing my ability to walk. I tried to combat this in several ways. I rarely used the scooter inside the university's public buildings, partly because it was too difficult to navigate around other people, through the lifts and tight halls, but mostly because I was determined to maintain some level of independent mobility. Moving between floors, I tried to use the stairs and handrail as often as I could manage, rather than taking the lift. However, over time I found myself tripping on the steps more and more frequently, as foot drop began developing in my left leg. Normally, when you walk, the toes on the advancing foot lift up and then come down again after you have placed your heel. With foot drop, your body may not lift your toes when you take a step forward, causing them to catch on stairs or ledges.

Muscle weakness and fatigue also continued to build, and although I was able to struggle up stairs if I fully focused on lifting my toes, I found it increasingly difficult to walk down again; my legs were not strong enough to support my weight in the step down, stressing them to the point where they would threaten to collapse under me — which they did on the odd occasion. Walking was hard enough without the foot drop — it felt as if I was moving through golden syrup, every step dragging, requiring determination to resist the lassitude that threatened to drown me. My foot drop continued to progress to the point where the toe of my foot would drop and, without warning, trip me on any surface, no matter how smooth.

I found I was also losing my ability to balance. Any uneven surface, even the sloping floors of an auditorium, became difficult to manage, requiring me to hold on to something. Walking through crowded halls was one of the most terrifying realities of my day. The unpredictable trajectories of students as they darted between classes was more than my foggy mind could handle, leaving me feeling entirely overwhelmed by what was going on around me. The only solution was to look down and just walk, monitoring only the patch of ground directly in front of me, without really taking account of where others were heading. This meant that people would often bump into me, throwing me slightly off balance — something that was terrifying in a crowded space.

The pressure of the situation also expressed itself through all kinds of weird sensory problems. I had numbness in my face, making it feel as if it was frozen and hard to move. Parts of my trunk and legs were continually hypersensitive, which meant that the brush of clothing or accidental touch of a person caused a feeling of searing heat. Tingling engulfed my face, feet and hands with increasing intensity, making it difficult to sleep. The intensity of the tingling was quite frightening at times, leading to an intensely claustrophobic sense of being trapped; there was absolutely no escape or reprieve. During these episodes I wanted to tear the flesh off my face, or just die.

I tried my best to adopt a healthy lifestyle. I knew that a good nine hours of high-quality sleep every night helped to minimise fatigue and muscle tightness, so I tried to go to bed before ten o'clock every night. I cut dairy products out of my diet and generally tried to eat as healthily as possible. However, the food served in the university dining room made healthy eating difficult and I had neither the money nor the access to a kitchen that would have allowed me to address this. Despite these attempts at a healthy lifestyle, the massive stress of this period meant that I was unable to halt the progression of my symptoms.

I was trying my best to hide my symptoms and internal struggles. The impulse for this arose, in part, out of a desperation to hold on to any modicum of strength and control, and thereby publicly maintain some level of social desirability or acceptance. This was a particularly strong impulse in an environment where outward conformity was so strongly emphasised and acceptance was based on performance. And discussing my symptoms could lead to talk of exacerbating factors, and potentially disclosure of the ultimatum I was under, which was something I wanted to avoid. It's amazing how, by adopting a bubbly persona, you can fool yourself into ignoring your own symptoms and signs. However, I also realised that keeping private and sublimating my feelings and the state of my health kept me from moving forward: ignoring a problem prevents you from developing a solution.

Nevertheless, and perhaps more often than I care to admit, I felt anger towards my body. Some of this rose out of the intense daily frustration of being unable to do simple things: type quickly, not shake while I held a glass of water, void my bladder fully, or do up a button on my shirt. At other times my anger was directed at those larger aspects of the disease: the unending tingling, the frequent tripping, and the overwhelming sense of fatigue. Whatever the case, it felt like the angry desperation of someone fighting for his life, as if I stood alone in the battle against the deepening darkness of decay. I felt justified in my anger at this brokenness, but I didn't dare express it. To express my anger would be to admit the presence of the disease, and I would not give it that pleasure.

During the months leading up to my February deadline, I realised how important it is to be surrounded by a supportive community, to not go at it alone. This realisation came through the friendship of three people — Jon, David and Joey — all of whom showed incredible generosity and acceptance.

Jon was a postgrad student who shared the same beliefs as me, and in the face of the university's apparent antagonism we became best mates. We spent many hours discussing, researching and thinking through the issues presented to us by our classes. Jon had a sharp understanding of theology and proved to be an excellent sounding board.

He also had a car, and was keen for any excuse to get off campus. This was a huge help to me, as it gave me an opportunity to be myself without the feeling that I was under observation, and to find freedom from the claustrophobia that came with being otherwise confined to campus. During the week we'd often spend our evenings at a Denny's diner. The plastic seats were never particularly comfortable, but Denny's was open until late and served unlimited cups of coffee — something of great appeal when you had an assignment to crank out. Saturday was the day for classier options: we'd head further out to the spacious booths at the Atlanta Bread Company, or the comfortable armchairs at Panera Bread. We'd stay all day, studying, eating and drinking coffee. We were like brothers, and these moments of reprieve were incredibly valuable, particularly for my mental health.

Then there were Joey and David, a middle-aged couple I had met a few months before I was presented with the university's ultimatum. Jon had known David and Joey for years and introduced me to them. They had gone through a process of theological ostracism not dissimilar to mine. Jon and I met David at a number of significant junctures to seek his advice, and I appreciated the wisdom and profound graciousness of his measured responses. Joey believed strongly in the benefits of a healthy lifestyle. She would often provide me with healthy meals to eat in the dorm, enabling me to move on from Pop-Tarts, biscuits and gravy, and coffee cake for breakfast, and she generally encouraged me to pursue a healthy and balanced lifestyle.

One of the things I particularly appreciated about being with Jon, David and Joey was the freedom to talk about my situation in its entirety. Instead of having to hide my symptoms and their deterioration in the face of the scholarship decision, I was able to

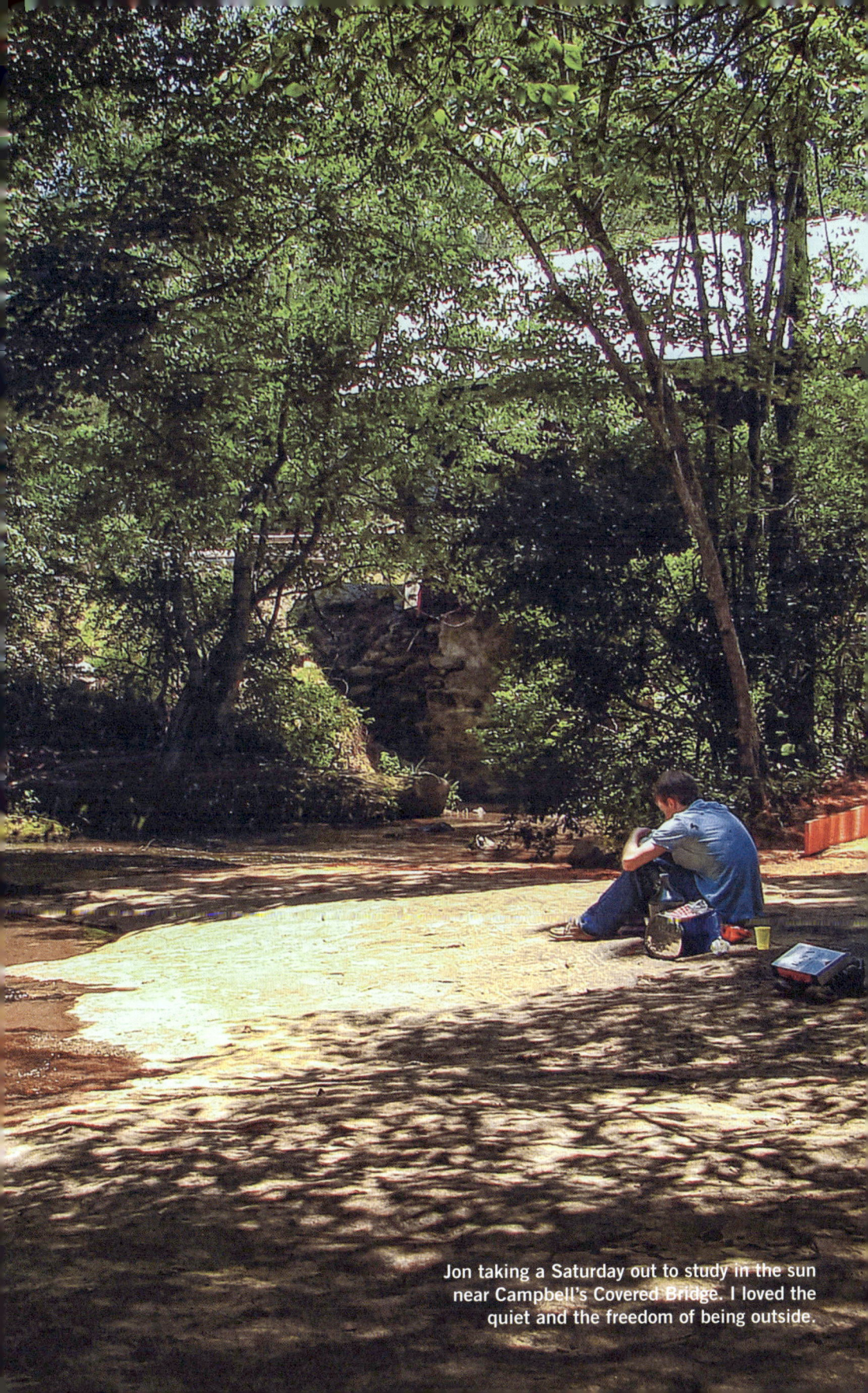
Jon taking a Saturday out to study in the sun near Campbell's Covered Bridge. I loved the quiet and the freedom of being outside.

talk candidly about how I was feeling, without fear of judgement or reprisal. Although this vulnerability was scary at times, with it came a sense of rest, freedom and acceptance.

The support I received from Jon, David and Joey was hugely significant, particularly when February arrived and I had to give my decision to the university. Wanting neither to be under the pressure of the scholarship nor to continue as a spineless coward, I told the university authorities that I could not, in good conscience, guarantee a change of perspective. The university quietly dismissed me from the scholarship programme.

I was entirely worn out by the experience.

Dismissal from the scholarship programme did not automatically mean I had to leave the university. Through the intervention of several key people, I was allowed to finish my second semester of study at no cost. It was very tempting just to leave, but despite all that had occurred I was loath to return home without a sense of purpose, and to leave the good friends I had made. Jon, Joey and David, and other friends had become an important part of my life.

However, my lack of purpose worried me; I was afraid of once again becoming encumbered by that heavy sense of not knowing what to do, of not knowing what direction my life should take. I was also frustrated by what dropping out of university signified. I felt as if withdrawal amounted to failure, and that returning home meant I was giving in to the disease.

But I did also realise that the life of a clergyman was not what I wanted, so I decided to transfer into the BA programme and take a bunch of general papers in a third semester at the university. I hoped that something in my philosophy, English literature or history classes might pique my interest and suggest a new direction. Jon got me a job for the summer, which would enable me to save some money, although it was obvious that finances were going to be very tight.

It was a cold, grey Saturday morning when David, Joey and I sat down in the IHOP restaurant just along the road from the campus. IHOP offered an all-you-can-eat deal on its pancakes and I ploughed in — something I felt slightly guilty about, but I was hungry.

'Nick,' David said quietly, 'Joey and I wanted to catch up with you today to ask you something.'

I looked up from my pile of pancakes.

'We have given it a lot of thought and we would like to make our home available to you, to come and stay as long as you like, and to support you for the rest of the time you're here.'

I had suspected this was in the offing, but I was taken by surprise nevertheless. I was deeply humbled by their generosity. I also found it difficult to accept their offer. I felt as if I did not warrant it, and should prove my suitability by showing that I could contribute. I tried to express my gratitude, then I opened my laptop and showed them a spreadsheet detailing my expenses and income.

'I've worked out a budget and figured out how much I could pay each week in board,' I said. I wanted to appear responsible and willing to put in the effort required to make this work.

David took a good look at the spreadsheet. 'I see here that this budget requires you to keep up your job on campus during the semester. Is that correct?'

'Yes, that's right. I think I should be able to keep up my job in the computer labs, which will provide an income. I'm not allowed to work more than twenty hours per week on my student visa, but I can certainly try to work as many of those hours as I can.'

Joey looked concerned. 'Nick, we want you to come and live with us without having to pay board. You have had so much going on lately — you're worn out. We want to help you get better by feeding you lots and lots of good food, helping you get lots of good sleep, and, well, just by supporting you while you study, without the stress of work and money.'

I didn't know quite how to respond. I knew that they were not particularly well off themselves and the big-heartedness of their offer shocked me. On the one hand it was confronting, because it acknowledged the full impact of multiple sclerosis on my ability to function — something I hated to admit and always tried to hide — yet the offer also embraced me as I was. The feeling of being fully known and also accepted was what made it so deeply humbling and brought an amazing sense of peace.

'Joey's right, Nick. We've given it a lot of thought and we want to do this for you,' said David. 'All we ask is that you participate in the life of our family and that you are willing to eat well and make the lifestyle changes you need to get better.'

I was overwhelmed by their generosity. 'Thank you so much. I don't know what to say.' I thought for a moment about what they were asking of me. David and Joey's kids, Heather and Aaron, were like a sister and brother to me. As for the lifestyle changes, I knew I needed to do this, to make those changes.

'I would gladly participate in the life of your family,' I said. 'I really enjoy being with you guys! And I want to make those changes. It might take a bit of practice, to break old habits and stuff, but I want to commit to change — I just need help to do it, that's all.'

'Wonderful. It will be our pleasure to have you, Nick,' David replied with a smile.

In the end I stayed with them for eight months, from May until December. David talked to the university's finance department and was able to get me a few small student-hardship scholarships, which helped financially. And over the next few months Joey slowly helped me to adopt a healthier lifestyle. Between banana-berry smoothies, vegan cheese and kombucha tea, I was amazed at how good healthy eating could be. There were times when I was secretly suspicious about a change in my diet, and I am sure Joey would say that I was often a slow learner. Nevertheless, under her care and away from the stress of the scholarship, my worsening symptoms plateaued and I found that I was able to enjoy slightly higher levels of energy.

With this increase in energy I felt as if I had regained a degree of agency again, and I was able to engage in short, controlled stints of exercise. This was huge for me, opening up the possibility of camping and very short walks, allowing me to get out into nature, something that had been painfully absent during my time at the university.

Permeating the life of David and Joey's family was an incredible sense of acceptance and encouragement. It took time to process all that had transpired at the university, as well as a second diagnosis of MS that I had received from a specialist. Their unstinting acceptance of me allowed me to fully acknowledge my struggles without fear and with the continued assurance of their support. Their confident realism helped me to avoid a blind optimism, and enabled me to engage with my struggles meaningfully. David and Joey's encouragement gave me the hope to keep on going, to not give up. It was in this milieu of gracious community that I found the support I needed to make changes, and where a strong belief in the benefits of a healthy lifestyle was seeded.

Gerwyn tackles a steep section of the climb.

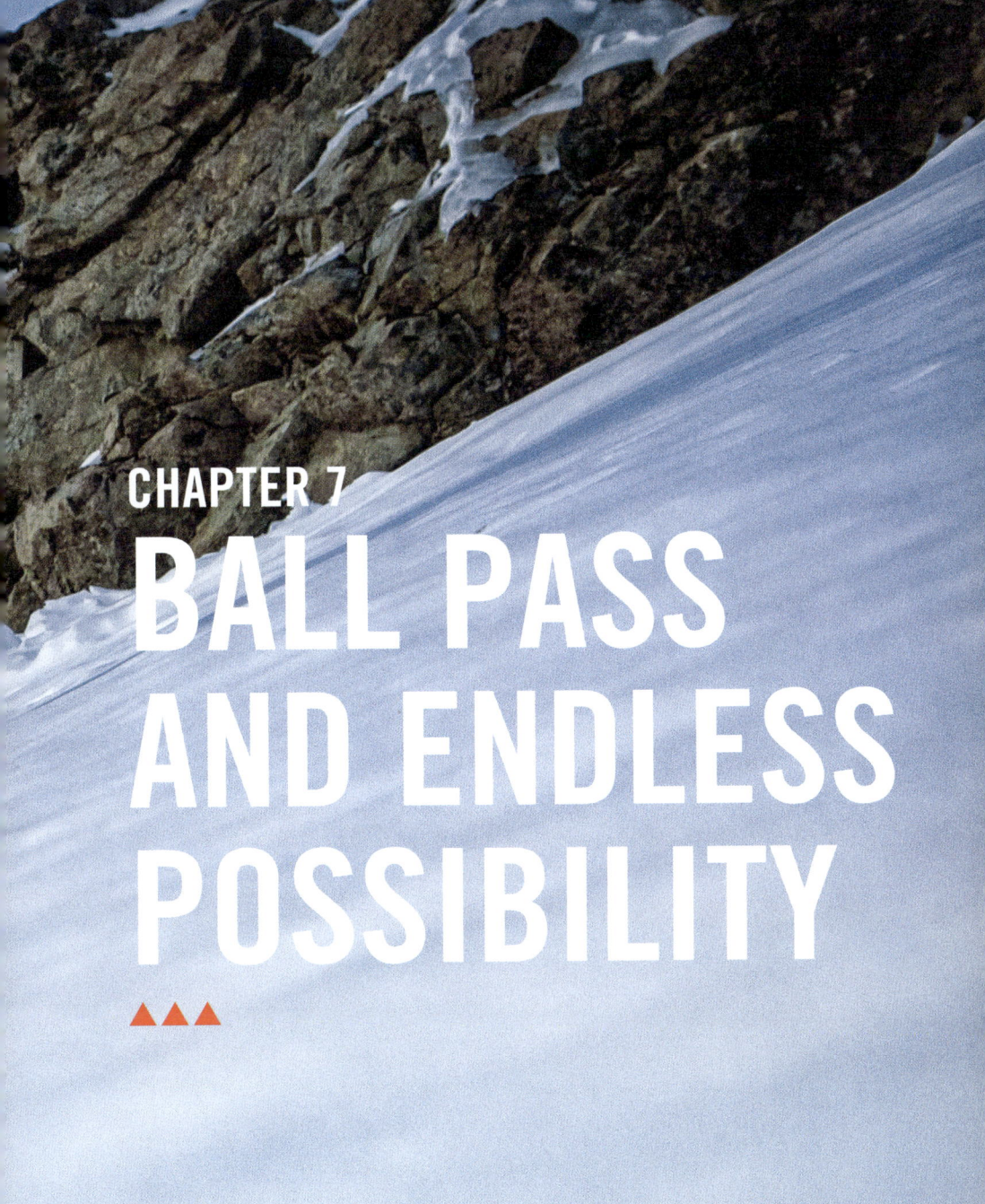

CHAPTER 7

BALL PASS AND ENDLESS POSSIBILITY

▲▲▲

August 2014
Mt Cook Village, New Zealand

My mate Gerwyn and I stood outside the Department of Conservation office at Mt Cook Village, waiting for it to open. It was a perfect morning to be outdoors, the air cool beneath a clear blue sky, with hardly a breath of wind. Snow lay in the shadows, in the garden and around the building, the remains of the big dump that had fallen a few days earlier.

Gerwyn and I needed to pop into the office to fill out an intentions form before setting off to cross Ball Pass. There were a few other people waiting to get in.

'So where are you guys heading?' I asked one of them.

'We're heading up to Tasman Saddle Hut, at the head of the Tasman Glacier, for a week of ski touring,' the guy replied, indicating three others who were with him. He sounded Australian. 'Should be awesome with all this fresh snow and beaut weather. What about you — where are you guys heading?'

'That'll be great,' I said, secretly jealous — ski touring had always interested me as a fun-looking intersection between exploration and mountaineering. 'We're doing Ball Pass, which should be a bit of fun.'

'Are you climbing or touring?'

'Climbing.'

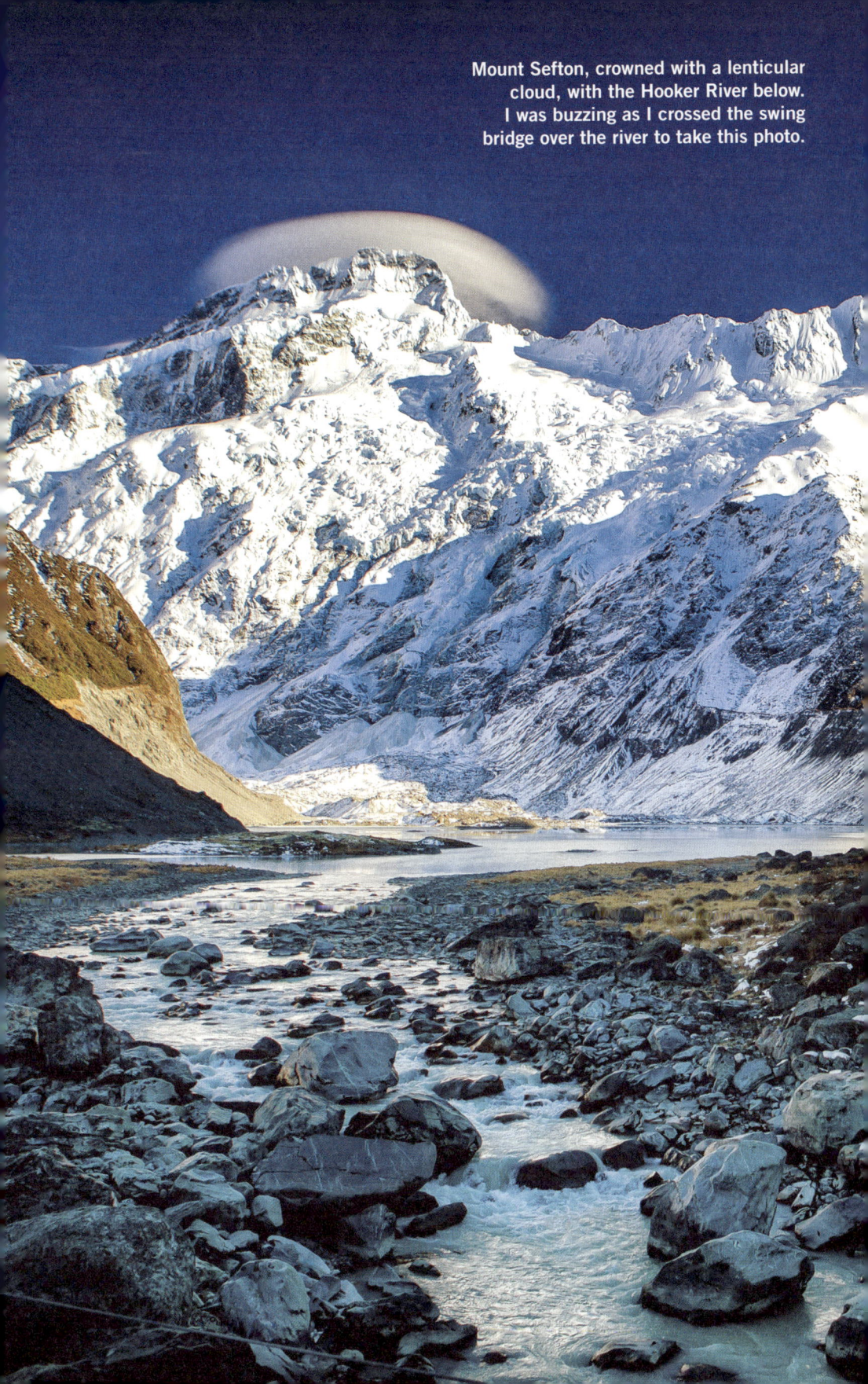

Mount Sefton, crowned with a lenticular cloud, with the Hooker River below. I was buzzing as I crossed the swing bridge over the river to take this photo.

'Shit,' he said with a smile, 'you must be pretty keen — it'll be a bit of a slog getting up there.'

'Yeah,' I laughed, unsure whether he regarded me as hard core or crazy, but I was happy with either. 'It will be a lot of a slog, but it should be good.'

Despite my apparent bravado, I knew attempting Ball Pass in winter was wildly ambitious for someone like me, and that left me feeling torn. On the one hand, I felt drawn to the hope of the credibility that would come with completing the pass — I wanted to be liked and accepted by guys like the one I was talking to — but the slog threatened my ability to achieve it. The snow was deep. What if I became too fatigued, I wondered, and had to come back down? And what if the trip made me overdo it and relapse?

Three years earlier, while on another road trip round the South Island, I had also walked through the doors of this DOC office. I'd made a lot of progress during those three years, and I loved the sense of freedom and the increased social access that came with that progress. The taste of acceptance and gracious community that I had experienced with David and Joey had left me hungry for more. Surprisingly, though, I kept gravitating towards a desire to prove my worth — which I thought of in terms of my ability to perform physically — missing the point of grace entirely.

Afraid of rejection or a loss of worth, I was petrified of losing all the mobility I had worked so hard to gain, of sacrificing all my progress on a hard slog through deep snow. Tempering this, however, was the equally scary thought of not trying, of stopping that flow of progress, and of being stuck in my current state. I knew that this drive to keep pushing was because I'd attached my identity to something as unfixed and impermanent as my ability to perform. I also knew that this sense of self-worth was screwed up, and that I would still be loved and accepted even if I was sick or in a wheelchair. Nevertheless, I wanted to secure my worth. Crossing Ball Pass would do that, I thought.

Going a bit deeper, at the root of my reluctance to accept grace, and fuelling the drive to establish my worth as a person, was a refusal to grieve. Implicit in the acceptance of grace is an acknowledgement that something is amiss or broken — which was an admission that I was not willing to make. By refusing to admit that something was wrong, I was able to fool myself into thinking that there wasn't anything to grieve for. While it was impossible to ignore the physical symptoms and signs of the disease, I was driven to distance myself from it through physical achievement, to hide my struggle from myself and others. I did not want to accept my inability. The appearance of any new symptom would invariably provoke fresh emotions — feelings that were quickly quelled. I thought it was more noble, more mature, to be brave in the face of adversity and to maintain a positive demeanour.

Not that it was easy to do so. There were many times when I was almost overcome by those emotions, filled with grief and sorrow at the progress of the disease. It is hard not to be: it feels like death is consuming your body, dragging you closer to an enveloping darkness. I felt scared of grieving, of what it might entail or bring up as I turned to look darkness in the face. It seemed too big, too hard and too scary. Better, I thought, to not go there; better to ignore it and run in the opposite direction, towards physical achievement.

Complicating this further, no doubt, was a relationship that had unexpectedly failed earlier in the year. I was head over heels about a girl who, one day, suddenly dumped me. I found this rejection devastating, especially as I could not help but wonder if she had passed me by because of my MS or, at the very least, because of the fact of my limited physical ability. I knew that I was stupid to invest my sense of worth in our relationship, but it was hard not to: I was in love with a beautiful person who made my heart sing.

After she had ended our relationship I had dropped her off at Auckland Airport and returned to my grandparents' place distraught. I tried to appear strong, but I think Grandma could tell that I wasn't. I stayed the night there but I needed to drive back to Palmerston North the next day. Grandma was obviously worried about me doing the trip alone, and she contacted my Uncle John to see if he could drive with me. I was deeply appreciative of this. I felt so low, as if the MS had won.

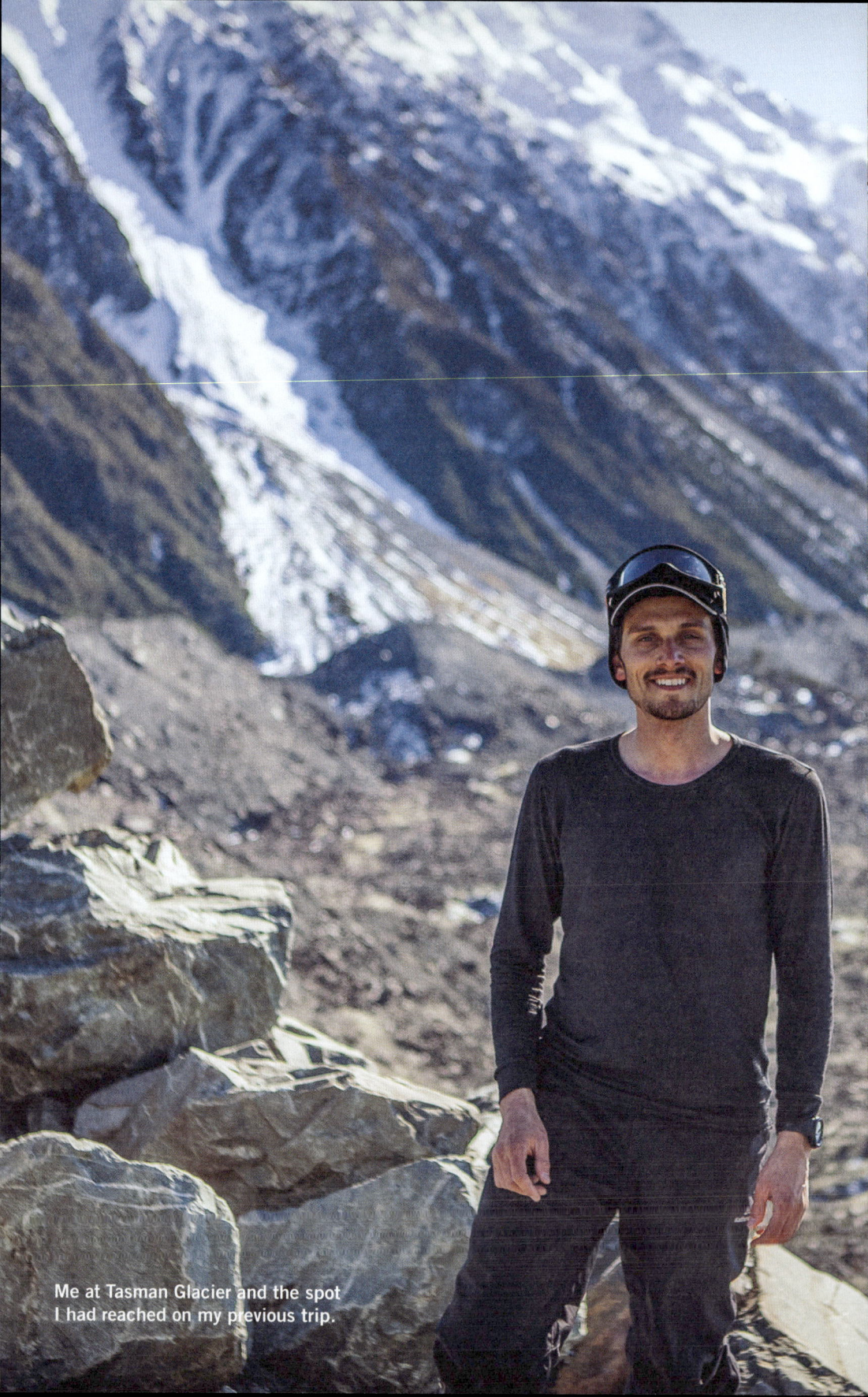
Me at Tasman Glacier and the spot I had reached on my previous trip.

Uncle John and I drove down to Palmerston North via National Park and the King Country. As we wound along the Mangawhero River and through the steep hill country that hems the river I had plenty of opportunity to think. I knew the guy for whom this girl had dumped me, and the thing I found most difficult was the fact that he was strong, muscular and athletic — things I was not, it seemed. I felt deeply devalued, undesirable and, once again, painfully emasculated. I felt the darkness of grief clawing at me, but I would not let it have me. Instead, I felt compelled to prove myself and the worth of my body as a man, to establish my desirability.

And now I was about to attempt Ball Pass. A photo of me on the top of the pass, posted to Facebook, would begin to establish my worth, I thought. I needed at least some recognition that her rejection of me was unfounded and did not reflect my value as a person, absolving me of the need to grieve.

Finally the DOC office opened and we all walked in. The Australians were first in line and started to chat to the DOC officer. Behind the counter was a large chart showing the capacity of each of the huts in the area, and how many people were in them. The DOC officer added four to Tasman Hut while one of the guys filled out the intentions book. I was pleased we weren't planning to stay at any huts on the Ball Pass route — tenting in the winter felt more adventurous, more hard core.

As I stood there waiting I looked out of the massive north-facing window filled with a view of Mt Cook and the Hooker Valley. It looked intimidating — as if it would require a huge amount of effort. It made me nervous and slightly fearful.

Slog, combined with boundary-pushing, can be a risky business — something I knew from my visit to this same place three years earlier. It was not long after my return from the US and my diagnosis of MS within the New Zealand medical system. As I had experienced previously, my return was difficult as I tried to figure out what I could and couldn't do, and what life back in New Zealand would look like as someone with multiple sclerosis.

My first plan of attack was to get walking. I had brought the mobility scooter back with me but I was desperate to get rid of it, so I sold it and bought my first digital SLR camera with the money. A desire to develop my skills as a photographer was a big part of the initial impetus to get outside walking again. I was living with my parents in a new subdivision on the outskirts of Taupo, and I started by wandering around the immediate area, on the footpath, snapping photos of fountains, birds and earthmoving equipment. After a while I started travelling further afield, camera in hand, through the tall grass and over the old farm fences that covered the undeveloped parts of the subdivision. I went down to the lookout on the corner of the main drag into town and Huka Falls Road, where there's a great view of the Kaimanawa Range and Ruapehu, standing proudly above the blue of Lake Taupo.

It was soon after this that I decided to take a short road trip through the South Island. I was desperate to get out into some big New Zealand mountains, so I took a camper van for a week. I wasn't able to drive very far each day, but I slowly made my way down from Blenheim to Mt Cook Village. The Mt Cook region is one of my favourite places on earth, and I was delighted to be able to stay there for a few days.

When I walked into the DOC office that February day I was looking for a short walk that would give me great views. I knew I could only handle a walk of about ten minutes. To my disappointment, there was nothing that fitted my criteria: all the options seemed too long and too strenuous. I walked out of the office feeling slightly defeated. I went into the Hermitage hotel, got a coffee and sat down for a while, intent on at least enjoying the view of the mountains from the safety and comfort of an armchair. It was pleasant and comfortable for sure, but the heavily mediated experience — the scented air expelled by the air conditioner, the background muzak — was no substitute for the feel of a fresh breeze on my face, the smell of the earth, the sounds of birdsong and nature. I wanted to be out there, even if it meant sitting in a carpark.

I drove round to the Tasman Glacier carpark, just to have a look and evaluate my options. There is a track that goes from the carpark to the top of the moraine wall forming the southern end of Tasman Lake. According to the DOC brochure it was 40 minutes return, and ascended 100 metres. I knew that 20 minutes each way would be a push, but I wanted to check it out, to see if it might be worth the effort. I could see that there were a lot of big steps, which made me nervous — steps were still very hard work, and 20 minutes of slogging up them would stretch my abilities.

Rationally, I knew I should probably walk away, hop back in the van and find somewhere else to enjoy the view. But I felt an overwhelming desire to walk to the top of the mound that was obstructing my view and to enjoy the immersive experience that the walk promised. What if I fell or tripped? There were plenty of people around and I was sure someone would help. What if I got to the top then didn't have the energy to get back down? I would cross that bridge if I came to it. Nothing ventured; nothing gained.

I gave Dad a call. After a quick catch-up I paused for a moment then said, 'Hey, Pa, the reason I called was to let you know that I'm going to do a short walk to the top of the moraine wall, to get a view of Tasman Glacier. I saw photos in the DOC office and it looks amazing.'

'Oh, OK,' Dad responded cautiously. 'How long is it — it sounds hard.'

'It's twenty minutes each way,' I replied, cringing slightly. I didn't want to be dissuaded.

'Are you sure you'll be able to do it? That won't be pushing it too hard?'

'Well, I'm not totally sure, and it is a bit further than I was hoping, but I really want to see the view. If I don't feel good I can turn round and come back. And I've got some lunch, so when I get to the top I can take a good break and enjoy the view while I eat lunch and recover.'

'OK, sounds good. And remember, Nick, it's OK to turn round — no one will judge you.'

'Yeah, I know.' I laughed. While I knew Dad was right, the real question was: How would I judge myself if I turned round?

'Anyway, the main reason I rang was to let you know what was happening, just in case anything goes wrong.'

'Oh, right. Well, flick me a text when you get back to the van.'

'Will do,' I replied.

It was an effort walking up the track to the lookout point and I found the steps hard. Harder still was being passed by fit young tourists who bounded up the hill while I slowly plodded along. It wasn't that I really cared about their opinions — they were strangers, after all — but it was hard not to compare myself with them as they walked briskly round me, someone who was in the way, and not feel different, abnormal, outside of the in-group. At times like this I kind of missed the scooter. At least it gave me an excuse to be slow, to struggle. Now, I was caught in the liminal state of being mobile but still not strong enough to participate as a normal person. I was grateful to have my new camera — at least that gave me a reason to take it slowly on the way up, under the guise of taking photographs.

As it approaches the top of the moraine wall the track zigzags through loose boulders and rock, between hebe bushes, matagouri and speargrass, and along a shifting surface that challenged my balance. It was the big rocks that I found most difficult. My legs quickly became tired and I struggled with the way the rocks rolled as I shifted my weight across each step. What made it worse was that I felt as if I had used up almost all my energy in the slog up the hill. This left me with a mental lassitude that made it hard to judge depth — everything appears flat in this state — and to maintain my balance and not trip on the rocks. My whole body felt drained. I needed to sit.

I looked down the path to see if anyone was coming. Some more fit young tourists were heading up, not far behind me, so I decided to struggle on for a bit longer, trying to look confident. They bounded past and I looked back down the track. There was an older couple coming up, slowly plodding along with their wide-brimmed hats, long-sleeved shirts and trekking poles. I didn't mind them seeing me rest, so I stopped and sat facing down the valley, watching the Tasman River as it wove down the flats alongside Ben Ohau to Lake

Tekapo. It was a beautiful scene, crowned with amazing lenticular clouds that looked like massive airships in the sky.

I turned round and looked up the track — the top was close. Not far to go. It's a tough spot to be in, without energy and yet so close to your goal. I knew I should probably turn back; to go on would risk overdoing it. But to go down would also be very draining. Damned if I did and damned if I didn't. Either way, I knew I would have to rest until I had recovered enough to go back down.

But sitting down just shy of the top was to leave a task undone. I also felt as if I was being cheated out of a fuller experience of the mountains; the unseen panorama tormented me, as if that view from the top was the only view worth pursuing. Resting up at the top would be so much better, I reasoned, so I stood up and slogged on.

By the time I got to the top I felt dizzy and had to lean against one of the large boulders to regain my strength. I looked up and along the shores of Tasman Lake, past the icebergs and the glacier's terminus, into the mountains that rose sharply like a white-crested wave above a steep, rocky beach. The view took my breath away: it was even better than I had hoped it would be. I felt elated. The struggle had all been worth it, despite the fact that I would have to sleep for most of the afternoon to recover. I clambered up on top of a rock and sat there for a couple of hours, resting and watching the mountains.

Now, three years later, I faced the same mountains, only this time we were going up and over them. I felt suddenly terrified, and the sight of the mountains — so huge and sharp — created a lurch in my stomach. The struggle of getting to the top of the moraine wall remained fresh in my mind. Was I crazy to think I could summit Ball Pass? The route was an overwhelming challenge, a prospect so much larger than anything I had contemplated since I had been diagnosed with MS.

'Bro, those are massive hills. I think we're a bit crazy,' I told Gerwyn.

'Nah. We're going to make it to the top and it's gonna be amazing!'

He slapped me on the back enthusiastically. Gerwyn was a Welshman who had moved to Christchurch not long after the 2011 earthquake, to help with the rebuild.

'Yeah, you're right,' I said, trying to psych myself up.

'Hey, don't let past experiences define your limitations. And remember, whatever happens, it's about the journey, not the destination.'

'That's true. And a lot has changed in three years.'

Not long after that first trip to Mt Cook Village I had started working with Freya Thompson, a graduate of Massey University's sports and exercise programme. Although I had not been aware of this, the Massey programme and the local MS society work together, pairing up students with people who have MS to help the students learn the process of rehabilitation. By then I had read a lot of the literature on MS, and much of it had emphasised the importance of exercise and the positive effect it can have in slowing the progress of the disease.

In time, and desperate to regain strength, I became convinced that gym work and exercise were going to be crucial if I was to arrest my body's steady decline. However, I was also aware of my natural inclination towards pushing my body too hard. I realised that I would only be able to make progress at the gym under the watchful eye of someone experienced in the rehabilitation of people with neurological conditions. Without this guidance I would simply crash and burn, and be unable to continue.

I had just started studying towards my honours in English literature at Massey in Palmerston North when I found out about Freya. I walked into the gym one afternoon and asked if there were any trainers who might fit the bill. The guy behind the counter recommended Freya, who was the most experienced trainer working at the Massey gym. 'Flick her an email,' he said.

One of my fears, going into the first appointment, was of getting assigned a regime that was too difficult, or that would cause me to become overly exhausted. My previous experience of gyms and exercise regimes was not all that positive, invariably resulting in high levels of fatigue, discouragement and eventual failure. These fears were quickly dispelled, however, as Freya set gentle but fun regimes that stretched me, but not to the point of exhaustion. I remember one of those initial consultations.

'OK, Nick, now I want you to balance on your left leg, with your eyes closed,' Freya told me. 'Our aim is for eight seconds this week. And remember, concentrate on being grounded.'

I closed my eyes for a moment, both feet on the ground, and imagined my legs as the trunk of a tree, its roots spreading, flowing into the ground through the soles of my feet, bringing a sense of stability. I lifted one foot off the ground. Freya started to count.

I began to wobble and thrust my foot down to prevent a fall. 'Six seconds — that's great! You've improved from last time, which is really great to see. Keep on working at it and let's see if you can crack eight seconds next time.'

This sense of progress was satisfying and enjoyable, even if it was just being able to balance three seconds longer than a month ago, or being able to complete a set of lunges without becoming fatigued. I tried to enjoy every step of progress as a privilege. More importantly, I found that the sense of progress motivated me to keep pressing on at the gym, even after a hard day of study.

I rarely found the gym easy. Not only is gym work often repetitive, boring and hard, but there were also many times when I did not feel I had the energy to work out. The gym feels like a drag when you are tired. However, my carefully set exercises made the times when I felt tired valuable learning experiences. Through them I learned to gauge my limitations and to pace myself appropriately, so that I could keep plodding, even when I was tired. Learning the art of pace-setting increased my stamina, enabling me to manage life better and maintain a more routine and predictable lifestyle, which in turn brought a sense of stability. I always tried to make it to the gym three times a week, doing as much as I was physically able to do.

Not that stamina through pace-setting necessarily ensured stability. There were times when, despite my best efforts, I experienced regression, a loss of strength and balance. These times were always frightening and disheartening. It was frightening because it often felt as if there was no coming back from that point of regression, as if I would never be able to recover and had to kiss goodbye to any hope of climbing and tramping. It seemed as if I was being pushed back to square one. Even more discouraging was the fact that these periods of relapse, when all my symptoms flared up and hindered my ability to be active, happened reasonably regularly. Nevertheless, it was comforting to know that progress was possible through gym work.

Interestingly, it was during these tough times that the prospect of grace also gave me the most hope. Knowing that grace would be there to give me strength and encouragement, even when I hit rock bottom, meant that I could keep plodding, even when it felt as if there was little other reason to hope. While I still tended to resist the process of grief, it was at those moments of grace that I felt most at rest, free from the tyranny of proving my self-worth. Resting in grace, accepting my strength and ability as a gift to be enjoyed, I learned to ride these troubling times and not to despair (not too much, at least).

I often felt exposed and weak at the gym. It felt a bit awkward to be struggling to balance on one foot or doing a one-arm row with a 4-kilogram weight and skinny white arms while the guy next to me had 30 kilograms in each hand, his muscular arms large enough to make Arnie feel threatened. I felt self-conscious about my weakness. However, under Freya's supervision, my weights and times slowly increased. With this came a sense of agency: I was not powerless against MS, and I could develop greater levels of strength.

This sense of agency had a profound impact. As I realised that MS did not have to limit me, and that I could slowly and carefully push the envelope, tracks and walks that had been off-limits gradually came within my grasp. At this point my gym work took on even more meaning. I asked Freya to customise my routines to meet specific challenges. To prepare for a walk that had more uphill sections, I would slog away at step-ups and squats. If I knew I was going to negotiate a rocky piece of track, I would do balance routines that focused on activating the muscles I needed for stability. This all gave me ample motivation to keep going and, with grace, a hope for the future.

Hope was important. When I was diagnosed with MS in the USA, and then had the diagnosis confirmed in New Zealand, I felt as if I had been given a death sentence. The prognosis given by my neurologist was not positive and spoke only of inevitable deterioration. A quick look online, and reading about the probabilities of various life expectancies, confirmed this. I felt as if I had little hope beyond being semi-comfortable throughout the inescapable decline, as if there was no chance of recovering that which I had lost.

And now I stood at the lookout at the bottom of Hooker Lake, staring across the turquoise blue of the frozen surface, up to the peppered terminus of the Hooker Glacier and on to the soaring peaks of Mt Cook, rugged and gnarly above the walls of snow, rock and ice. It was an incredibly intimidating view.

'Ball Pass must be that little dip there,' I said to Gerwyn, pointing to a ridge coming off the side of Mt Cook, 1100 metres above us. I examined my map. 'And the playing fields must be that little flat area there, halfway up.'

'Really?' Gerwyn responded. 'It looks amazing! But this section up to the bottom of the playing fields is going to be a bit tough.'

'Yeah, and the snow's pretty deep in some of these dips, and between the rocks,' I said, plunging my walking pole into the snow as I spoke. 'We'll have to be careful not to fall through the rocks.'

'Definitely,' Gerwyn agreed. Then he clapped his hands together and shouted, 'Woo! Let's do it!'

We began our journey up the side of the Hooker Valley, alongside the lake, heading for a gully past the terminus where we would begin our ascent proper. It was cold and everything was frozen. The glacial lake below us was covered with thick ice and the sheer scale of the scene became apparent when we realised that the three small dots on the surface of the lake were people having a photoshoot. But Gerwyn's enthusiasm was infectious. He helped to me focus on allowing a positive emotional response that would override my more

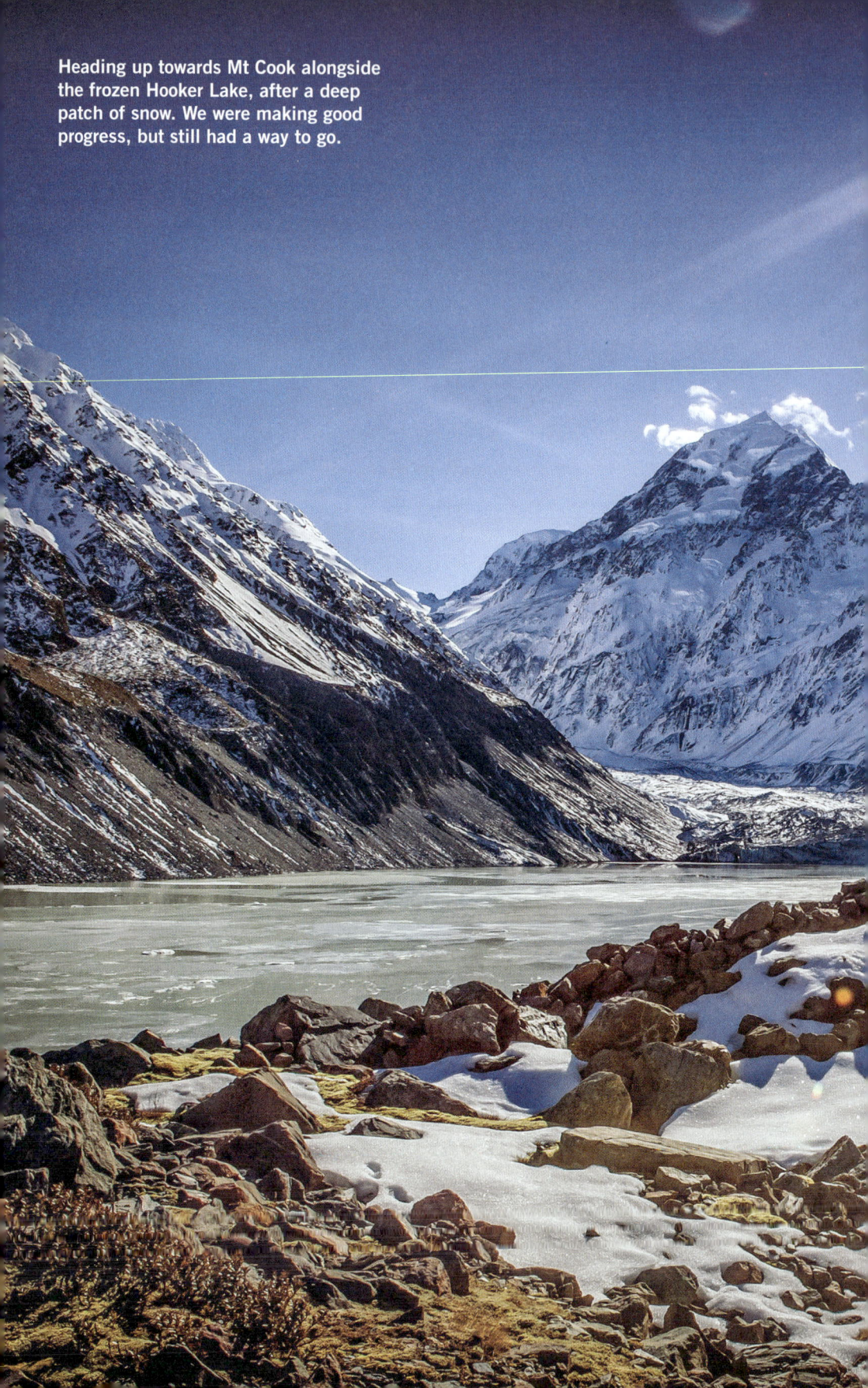
Heading up towards Mt Cook alongside the frozen Hooker Lake, after a deep patch of snow. We were making good progress, but still had a way to go.

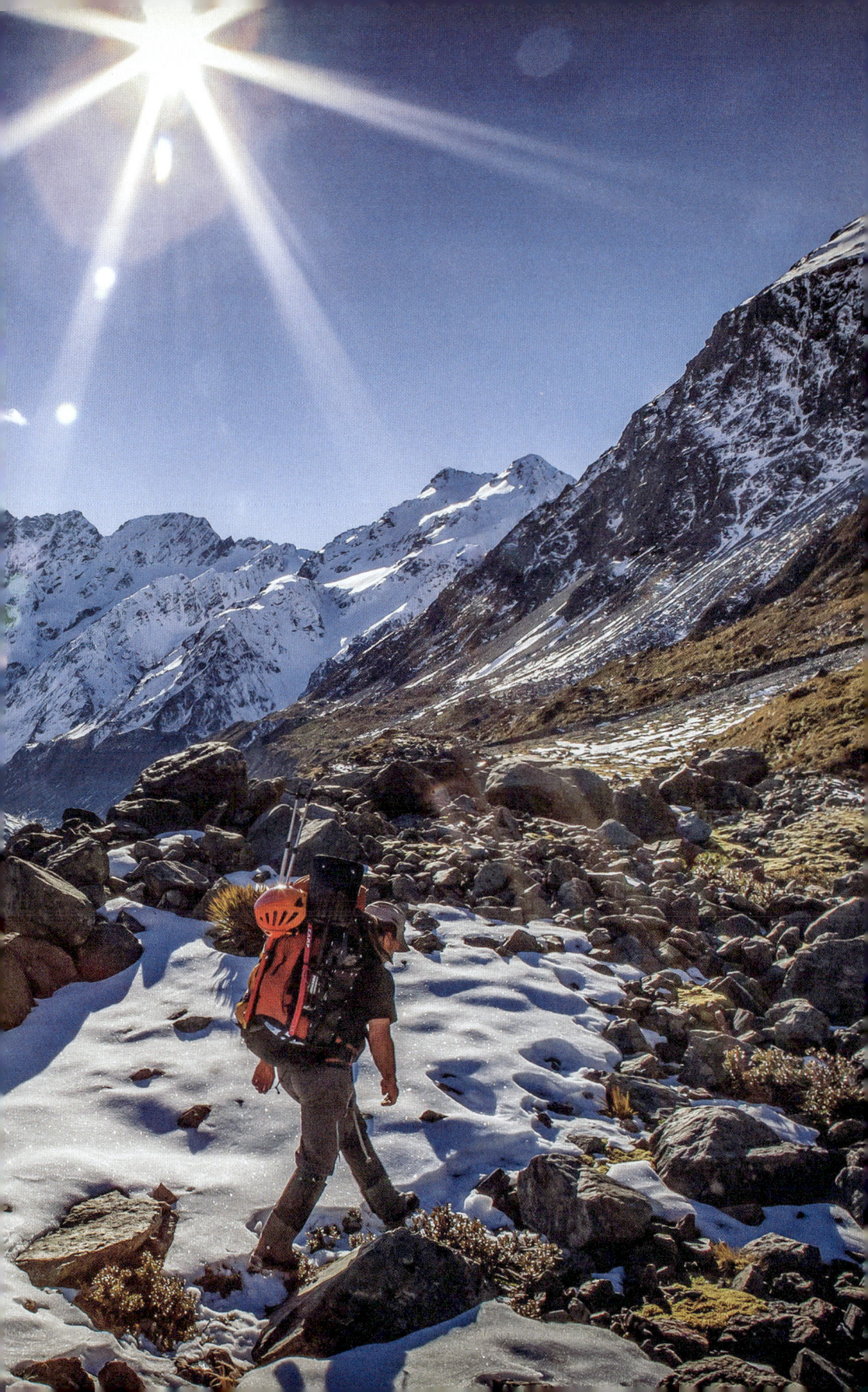

rational moments of wondering what on earth I was doing.

There was no denying that it was tough going. First, there was no discernible track to follow — most of the tracks we found were soon lost beneath the snow. We had to crash our way through the bushes and grasses that filled the valley floor and often obscured the rocks and holes beneath. The deep, wet snow was at times impossible to avoid, and we'd sink up to our knees in it.

We finally arrived at the bottom of the gully in time for a late lunch — much later than we'd anticipated.

'Hey, Gee, how about we just aim for the playing fields tonight, rather than the top of the pass? It's one thirty now and I feel like I might have to bust my burner to get to the top tonight. It's been a lot of hard work so far, and we're quite a bit behind schedule.' I pulled out the stove to cook up some lunch. 'We can relax here for a while, enjoy our lunch, and take a more relaxed pace up there.'

'Yeah,' Gerwyn replied. 'This has been a lot harder than I thought so far and it'd be pushing it to get up to the top, it would. We'll just take it easy. I'm feeling a bit tired myself.'

'Awesome.' I was relieved. We sat down on top of a big boulder to rest while the water boiled. Resting felt good, and taking it a bit more slowly meant I could plod up the gully rather than rush. It would make a big difference.

'So what you got for lunch, then?' Gerwyn asked, as I poured boiling water over my meal. Gerwyn is a trained chef and we frequently exchanged ideas about food.

'Well, this one uses a rice-flake base — it's so easy, you know — and then a couple of tablespoons of ground almond, a sprinkling of pine nuts, a couple of tablespoons of dehydrated veges and a bit of curry for flavour. Hopefully the rice will act as a slow-release energy source, and the nuts give a bit of protein, without ending up as stodge in the stomach. It's an experiment.'

'Too easy,' Gerwyn replied with a smile, patting me on the shoulder. 'You know, something like that would be good when we go to Nepal, except that I would probably grind all the nuts a bit finer — it'll require less energy to digest. But, otherwise, it sounds like you got it all sorted.'

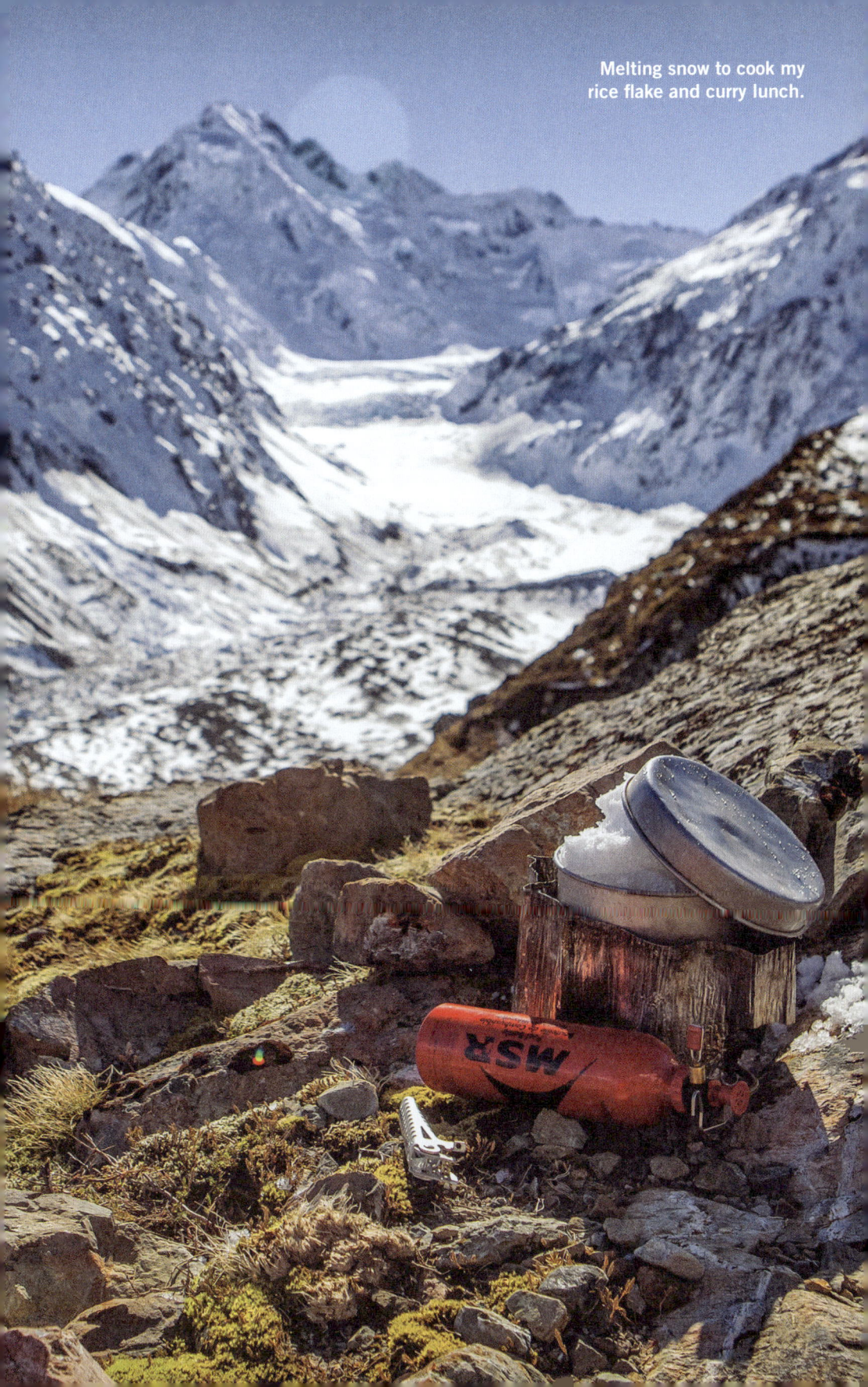
Melting snow to cook my rice flake and curry lunch.

I appreciated his confidence, but inside I was hoping like crazy that my recipe worked. My experiments with food have not always been a success. The first time I experimented, when I was about 18, all my pasta turned into one massive lump and the tinned stew I used as a base turned into a wobbling mass of jelly-meat. The texture of the meal was so disgusting that my friend and I gagged on the first few mouthfuls and couldn't eat it. Instead we decided to lure possums with the dinner and try to catch them. Then there was the corn couscous that I tried to eat with cold water and tuna — that wasn't so great either. Fingers crossed, my latest concoction would not only be edible, but it would also taste OK.

Getting my food sorted is crucial for success not only in tramping but also in everyday life. When I was on my way back home from the US, Mum did some research and found out about a diet specifically for people with MS, designed by a guy called George Jelinek. Initially, I was pretty opposed to it, as it meant an end to a lot of foods I really liked: steak, pies, McDonald's hamburgers, pastries, cakes, potato chips, deep-fried food, lollies, chocolate bars and a lot of other things. I already knew I had a dairy and gluten allergy, so Mum encouraged me to give those up too. With the exception of red meat, I did not eat any of those things very often, but it was tough trying to cut out so much deliciousness at once. Despite what I had learned from Joey, I was not *that* into the concept of healthy eating.

Perhaps my slightly uneasy relationship with what seemed to be a hard-core eating regime was rooted in a denial of the seriousness of my diagnosis. I had hoped that everything would just get better without my having to put in too much effort. But that was before the tingling became a big problem. I could almost tolerate the sensation in my hands and feet, but it was the tingling in my face, around my lips and nose, that I found most difficult to handle. It was often so intense that I wanted to tear the skin off my face to gain relief. It kept me awake most nights, and I felt exhausted.

One night, I hit rock bottom. I was driving back from Massey University, out along the edge of town to the place where I was living, when I decided to wrap my car round a tree. It had felt as if my face was being relentlessly shot-blasted for several days straight. I could no longer fight through the pain to retain a clear focus: it was consuming every part of my mind. I felt trapped inside my body, trapped inside the pain, and as if there was no other path to relief.

I was screaming, frightened, beating the steering wheel with my fist, when the thought occurred to me. I saw a sturdy tree and started driving towards it at speed. It was a few metres away when I looked down at the speedo. I was doing about 120 or 130 kilometres per hour. I looked up at the tree. It occurred to me that I was not really going that fast, and that I had bought the car because of its five-star safety rating. In all likelihood I would survive, but probably as a quadriplegic, which would totally suck. I swerved away from the tree, narrowly missing it. I pulled over and stopped. That's when I realised I needed help, and that I needed to get radical with my lifestyle, if I wanted to survive.

I told my parents what had happened and asked for their help. They were amazing, dumping everything and moving from Taupo to Palmerston North to help get me back on track and to support me while I continued studying. I decided I needed to get real about my diet to see if that would deliver the benefits Jelinek promised. Mum and Dad agreed, and in order to help me they adopted the diet as well.

One of the difficulties I'd had when I first tried the diet was the feeling of missing out. My parents might have a nice Scotch fillet, which I love, while I was stuck with a watery piece of defrosted fish. I knew it was a bit of a spoilt attitude, but that was the reality. Once Mum and Dad were on the same diet it was much easier to stick to it. We all struggled at times to make the required changes, and being able to talk about the difficulties was hugely beneficial. It didn't take us long to decide that it was pretty hard to kick everything at once, and so we decided to introduce the changes gradually over the space of a few months.

With time, I started to notice a difference. Sugars made me

lethargic, gluten made me sick, red meat sat like rocks in my stomach and drained me of energy, and potato chips and deep-fried foods made me feel bloated. I noticed that my dietary changes were making a big difference at the gym, supplying me with the energy I needed to keep progressing. It became increasingly easy to make healthy choices, and I spent a lot of time experimenting with ways to tailor my diet to specific situations, just as I did with my gym routines.

▲▲▲

After our lunch Gerwyn and I lay in the sun on the top of a big rock, resting. There was the familiar sense of being deep in the mountains, completely cut off, as we sat overlooking the glacier. I felt deeply rested and at the same time deeply invigorated. I have heard it said that true restedness is a state of grace. This was definitely a grace, a gift, the kind of scene and situation that most thrills me, that satisfies a deep longing to be enveloped by something awe-inspiringly beautiful and majestic. I soaked it in, thrilled to have made it this far. Although the morning had been hard and I wanted to be careful not to push it, I felt quietly encouraged by how well I had handled the challenge of getting to this point. I knew getting up the gully would be hard work but I felt confident I'd be able to make it to the top.

The gully faces south and it was very cold in there. Gerwyn and I plugged our way through the snow slowly, zigzagging up the steeper sections. The snow conditions were safe enough but not ideal. Because of the recent dump of snow there was a fair amount of wind slab on the leeward-facing slopes. Wind slab manifests as a crusty layer of hard snow on top of a much thicker layer of soft snow, formed by a rapid accumulation of wind-blown snow particles. Walking through wind slab is hard because it often supports your body weight when you initially step on it but then breaks as you shift your weight on to the leading foot. As this layer of hard snow breaks, you drop down, in our case bringing the snow up to our knees as we compressed the snow beneath. A couple of hours of repeatedly falling through the snow and then having to

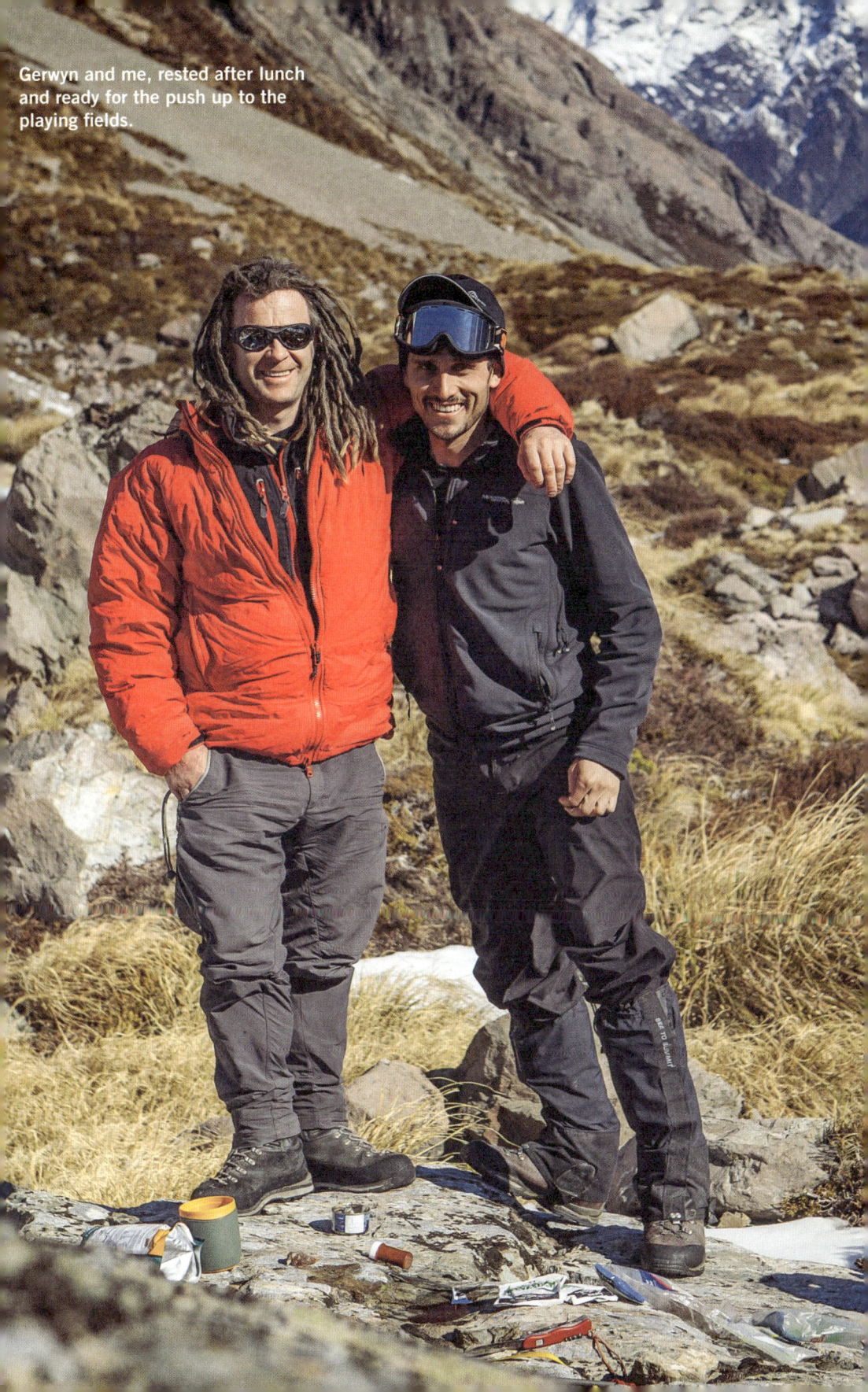

Gerwyn and me, rested after lunch and ready for the push up to the playing fields.

lift our legs high to step out of the hole was pretty tiresome. As the slope got steeper, the snow slab sometimes made it difficult to get a solid stepping platform — somewhat unnerving when there is a very large, icy chute beneath you.

We'd been huffing and puffing our way up the face for nearly three hours when I began to falter. I was a bit behind Gerwyn, my legs were burning, and I felt wiped out, running on fumes. I thought about calling out to him, to ask if he could help me with my pack, but my face was so numb that I was past being able to articulate my words, much less shout intelligibly to him. I knew I was close to the top, just beneath the part where the steep gully tapers off and becomes the level area just below Mt Mabel, commonly known as the playing fields. I wanted to finish this, to do it on my own, to prove to myself that I was able.

I rested for a bit. I'm going to make it, I told myself. I looked at my watch. It was five o'clock. We had left the carpark over seven hours earlier. My legs had been cramping from the fatigue and cold for the last hour or so. I had to be careful not to straighten them or the muscles would lock up, which in itself was exhausting, since it meant I didn't have the option of resting on straightened legs.

I picked myself up and continued through the deep snow. I thought I'd try to use Gerwyn's tracks to make it a bit easier. A couple of footsteps in, his tracks collapsed and my leg slid downhill. I plunged the shaft of my ice axe deeper into the snow, using it to help me up again. I stood, stopped and kicked a new, solid platform into the snow. I rested for a moment. My feet were numb. I gave up on Gerwyn's tracks and forged my own path once again, not without difficulty. This last hundred metres seemed to take every ounce of energy to complete.

I finally reached the level area, where Gerwyn was already at work on a spot to pitch the tent.

'Wow,' I mumbled with numb lips as I dumped my pack on the ground.

'How you doin'? All right?' Gerwyn asked, also struggling to sound his consonants. I could tell he was tired too.

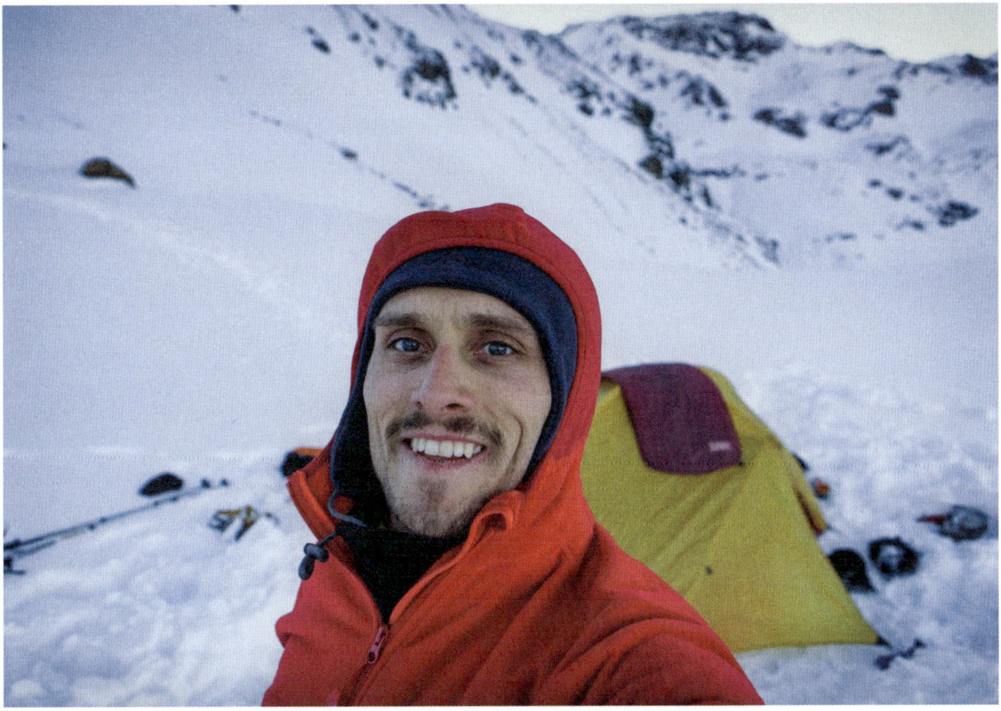

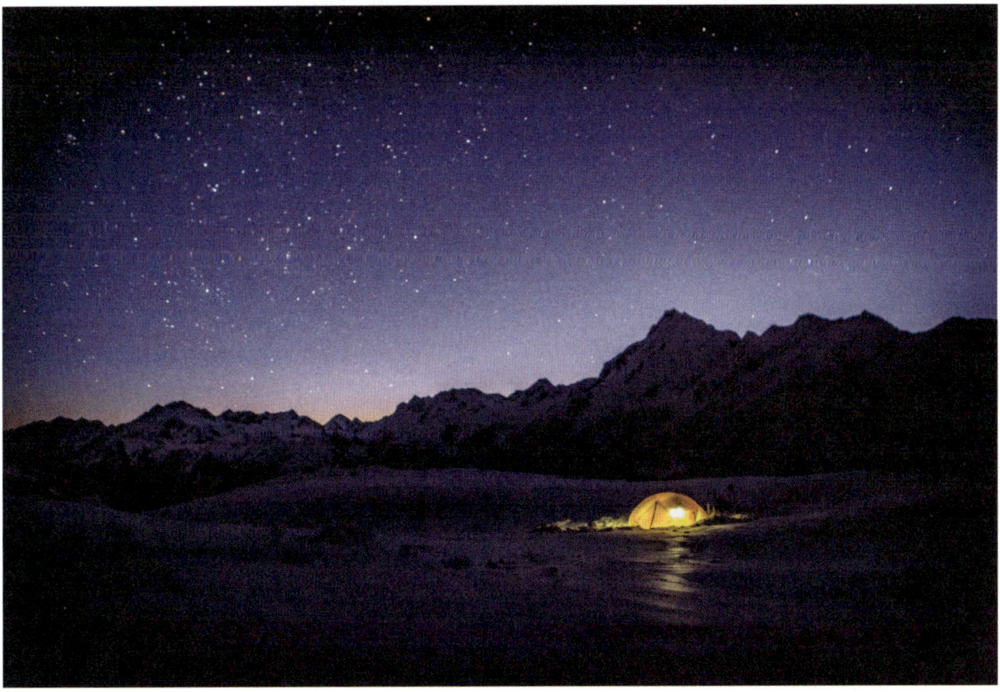

Top to bottom: Me, in some fresh warm clothes, having just finished setting up the tent — my Therm-a-Rest mattress was on top of the tent, waiting for Gerwyn to get changed; Our tent and the stars.

'Dude, I am totally spent. That was hard work.'

'Brutal, that was. And cold. But what an awesome spot this is, in't it?' he said triumphantly.

It *was* an amazing spot, a nest in the mountains. The delicate contours and fine wind-sculpted edges of the playing fields were lit with orange as the sun began to disappear behind the peaks across the valley. I was suddenly overwhelmed by what I had accomplished, by the realisation that I had got this far, and that even if I went no further this was enough. I let out a loud whoop. Gerwyn laughed.

We pulled out our shovels, cut through the wind slab and made a level place to pitch the tent, all the while watching the blue shadows creep up the fire-capped, snowy summit of Mt Cook. There was something magical about the light, the stillness of the air, and the fact of being perched on the side of a mountain. It was a truly amazing experience, the kind of evening I had always dreamed about, the kind that epitomised, to me at least, the beauty of mountaineering. A Brian Turner poem that I'd always loved called 'Place' came to me.

> *Once in a while*
> *you may come across a place*
> *where everything*
> *seems as close to perfection*
> *as you will ever need.*
> *And striving to be faultless*
> *the air on its knees*
> *holds the trees apart,*
> *yet nothing is categorically*
> *thus, or that, and before the dusk*
> *mellows and fails*
> *the light is like honey*
> *on the stems of tussock grass,*
> *and the shadows*
> *are mauve birthmarks*
> *on the hills.*

The golden lick of light slipped up, off the top of Mt Cook's summit, and I returned to the tent to get warm. Out of the sun I could feel the temperature dropping, so I put on some warmer clothing and made a start on preparing some hot food. The stars were beginning to appear as we finished our meal. I went outside briefly, to look at the stars and take a few photos. The night was as stunning as the sunset had been, perfectly clear and without a breath of wind. It was astounding.

Our alarms went off at 6 a.m. Our plan was to get an early (but not too early) start while the top layer of ice was frozen and firm — it would make progress a lot easier. I climbed outside to light the cooker and warm up some food while Gerwyn packed his gear. As I opened the tent, I noticed that the moisture from our breath had frozen on the inside. It was cold. I tucked my chin a little deeper into my down jacket to try to get warm, and turned off my head torch while I waited for the water to boil.

I looked across at the mountains, silhouettes on the horizon, as the sky slowly lightened in anticipation of the morning sun. I could see head torches, climbers across the valley, lighting up a face as they approached the summit. Again, a flicker of envy strengthened my resolve to make it to the top: I would prove that I was physically capable as well. I would post that picture.

'How are your boots?' Gerwyn asked, as I took my turn to pack up my gear in the tent.

'Frozen solid, unfortunately. I think I need better boots for this. Standard leather tramping boots don't quite cut it — they get wet and then have little insulation.'

'When we go to Nepal, you'll want better boots — something a bit warmer. Mine are three-season mountaineering boots and they're brilliant, they are. I've done three trips in these.'

Gerwyn is a stocky guy, with a full head of dreadlocks. I first met him in Arthur's Pass, at Edwards Hut, in November 2013. He'd been up since the crack of dawn and had crossed the Polar Range, via

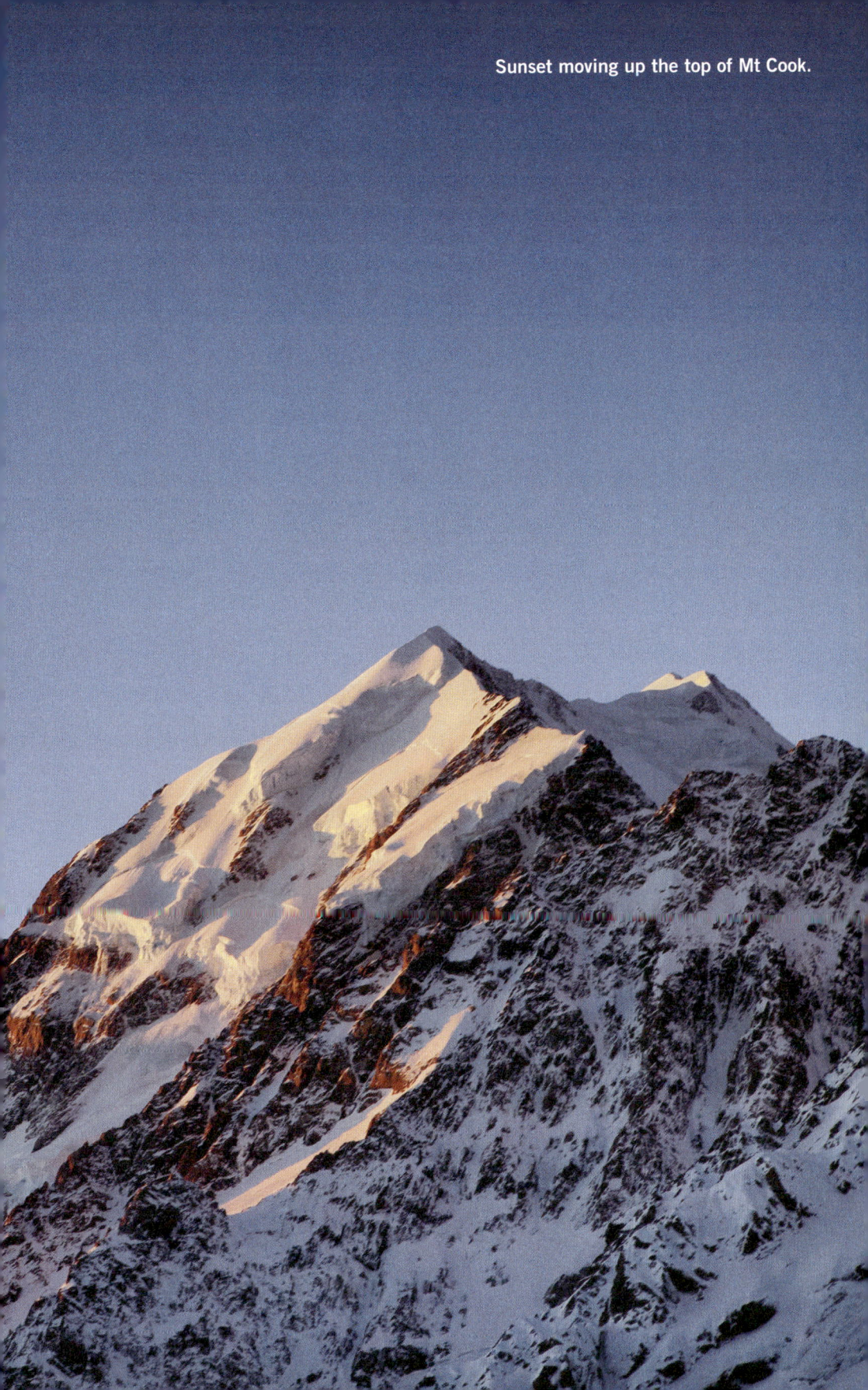
Sunset moving up the top of Mt Cook.

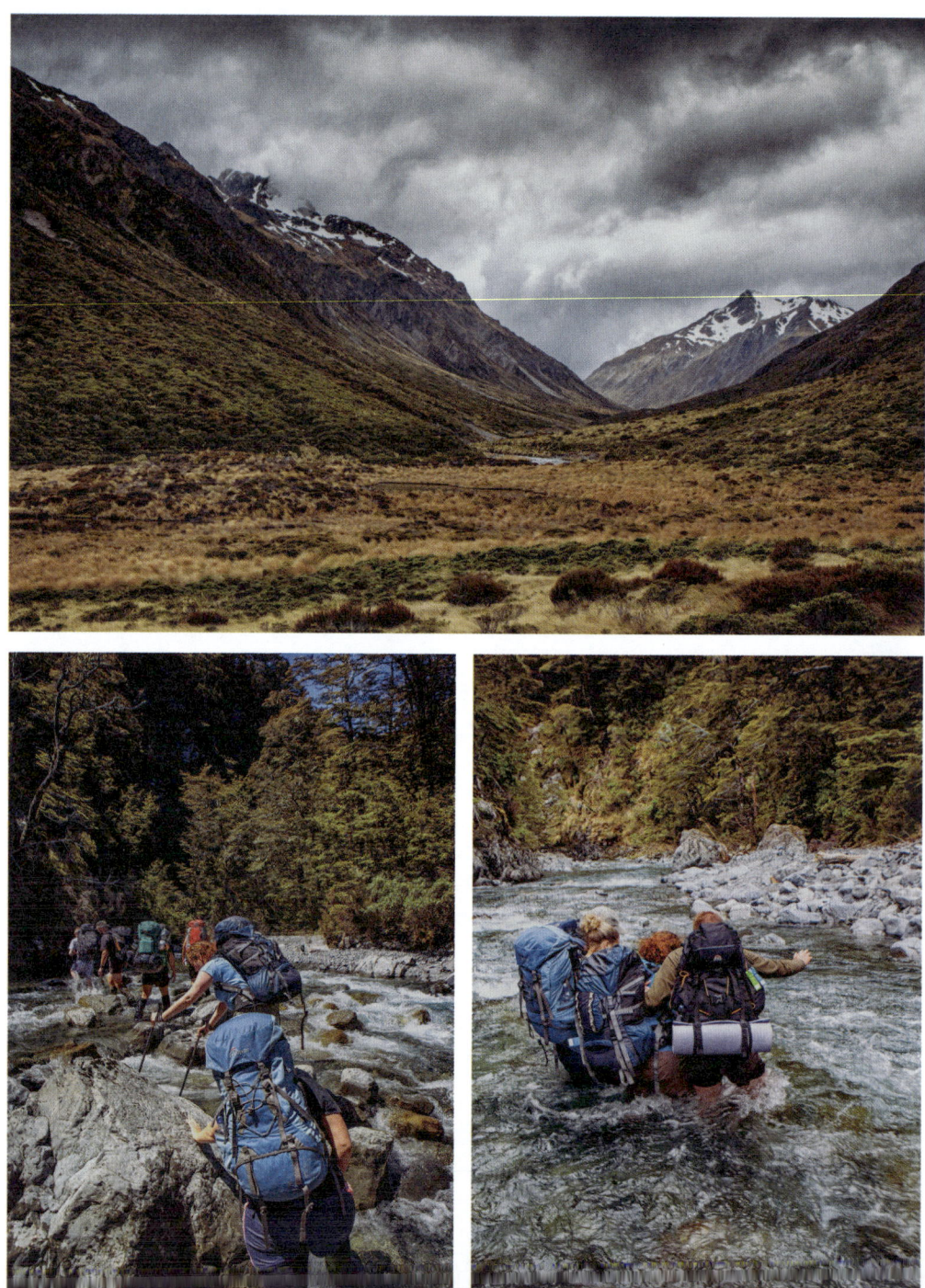

Clockwise from top: A stormy afternoon looking up the Edwards Valley from Edwards Hut, waiting for the rest of the party to get back; Walking down the Edwards River, the only 'track'; Crossing the Edwards River, which was slightly swollen with rain from the previous day.

Amber Col, and was heading down the beech-laced Edwards River the next day. It was a rainy, windy weekend and he arrived sodden and cold. I offered him some salmon jerky I'd made. We got chatting about food and then hit it off as he told me about his trips to Nepal.

Nepal has always been a place that has interested me, holding the mystique of massive mountains and brave mountaineers, and I'd been transfixed by his descriptions of the place and of his adventures.

'So, when are you going then?' he had asked.

'I wish!' I laughed. 'It'd take me a couple of years to save the money.' Nepal seemed an impossible dream.

My 2013 trip to Edwards Hut had been my first attempt at a tramp longer than three hours. I'd gone with a group and it had taken us five hours to get to the hut, a monumental achievement for me, particularly as it involved several hours of travel along riverbed, around boulders and through beech trees into a tussocky valley nestled beneath the high, snowy peaks. The trip was four days long and some of the party, having spent the first night at Edwards Hut, had gone on to Otehake Hut for the second night. Anxious not to push my limits, or my luck, by going over the rocky Taruahuna Pass and beneath the ominous-sounding Falling Mountain, I had opted to stay with a couple of the others for a few nights at Edwards Hut. I wanted to use the time to recover and rest in preparation for the trip out.

The trip up to Edwards Hut was also significant in that it was my first tramp with other people since my diagnosis. As I slowly built up my tramping times and distances, I always tramped solo. To begin with, the reason was that I tramped so slowly; on those first few tramps, I would walk for about 20 minutes or so, then sit down to rest or sleep for a few minutes before continuing for another 20 minutes. I thought that anyone tramping with me would be driven mad by my frequent stopping. Even as my stamina increased I remained afraid of holding people up, and of not being able to keep up with them. I hated to be an inconvenience so I continued to go solo. I found this social isolation difficult, and I also realised that to learn the skills I needed to progress I had to start tramping with more experienced people.

It was a scary prospect, getting involved with experienced trampers. Because of my social isolation and without others to compare myself to I never knew how fit — or not — I actually was, and I just assumed that I was slower than everyone else. I had chosen to go on the Edwards Hut tramp only because I knew there were a number of slower people going, and because the trip leader had assured me that they would be able to accommodate me, even if I had to go more slowly.

That's why, when Gerwyn, an obviously fit, fast and experienced tramper, suggested that I should go to Nepal I did not seriously consider it as an option.

'You should just do it,' Gerwyn had said with his cheeky grin. 'It'll be a life changin' experience, it will. I promise you, you'll never look back.'

'Yeah.' I'd shaken my head, sure he was right. 'I would love to go, but I'm just not sure I could handle the physical demands of a trip like that.'

'Nah, you can do it. If you can do this, you can do it.'

I'd found Gerwyn's reassurance unexpectedly affirming, and it seeded the idea of moving towards a goal much greater than I had ever thought possible.

'Well, when you decide to go, let me know and I can give you contacts, suggest treks, recommend equipment, whatever you need. Just give me a call,' he said, writing down his number on a piece of paper. 'And if you are ever in Christchurch and need a place to stay, or want to go on a tramp, let me know.'

We kept in touch over the intervening months and caught up once when he was passing through Palmerston North. I was keen to do something around Mt Cook, and when I talked to Gerwyn about it he suggested Ball Pass, which he had done a couple of summers earlier. That's how we'd ended up here, climbing a ridge that leads to Mt Cook.

'Would you buy the boots here, or can you get them more cheaply in Nepal?' I asked him as we packed up the tent in the snow.

'Nah, I'd get them here. You need to be a bit careful in Nepal, of fakes and stuff. And the prices are actually not always much cheaper in Kathmandu, mind.'

After we'd eaten breakfast and packed up our gear we headed off. We could see tracks in the snow where someone had done the pass a few days before us. There were a couple of ridges to traverse and a large snow-filled gully to cross, making the route a little bit tricky. The snow cover meant it was not immediately obvious where we could traverse the ridges without getting caught in dangerous bluffs. The person before us had evidently found it difficult too, their tracks working their way up and down the ridge, trying to find a place to cross. We had the benefit of their experience and were able to head straight to the crossings. That gave me a good deal of confidence.

A sharp ridge comes down the mountain between the peaks of Mt Mabel and Mt Rosa. Gerwyn and I were following a ledge around this ridge, but as we approached the crest of the ridge the snow became increasingly steep and icier. We stopped right beneath the crest, below a big rock, on a small, flattish spot carved out by the wind.

'Bloody hell, this bit's gonna be steep,' Gerwyn said, turning to me.

'Shoot. You're right.'

The wind, swirling around the ridge, had carved out a very steep section of snow that morphed into an extended section of steep snow with an icy crust. To cross the ridge we would have to traverse out on to it. It was terrifyingly exposed: ice and large rocky bluffs loomed beneath us.

'You feel OK doing it?' I asked.

Gerwyn took a deep breath. 'Yip. It'll be fine, it will. The exposure makes me nervous, that's all.'

He plunged his ice axes through the ice and into the deep snow beneath, committing himself to the move. It made me nervous to watch him.

Once he was round the corner I began to follow, using his steps. I focused only on what was immediately in front of me. Transitioning from the initial, near-vertical section to the next, less steep section was difficult as there was a sharp edge. I looked down between my legs, and felt a rush of fear as I realised how precarious my position was. I stopped for a moment, closed my eyes, took a couple of deep breaths, and focused on the security of my ice axe and crampons in the icy snow.

At that moment, I was very grateful for the training I'd received through the Palmerston North Tramping and Mountaineering Club just a few months earlier. The club runs three snowcraft courses each year and I had decided to enrol in the first two to keep myself motivated in my work at the gym. I didn't think I'd be able to handle the final, most advanced mountaineering course and, as before, was afraid that my weakness or slowness might reveal the presence of MS, resulting in a loss of acceptance in the group.

However, I was surprised by how well I managed the first two courses, and I was encouraged to participate in the third. This was a huge confidence booster for me, and one that could only come through participation in a group. I could see that by remaining in isolation from everyone else I had adopted an unnecessarily negative view of myself and the impact of the disease. I also really enjoyed the friendly atmosphere and camaraderie of the group — something else that is missed by being reclusive.

I repeated the mantra I had learned on the course as I traversed this difficult section of the ridge — kick-step, kick-step, plunge. I plunged the shaft of my ice axe into the snow with all the vigour I could muster, and kicked the toes of my crampons into the ice as deeply and securely as I could.

'Phew!' I laughed as we got to the end. 'Well, that was a bit of fun, eh, Gee.'

'Nah, I was scared, I was,' Gerwyn replied, shaking his head. 'I really don't enjoy exposure like that. We probably should have roped up, mind.'

'Yeah, true,' I agreed, turning to look at the view ahead. We were now on the large north-facing slope, an icy area that would take us to the next ridge, running off Mt Rosa. The sun had just broken in over the ridge, spilling warmth and long shadows over the icy snow, the frozen product of a day's thaw–freeze cycle. It provided a solid, albeit exposed footing, and as I turned I tried not to think about the slope

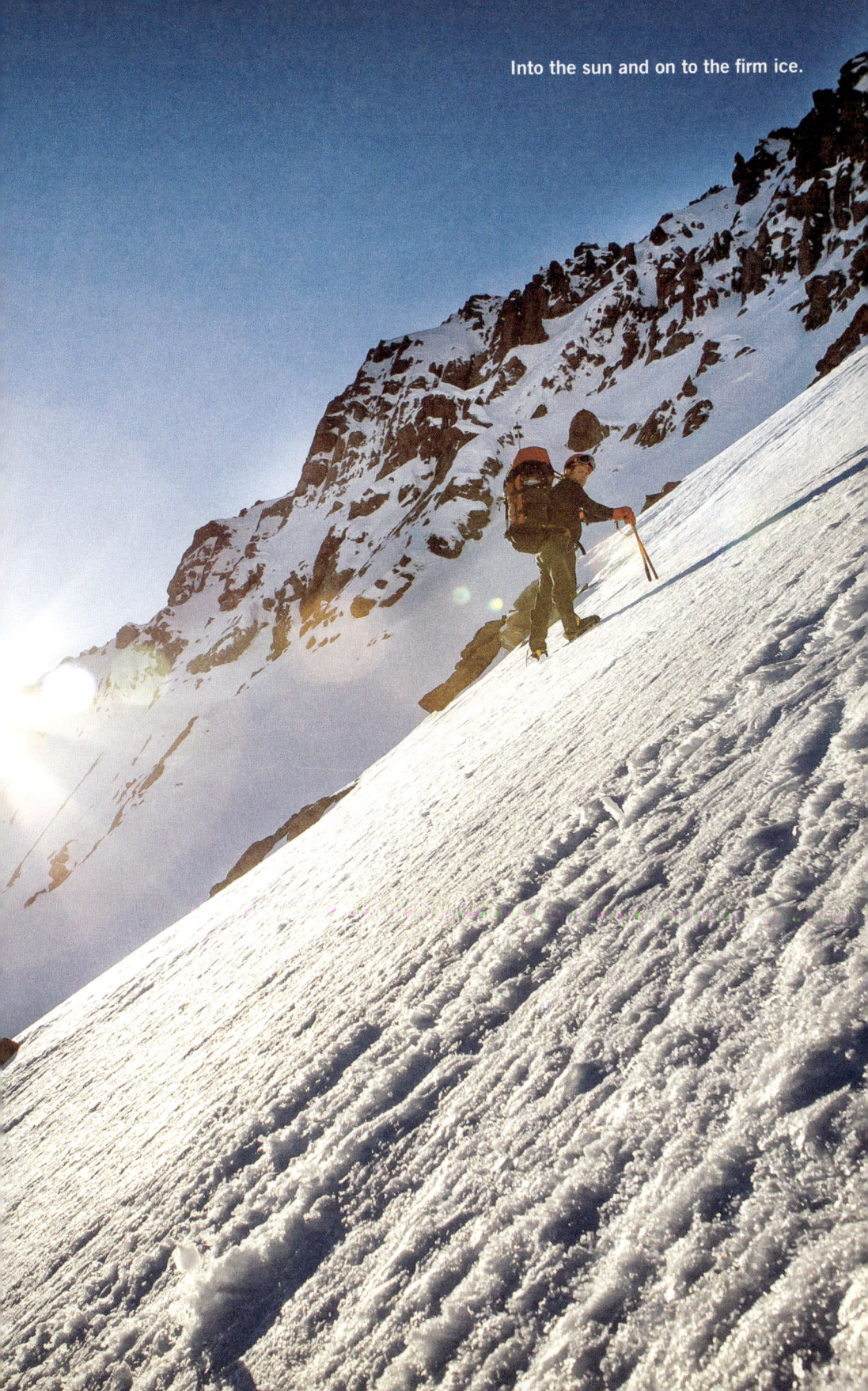
Into the sun and on to the firm ice.

beneath me, dropping 800 vertical metres into the Hooker Glacier. I plunged my crampons hard into the ice to get a good bite, causing the brittle layer of surface ice to shatter and skim down the face, playing the other pieces of ice like a xylophone. The music cross-faded into the silence of the still sky. I stood, closed my eyes and felt the warmth of the morning light spreading through my body — this too was a grace, a moment of deep rest.

Then I felt the urge to capture the moment with a photo. I took off the lens cap and tried to stick it into my chest pocket, but my hands were cold, and as I fumbled with my gloved fingers I dropped the cap. I gasped as I watched the cap shoot down the slope, past Gerwyn, accelerating at a frightening speed towards the glacier beneath, lost forever. While I was annoyed about losing the lens cap, there was also something strangely comical about watching it skittle along the ice — I am not sure what, exactly — and I laughed.

'You all right?' Gerwyn asked, trying to turn up the slope towards me.

'Yeah, I'm fine. I just dropped my lens cap and it shot off down there.' I pointed towards the glacier beneath.

'Oh,' Gerwyn said, looking at me quizzically. 'Your camera's going to be all right?'

'Yeah, it'll be fine. I'll just have to be careful with the lens, that's all.'

'Right. You want to go first for a while?' he suggested.

'OK,' I said, and I began to move carefully forward into the cold, long shadows, towards the pass.

We plugged away for a while then rounded the final ridge and began the slog up the slope toward the pass, sitting above us in plain sight. We'd been going for a couple of hours and I was feeling pretty good, only slightly tired. Knowing that I had been able to make it up to the playing fields had increased my confidence, and I felt good inside myself.

Gerwyn was a fair way ahead of me now and, apart from my rhythmic step-step-plunge, step-step-plunge, there was perfect silence, interrupted only by the occasional screech of a kea. As before, I felt a deep sense of rest, enjoying the enveloping enormity of the peaks and the pure splendour of the white snowscape. Light was falling parallel to some of the faces, illuminating the lines brushed into the wind-sculpted contours of the snow. There was something particularly sensuous about the way the light fell across these lines and contours, drawing me in, inviting me to stand, stare and enjoy.

The final push to the top of the pass was tough. The surface was frozen-solid snowmelt, and steep enough that we had to front-point our way up to the top. Front-pointing is where you use only the front few points of your crampons to climb, your heels floating in midair. With entirely ridged mountaineering boots this is not too difficult, allowing you to stand on your front points without too much strain on your calves. However, my boots were not proper mountaineering boots and allowed a bit of flex in the toe to make walking more comfortable. This meant I had to work my toes to keep the boot as straight as possible if I was to keep my crampon points from popping out of the ice. Trying to do this for 10 minutes straight was brutal on the calves and they burned. I had to stop often.

The view opened before me as I approached the top of the pass. It was astounding. I felt as if I was on top of the world, looking down into the Tasman Glacier and up into the white expanse of the bowl that feeds it. I gazed at the white peaks soaring out of the green and turquoise valleys below, and up at the rugged Caroline Face of Mt Cook with its massive hanging ice sheets. I felt an amazing sense of opportunity and potential. It blew me away.

The exhilaration of making it to the top was intensified by the fact that I had achieved something I'd hardly dreamed possible. The peaks around me were no longer off-limits, no longer monuments to remind me of all that I had lost. Now they represented possibility, places to explore, worlds of opportunity. In that moment, I felt as if the MS had faded away, as if I could do anything I set my mind to.

'This is amazing!' I yelled.

'Not too shabby, in't it,' Gerwyn replied with a told-you-so smile.

'Man, I don't think I could ever get enough of this,' I laughed. 'This is totally mind-blowing.'

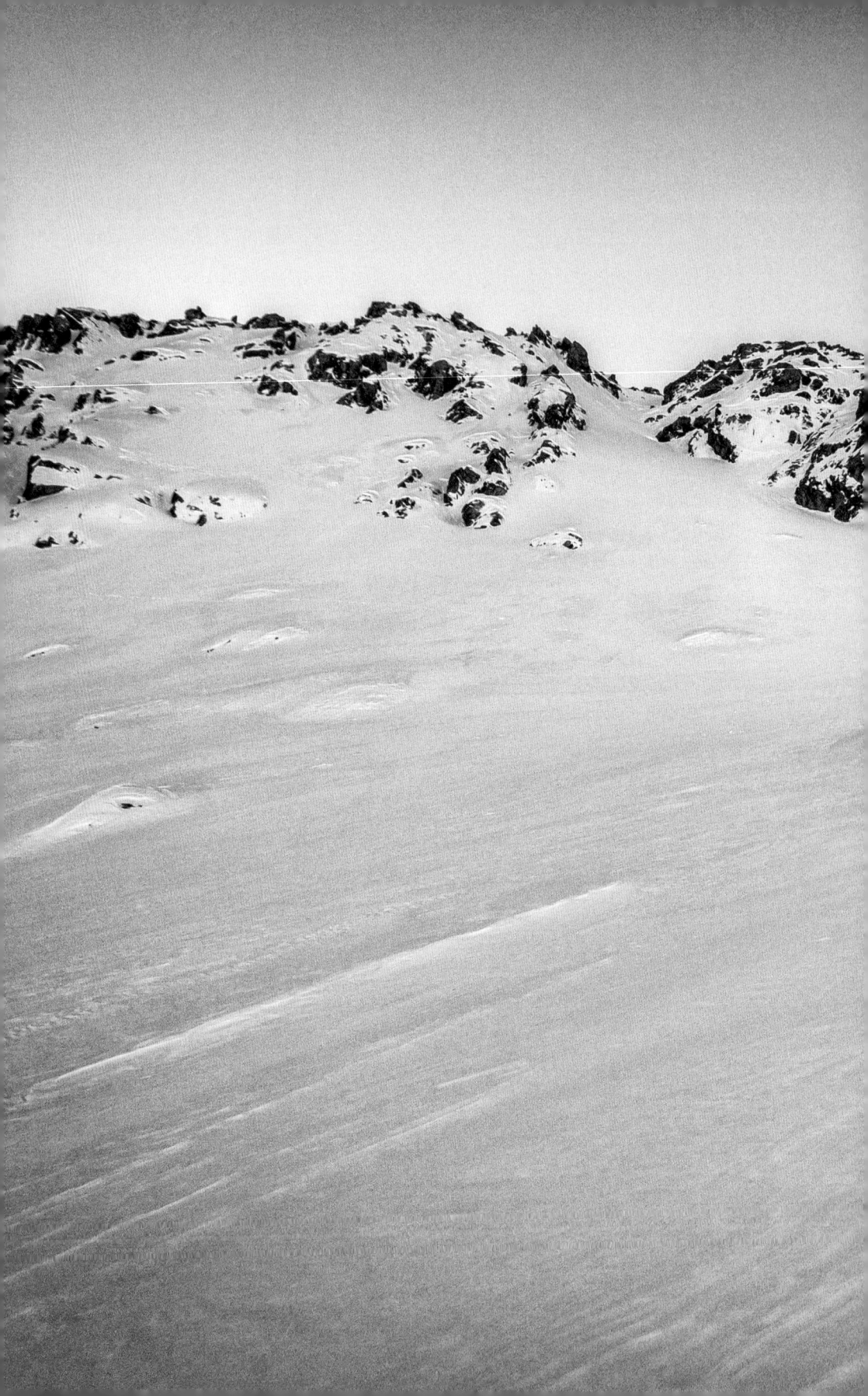

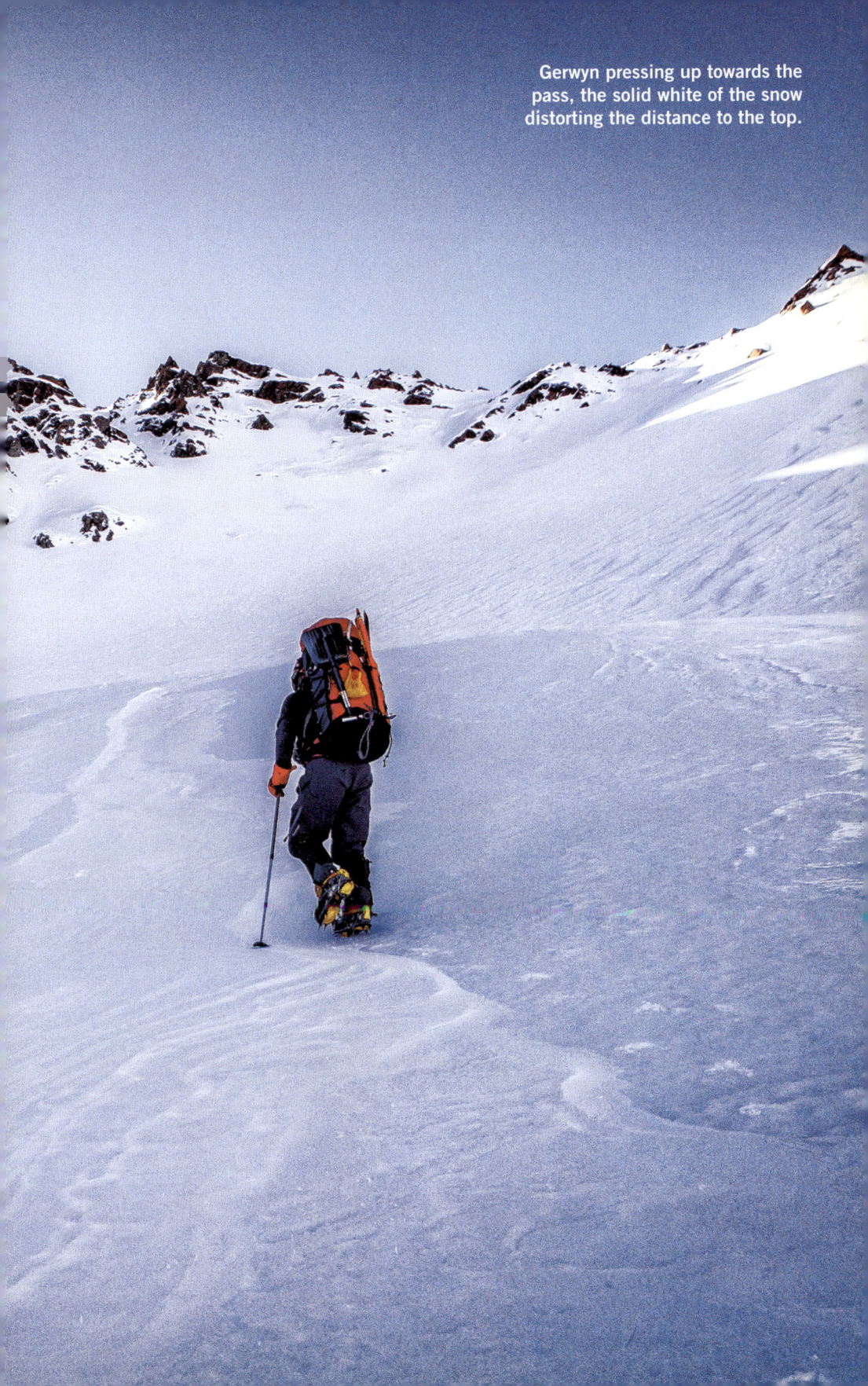
Gerwyn pressing up towards the pass, the solid white of the snow distorting the distance to the top.

Happy to be at the top of Ball Pass, surrounded by all that snow: a photo for Facebook.

'Imagine what it is like in the Himalayas, top of Rengo Pass, with 8000-metre peaks around you, rising up a whole 3000 metres above you. This is amazing, but over there —' he paused for a moment — 'it's unbelievable.'

'I bet,' I said, struggling to comprehend something more stunning than the scene before me. I looked over to Mt Cook, rising 1500 metres above us, and tried to envisage a mountain peak twice that height. It was almost inconceivable.

'Well, if you come with me next year, you'll see it with your own eyes.' Gerwyn laughed. 'Are you keen?'

'Hell yeah! I am so keen,' I said, handing him my phone. 'Hey, would you mind taking a picture? It's for Facebook.'

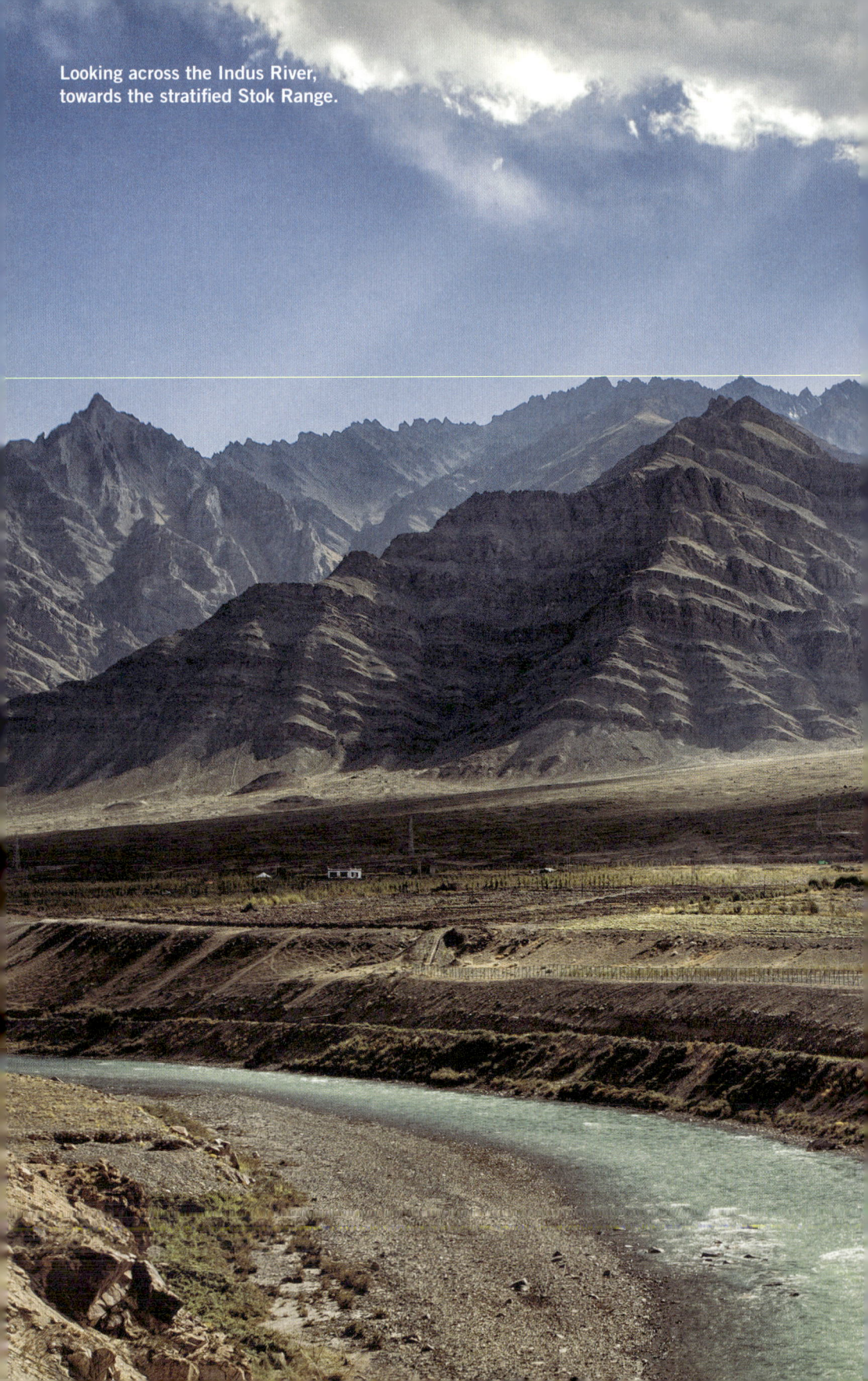
Looking across the Indus River, towards the stratified Stok Range.

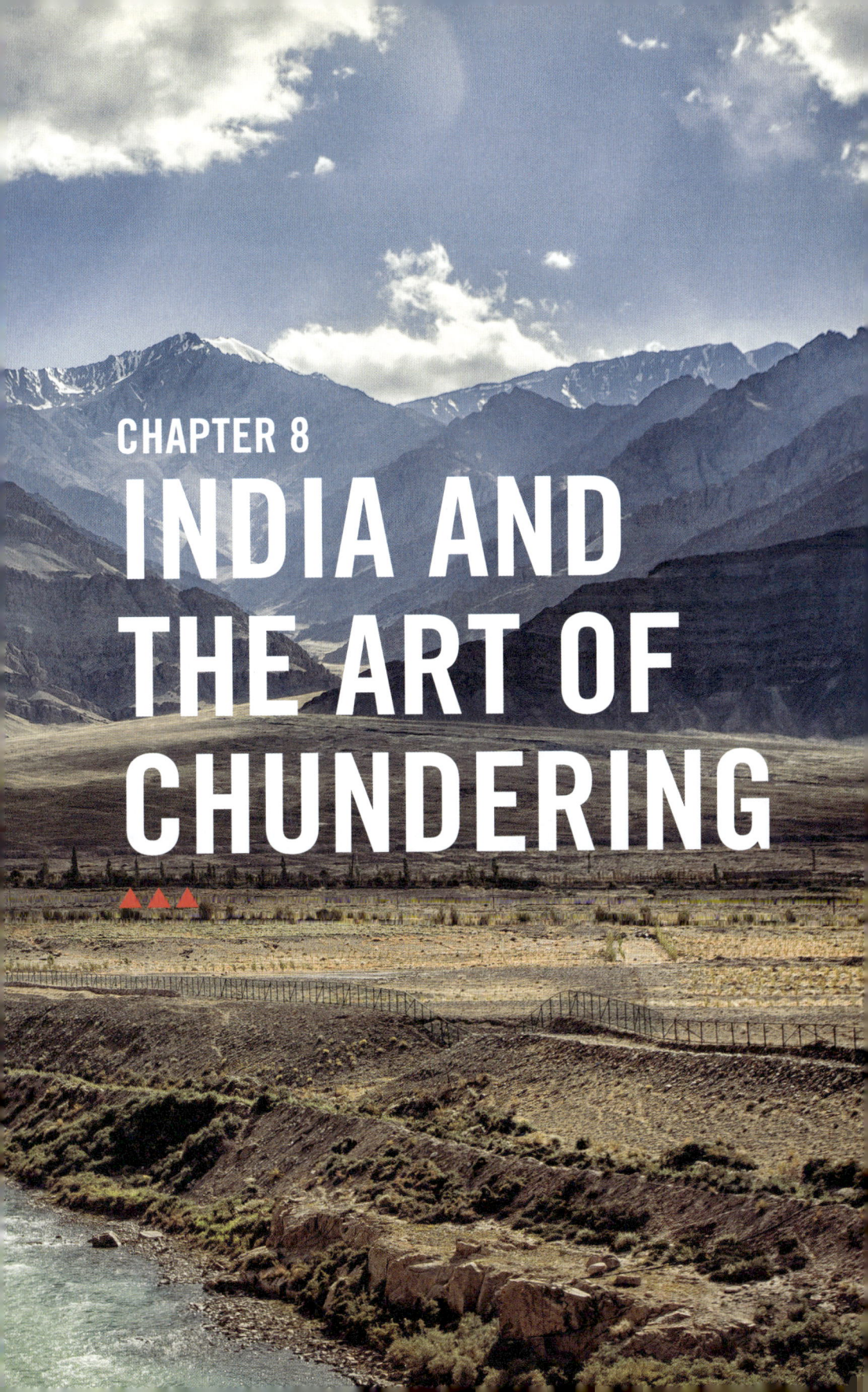

CHAPTER 8

INDIA AND THE ART OF CHUNDERING

September 2015
Ladakh, India

The first sight of the Himalayas on the flight from Delhi to Leh caused quite a stir on the plane. The range was breathtakingly impressive — awesome, in the truest sense. The snaking glaciers, fed by giant snowfields, hung precariously from rugged peaks and seemed to defy both sense and the laws of gravity in their immensity and steepness. The landscape, or, more specifically, the angles and lines of the ridges and peaks, looked unreal, an impossible pile of crustal fragments tossed carelessly on the ground. The view and the sheer enormity of the whites, blues and snow-dusted greys were mesmerising; once your gaze locked on them it was hard to turn away.

As I stared out of the window of the plane I once again wondered what on earth I was getting myself into — the Himalayas were huge, and we had set ourselves no small task. Our goal was to climb Stok Kangri (6153 metres), a non-technical peak a short distance from Leh that offers an introduction to high-altitude mountaineering. Gerwyn wanted to check a 6000-metre peak off his bucket list; I wanted to climb Stok Kangri as preparation for the more difficult climb I was then planning to do in Nepal. After climbing Stok Kangri we planned to make the 1000-kilometre journey back to Delhi by bus and train, doing a bit of trekking along the way, before flying on to Kathmandu.

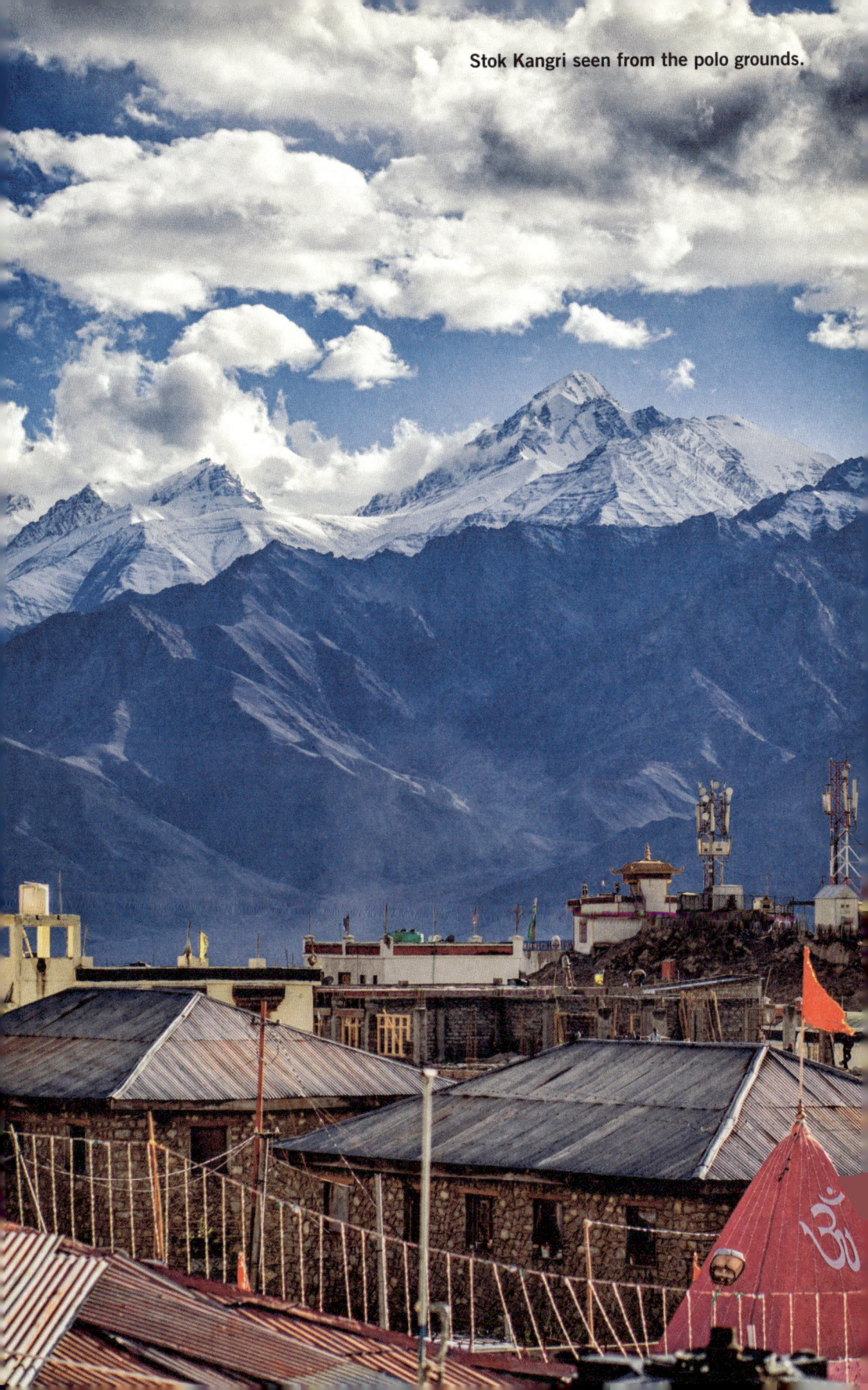
Stok Kangri seen from the polo grounds.

It was going to be a big journey.

Leh is the biggest city in Ladakh, a region in the Indian-administered Jammu and Kashmir, sandwiched between the northern slopes of the Himalayas and the Tibetan Plateau. It is an arid region, the mountains bare, the valleys filled with fanning skirts of scree. The morning we arrived in Leh there was just a smattering of cloud about, creating a beautiful dappling of blue shadows that slowly drifted across the hillsides. It reminded me of Central Otago on a clear autumn day, with dry hills, a stunning blue sky, crisp air and that amazing quality of the light.

Outside the airport terminal the scene was chaotic — people jostling for taxis, the banter of negotiation, the throw and thud of bags lifted for tourists who were struggling with the sudden gain in altitude. Leh sits at 3500 metres above sea level — a big change from Delhi, which is at 200 metres — and you definitely notice it when you arrive; you feel slightly out of breath and dizzy. I felt proud that I had managed to lift and carry my bag without help, a good sign of a positive response to the altitude, I thought.

Next to us was a cluster of Indian Army soldiers, guns slung over their shoulders, on the alert and checking passports and visas. I was surprised at the military presence; there were guards with guns everywhere, it seemed. Perhaps this was understandable; Ladakh borders China and is close to Pakistan, and is a potentially volatile area. The airport also supports a large air-force base, and fighter jets were taking off with a deafening roar in between the commercial flights. Flights in and out of the airport can only take place in the early morning, before the mountain winds rise and make landing dangerous.

Ethnically, the Ladakhi people belong to the same group as the Tibetans, and they have their own language, as we were about to discover. A tiny Maruti Suzuki minivan with dinner-plate wheels pulled up in front of us.

'Shaolin Guest House — can you take us there?' I asked the driver.

I had no idea what he said in response — I assumed he was speaking in Ladakhi — but he looked confused.

'Sha-o-lin Guest House?' I repeated.

The driver pulled out a map and pointed at it blankly, muttering, inviting me to tell him where to go, I assumed.

I shrugged my shoulders in a purposely exaggerated gesture. I had no idea whatsoever where Shaolin Guest House was.

'Um, Shou-lin Guest House?'

'Ooh! Shao-lin,' he replied, adding a bunch of other stuff that I didn't understand. He picked up the government-issued charter of taxi fares, looked at the map again, figuring out the distance, and pointed to the relevant fare: 600 rupees.

'Nah, mate,' Gerwyn said. 'Too expensive. Four hundred rupees.'

The taxi driver shook his head.

'Nah, mate,' Gerwyn repeated, slightly peevishly. 'Sorry — too much.' He turned to me. 'C'mon, Nick, he's too expensive, let's find someone else.' He began walking away.

I was not entirely sure what to do; I'd spoken to a couple of other drivers earlier and knew they were charging more.

'Ah!' The driver shouted, waving at us. He held up a hand, signalling 'five' with his fingers.

'Hey, Gee! He's saying five hundred rupees,' I shouted. Gerwyn paused for a moment and looked at me. 'That's a really good price. The others are charging seven hundred,' I said.

'Are they?' Gerwyn turned round and faced the driver again. 'What about four fifty?'

The driver shook his head and held up five fingers again.

'Gee, let's just go with it. Five hundred is a good price. It's not worth the hassle — we're talking about a dollar's difference.'

We had woken up at 4 a.m. in order to catch our 6.30 flight, and we hadn't slept well the night before. We were both a bit tired and irritable.

'OK. Let's get on with it, then.'

I gave the driver a nod.

'You're ripping us off, mate,' Gerwyn grumped as the driver picked up our bags and threw them on the roof — there was not enough room inside the tiny van for the two of us and our bags.

I was a bit nervous as we bumped along the empty streets. I was not entirely convinced that I had managed to accurately convey our destination — the language barrier made it difficult to tell. Maybe there was more than one Shaolin Guest House. This sense of uncertainty was not helped by the fact that Leh appeared to be deserted. It was about 8.30 and the streets were empty. It was only later that I found out that the shops don't open until 10 a.m.

I was also very conscious of the fact that our bags were held in place only by the tiny edges of the roof rack. I couldn't help but wonder if a bag might bounce off given the rough, potholed road.

We passed through the town, up the main drag, and out into the countryside. That's when I really began to worry. Had I told him the right place?

Despite my anxiety it was a lovely drive as we wound up the poplar-lined roads, beside stone walls and fields. We finally came to a stop and were enveloped by a thick cloud of dust, which we let pass before opening the door. Beside us was the iron gate of a beautiful house in the traditional Ladakhi style, intricately designed, and surrounded by a well-maintained garden filled with colourful flowers and vegetables.

I climbed out of the van and stood for a moment, taking in a deep breath. The air was cool and clean. There was silence, apart from the swishing of wind in the poplar trees and the burble of a small, clear stream that ran beside the house. It was so different from Delhi, where we had spent the last couple of days. The city had been incredibly hot, the air smoggy and foul, and there was the continual bombardment of noise and people thronging around you. This was magnificent, lovely, a place of rest.

We knocked on the door and were greeted by Sonam, who turned out to own not only the guest house but also the only ice-cream factory in the whole of Ladakh.

'Welcome!' he said, with a friendly smile and a warm handshake. 'Come in. Let the boy carry your bags.'

A young man appeared and took our packs while we followed Sonam to our room.

'Wow — great room!'

'Yes please, thank you. This is a good room,' Sonam replied.

'It's so bright with those big windows. And the view! Is that the Stok Range, across the valley?'

'Yes please, it is.'

'We are hoping to climb Stok Kangri,' I said, gesturing towards Gerwyn. 'Are we able to see Stok Kangri from here?'

'Yes please, you can,' Sonam replied, walking to the big bay window. 'See the big poplar tree — it is the tallest peak just to the right of it.'

I was not sure what was up with the 'Yes please' response, but it was strangely endearing.

'Wow,' I said, my stomach suddenly churning with nervous excitement. 'It looks pretty intense.'

The cloud had only just lifted off the range and it was covered in a thick dusting of snow, accentuating the sharp ridges, hanging snowfields and steep gullies. It looked hard — much harder than I had imagined.

'You'll be fine. It will be bit cold these times of the year. But you will be fine. You are strong,' Sonam said, laughing.

After we'd unpacked, Gerwyn and I decided to walk into town, ambling along at a deliberately slow pace in the hope of avoiding altitude sickness. Before long we came to the first strand of shops, which were just beginning to open. I popped into a rug shop to have a look, and was surprised at the massive variety of rugs, carpets and tapestries on offer.

'As-salamu alaykum,' the owner greeted me, bowing slightly, his right hand raised to his chest. He was a clean-shaven Kashmiri gentleman with slicked-back black hair. 'How can I help you today?'

'Hi,' I said. 'I am just looking at rugs, to get an idea of prices.'

'Certainly,' he said with a friendly smile, gesturing at the couch. 'Please have a seat. Today, are you buying for you or is this a gift for someone else?'

I was surprised at his excellent English. 'It's for me — I am thinking about getting a rug as a souvenir of my trip.'

'That is a very fine idea! Now let me show you what I have on offer.'

The rugs he pulled out were absolutely magnificent, and it was fascinating learning about the different varieties of rugs and tapestries. It was an incredibly sensory experience, with the beautifully musky smell of sandalwood burning in the corner of the room combining with the smells of the dyes and wools. Then there were the vivid golds, scarlets and blues of the tapestries on the walls, the soft touch of the wool-silk carpets that changed colour as you viewed them from different angles, and the pleasantly coarse feel of the woven carpets. The only problem was, they were also very expensive.

'It's an investment you'll never regret,' the owner assured me, as I eyed a particularly attractive rug. 'And you had better purchase it now, because this is very popular design and there is no other rug like this in the whole world. It will sell very fast. And we have credit card facilities,' he said for about the third time.

Just then Gerwyn walked in the door. 'Nick, mate, we need to go.' He sounded impatient.

I thanked the shop owner and shook his hand. 'I'll have a think about it and maybe pop back in a few days,' I told him.

'Khuda hafiz,' he replied as we walked out.

'Thanks for that, Gee,' I said. 'That was perfect timing — I was just starting to feel the pressure there! How are you feeling?'

'Like shit, I am. All short of breath and dizzy, like — it's the altitude, it is. I need to sit down.'

We walked across the road to a German bakery and sat there for a while.

Unlike Gerwyn, I was feeling great, albeit slightly tired and hungry because of our early-morning start. I was encouraged by my body's response to altitude and felt pleased that the months spent on altitude training in New Zealand had not been wasted. While Gerwyn felt increasingly ill and wanted to get back to the guest house to lie down, I was feeling increasingly hungry, ready to get some food. The German bakery also sold regular meals, and since it was approaching lunchtime I ordered a chicken masala curry to take away.

My mouth had been watering from the smells coming from the

open kitchen. I was looking forward to an authentic Indian meal. So I was slightly surprised when they delivered my chicken curry to me in an empty potato-chip packet, the salt and oil still stuck to the silvery inside of the bag. Up-cycled chip packets — what a resourceful idea, I thought.

We caught a taxi back to the guest house, me carefully nursing my curry to make sure it didn't spill. I devoured it as soon as I was back in our room, and I was not disappointed. It was exceptional, even if it was eaten out of a used chip packet, and I felt totally satisfied. Gerwyn also improved over the course of the afternoon, and we took an early night.

Around midnight I woke up under a wave of nausea, my stomach uncomfortable, gurgling noisily. I felt sick, which was strange, I thought. I sat for a moment on the edge of the bed, trying to process what was happening with my groggy mind. The nausea seemed to be easing slowly so I lay back down again, only to be hit by another wave. Once again I sat bolt upright in bed. Then I felt it at the back of my throat, the warning that my lunch was about to come up. I leapt out of bed and ran for the bathroom, making it just in time and planting my face in the toilet bowl. So much for enjoying the chicken curry, I thought, as curry and bile burned their way back up my throat and through my nasal passages. Then I thought, thank God this is a clean toilet bowl. It was going to be a long night.

I sat resting in the morning sunlight as it streamed through the bay window of our room. 'To be honest,' Gerwyn was saying, 'I don't really like it here in Leh, and unless we can climb Stok Kangri in the next day or two I don't really want to stick around.'

'Fair enough — and, hey, you didn't fly all the way over here to sit around doing nothing.'

'Yeah. You know what I mean?'

'Of course,' I replied. 'But I feel like this food poisoning has really knocked me — I feel totally smashed, which makes me really worried.'

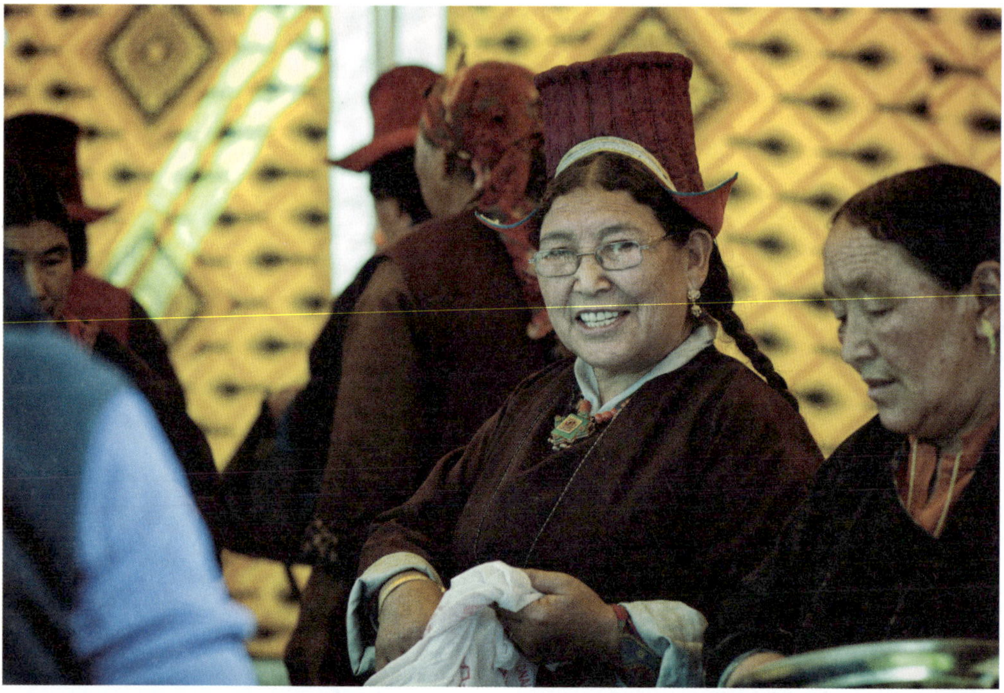

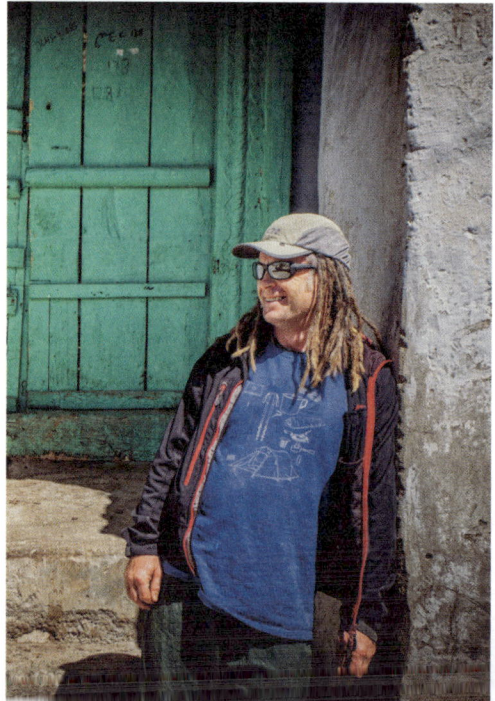
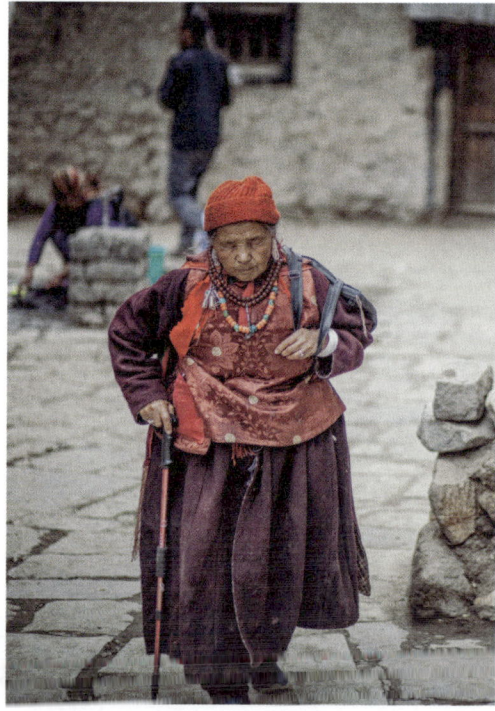

Clockwise from top: A woman in traditional Ladakhi dress serves food at a small fair celebrating Ladakhi culture; A woman walking through the back streets of old Leh; Gerwyn taking a break on our way into town, trying to acclimatise.

The last time I got food poisoning it had triggered a minor relapse of the MS and knocked me out for a couple of months. I explained this to Gerwyn, and my anxiety about the situation and about potentially being unable to climb in Nepal.

'I mean, climbing there is my number one goal, so I really feel I need to be careful not to mess things up by pushing it too hard. That's why I'm keen to continue resting, and why I'm worried about travelling back to Delhi by bus — I find travelling really draining.'

'Fair enough.' Gerwyn nodded.

'The best thing for me, I reckon, will be to stay here and rest. And I love it up here in Leh. I also see it as a strategic place in terms of acclimatising for Nepal. But why don't you climb Stok Kangri by yourself?'

'Yeah, but the only reason I wanted to do Stok Kangri was to say, like, that I have been above 6000 metres. You know, bragging rights,' Gerwyn said, laughing. 'Otherwise, I'm not really that keen. You know, I'm more of a trekker than a climber. I just can't wait to get down to the Hampta Pass and Himachal Pradesh and do some trekkin'. For me, that's the main goal of the trip — from the pictures I've seen and stuff, it looks amazing down there, it does.'

'Makes sense, Gee.'

'See, and I'm getting really restless with all this sitting around — it's bad for my energy and I start getting irritable and stuff,' he said, scratching his head. 'Are you OK if we split up and I go south? I just can't hang around any longer, mate. What, and will you fly down to Delhi, like? We could meet up there.'

'Yeah, I was thinking that I could book a flight back down at the end of the month.'

'OK, too easy. Let's do that then. I'll catch the bus south to Manali tonight,' Gerwyn said. 'And what do you think you will do in the meantime?'

'I think I'll definitely rest for a few days, to build up strength again, and then aim to climb in a couple of weeks' time, at the end of the month — if I'm up to it. In the meantime, I'll definitely catch a taxi up to the top of Khardung La, to begin the acclimatisation process. If

I'm feeling OK, I may hire a motorbike and travel to Pangong Lake or something.'

'Too easy. I hope it all works out, mate,' Gerwyn responded, smiling. We were both relieved to have come to a decision. 'And now I had better get packing,' he said.

▲▲▲

I enjoyed a few days of slowly wandering around Leh as I tried to rebuild my strength. I particularly liked the genuine antique shops: little caves filled with artefacts that gave a glimpse into the past. I tried to imagine the unspoken history behind the dusty tools, wooden bowls, worn horse tack and used butter churns. There was something special about picking up an 80-year-old butter churn, for example, and examining it under the orange glow of the single, naked incandescent bulb.

The shops were often long and narrow, any outside light that could have illuminated them blocked by all the merchandise stacked on the shelves in the small front windows. I'd strain to see in any sort of detail the years of fat solids caked on the inside of a wooden churn, the handle worn smooth through use. I would run my fingers over the dings and cracks, imagining how they might have been created, by whom and when — the churns told a story that I could not decipher.

I loved the smell of the shops as well, the musty scent of antiques mixed with the smell of old horse rugs, caught up with the smoky perfume from the incense. Some of the oldest shops had exceptionally low studs; the ancient door frames and hand-hewn rafters posed head-hazards as I traversed the creaking floorboards.

Above the city, on a rugged granite ridge, the royal palace dominated the skyline — a huge structure, modelled on the Potala Palace in Lhasa, Tibet, that soared nine storeys above the town. It was built in the seventeenth century, and the skill and manpower that must have been involved was staggering to consider; millions of bricks were cast or individually hand-hewn from granite, carried

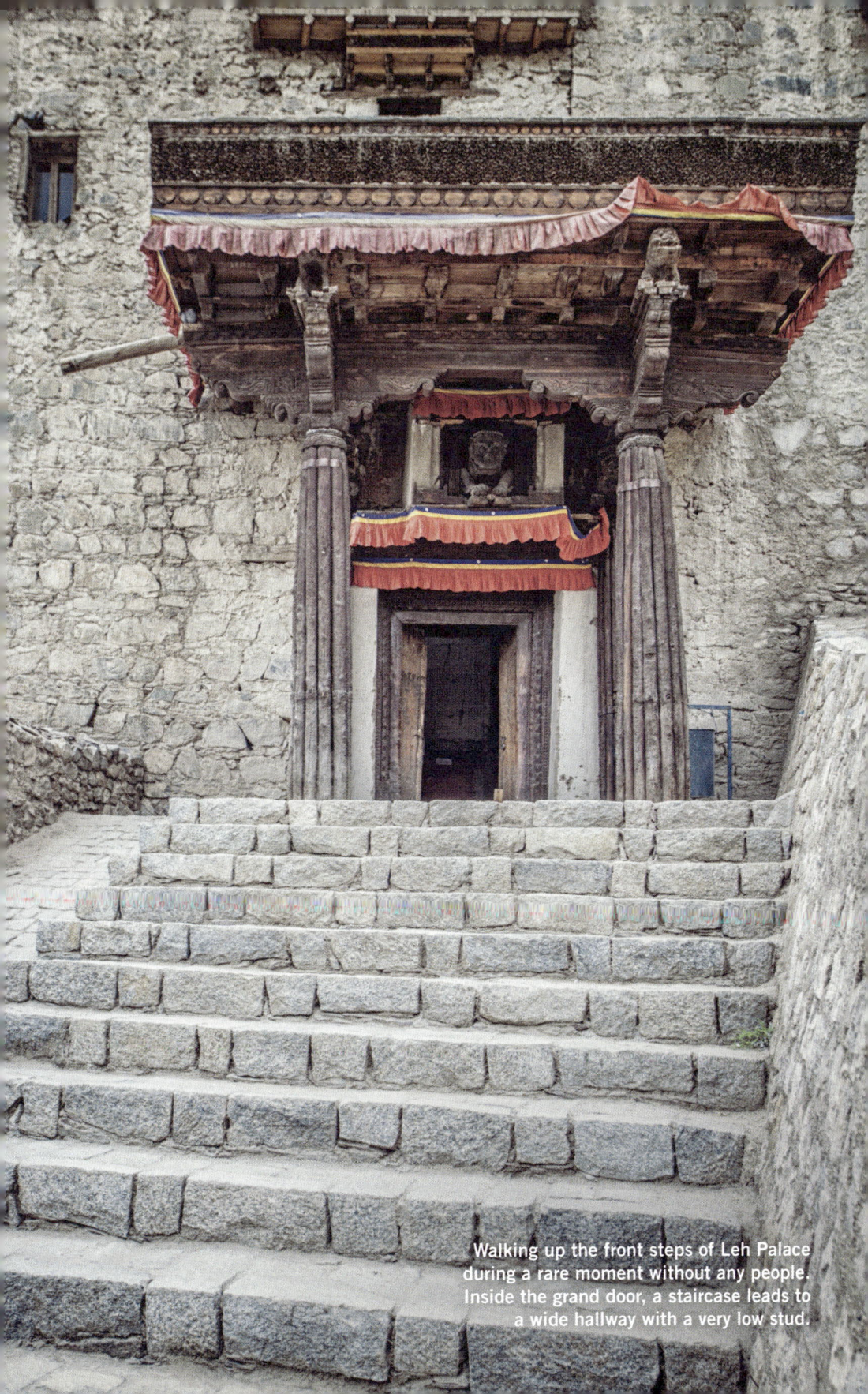

Walking up the front steps of Leh Palace during a rare moment without any people. Inside the grand door, a staircase leads to a wide hallway with a very low stud.

up the cliffs and laid with precision, and all without modern machinery.

The lower levels of the palace went deep into the darkness of the hillside, accessible through tiny doors, and filled with dirt and debris. The upper levels were suffused with a sorrowful beauty. The remains of magnificent frescoes could be seen on the plaster that had not crumbled; the ornate capitals crowning the pillars in the rooms bore the marks of past glory in their now faded greens and pinks; the massive walls, once proud and strong, had been crumbling ever since the royal family was exiled in 1830. They had been displaced to the town of Stok, where their descendants still live today.

There was an amazing view from the roof of the palace, over the whole of Leh and across the Indus Valley. Leh is not a big city, supporting roughly 30,000 people, and from the palace you could see how it was nestled in the valley, backed into the mountain walls. Directly below the palace was the old city, with its maze of narrow alleyways and crumbling mud-brick buildings. The scene gave off a sense of exhaustion and struggle — signs of the battle generations had fought to survive in such a barren land.

The Stok Range loomed above the city, across the Indus River. I'd look at Stok Kangri every morning as I walked the kilometre along the dusty backstreet into town. I'd go in early, before things got too busy, when the quiet was disturbed only by the distant bark of a dog or an occasional motorbike idling past. As I glimpsed the mountain rising above the minarets and green dome of the mosque, framed by the mud-plastered walls and poplar trees, I felt a momentary thrill, a strong sense of serenity, and occasionally a slight feeling of terror.

Down past the mosque and the fruit-sellers sitting on the shaded corner of Fort Road was Leh's Main Bazaar. Here, the Stok Range could be seen between the crudely built multistorey buildings, through the chaotic tangle of fluttering prayer flags and the cross-hatching of the power lines.

Stok Kangri was the pinnacle of the range, and the view of it from the mosque was my favourite. From there you got a sense of the mountain's scale, as your eyes were drawn up along the slender minarets and on to the sharp ridges that feed into the ice-capped peaks 3000 metres above the floor of the Indus Valley.

But the view was also intimidating — almost terrifying — if I thought about it too much. The dark, sharp ridges seemed formidable barriers to the would-be climber.

The range consists of sedimentary rock, expressed in thousands of layers, once horizontal but now vertical or near-vertical. The harder layers of rock have been thrust upward to create gilled multicoloured ridges, their sharpness accentuated by the softer, more easily eroded layers of shale. Impossible to traverse, in ancient times the ridges functioned as natural palisades, protecting the Stok heartland from invaders. Ancient rulers used the rock formations to create unassailable forts from which to fight the invading Mughal war parties. Now the sad beauty of those crumbling forts, and the ruined farms that once supported them, speaks of the inhospitality of the place.

The ice-capped peaks above the crumbling forts sit around or above 6000 metres. Operating at these altitudes, a climber has less than 50 per cent of the oxygen enjoyed at sea level, which means you have a lot less energy and a decreased ability to stay warm. This was a worry, given that I was already wearing a jersey in town during the day. Mentally I was prepared for the fatigue, but I was concerned about the cold, particularly as the climbing season was drawing to a close and it was getting colder every day. Generally, the climbing season ends either when the streams freeze on the mountain, causing the loss of the water supply, or with the celebration of Bakr Id, the Muslim festival that commemorates the patriarch Abraham's willingness to sacrifice his son. In fact, the whole town of Leh closes down for the four days of Bakr Id and doesn't reopen until the spring of the following year.

Adding to my concern was the fact that I'd picked up a lot of talk about climbers unprepared for the extreme cold having to turn back, frostbitten. As I set about finding a guide to take me up Stok Kangri, I was determined to do my homework and find a good one

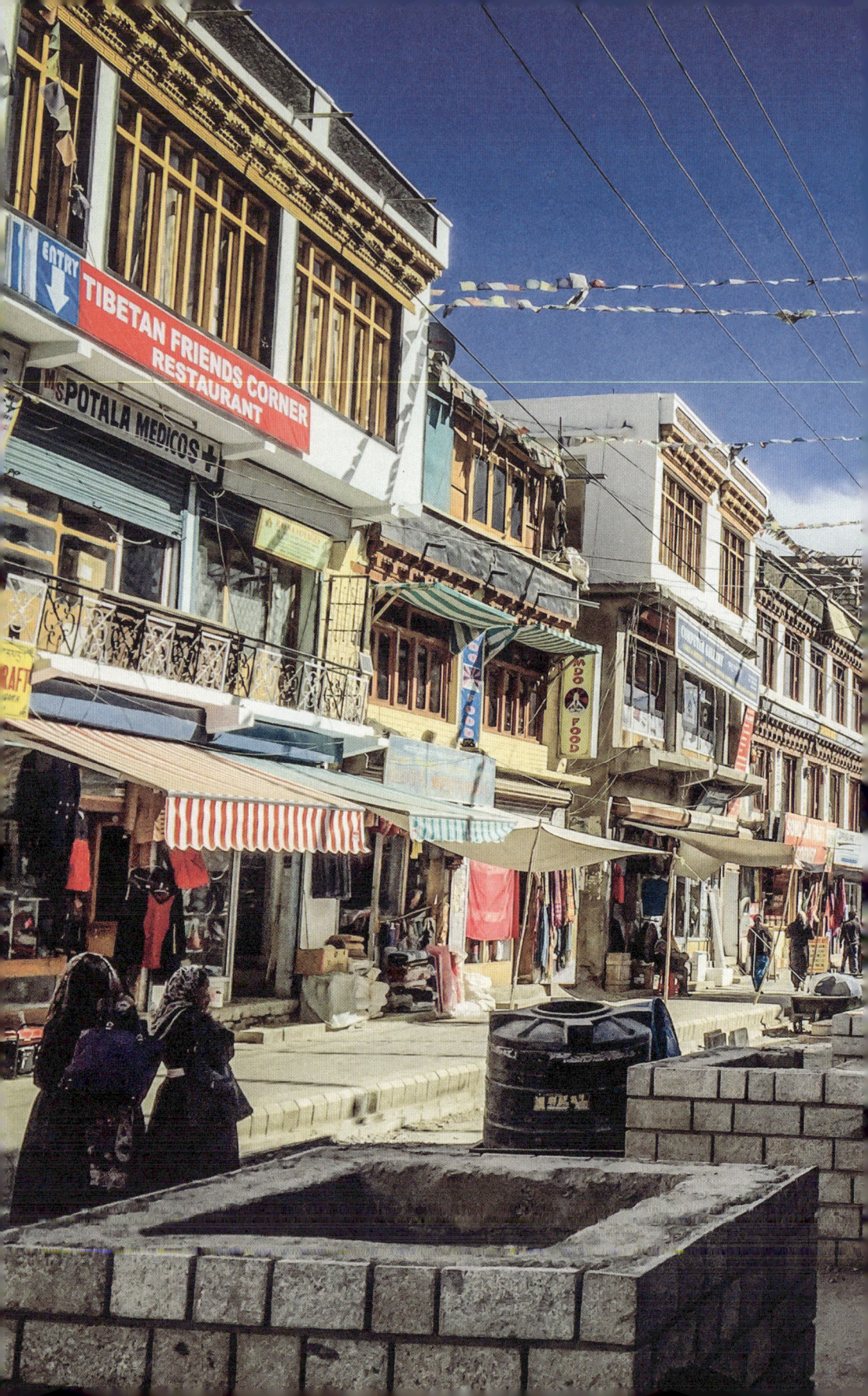

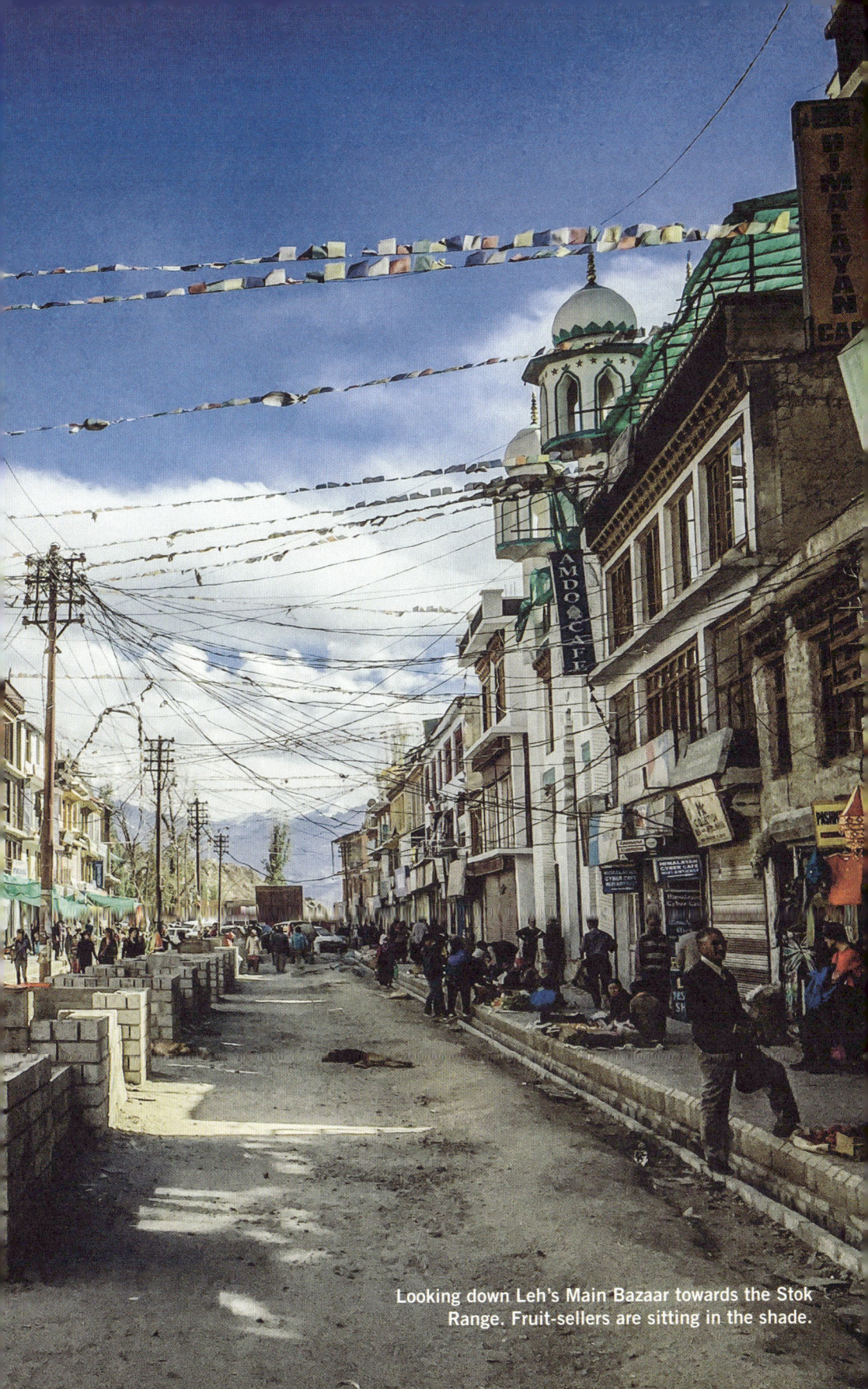

Looking down Leh's Main Bazaar towards the Stok Range. Fruit-sellers are sitting in the shade.

— someone I could really trust. I'd already spoken to a number of guides and guiding agents, which is where I'd first heard about the struggling tourists and their frostbitten toes. Some even spoke about two climbers who, earlier in the season, had died on the mountain because of the weather. Then there was the German guy I sat next to in a restaurant one day, who told me about the cold, about how it was −20°C when he left Base Camp, not including wind chill. The summit was bitterly cold.

Stok Kangri was a daunting prospect: thrilling but terrifying. Almost as horrifying as your guide pulling out and going home the night before you set off to begin climbing the mountain.

'Gidday, Jigmet!' I said as I walked through the sliding door into his office.

'Hello, Nick. How are you this morning?'

'I'm very well, thanks. Although maybe a little bit worried about the weather front that's on its way. I think tomorrow is definitely going to be the day to begin the climb, before the weather comes in. It looks like Sunday evening and Monday will bring a dumping of snow. Hopefully summiting on Sunday morning won't be cutting it too fine.'

Jigmet was a young guy and owned his own guiding company, Mountain Express Adventure. He had impressed me from the very beginning. We had spent a lot of time talking about climbing and mountaineering, of peaks we had climbed, and favourite adventures. We got on well and I could tell he knew what he was doing, was competent and trustworthy.

'Anyway,' I continued, 'I was on my way into town for lunch and thought I would pop in to talk about tomorrow. What time shall I be here to meet the guide?'

'Um, what do you mean?' Jigmet shifted uncomfortably in his seat.

I was confused by his question.

'You know, when I came in yesterday, we talked about a guide for tomorrow? Because tomorrow looks like the day to begin the climb up Stok Kangri. Any later and we're going to get caught in the snowstorm.'

'Oh. Yes. Well, unfortunately, the guide decided to go back to his home this morning. I only just found out.'

'Oh?' I said.

'It is getting too cold, and he wanted to get home before the mountain roads become closed by snow. He is from a very remote part of northern India, from the Zanskar Range, and after this snow the roads will be closed for the rest of the winter,' Jigmet said apologetically.

'I see,' I replied, looking at the ground. This was a very awkward situation to find myself in, particularly when the weather was forecast to deteriorate, signalling the official end to the season.

'So there's no one you know of who can guide me up Stok Kangri tomorrow?'

'No, all the guides are gone. I am very sorry. But perhaps you can find another guide through a different company?'

News of the guide's need to get home was a total surprise, and I was slightly shocked. My mind started racing as I faced the thought that I might miss my opportunity to climb.

'OK, all cool. Well, I'd better get cracking then!' I said, standing up. 'Hey, but I'll pop in after the trip and let you know how it went.'

I shook Jigmet's hand and headed back out to try to find a guide.

Travel agents, who sometimes offer guiding services, and the more specialised guiding companies were scattered around the centre of town. I rushed around as many of these as I could, trying to find someone who would take me up the mountain. Most of the companies did not think it was feasible to find a guide overnight, particularly as many of them had left for the season.

Only three of the companies said that they could provide a guide for the next day. Two of these did not inspire much confidence. The first, on Zangsti Road, across the street from the back door of the German bakery, had a pair of white climbing boots displayed in the window, which drew me in. The guy behind the desk — young, with

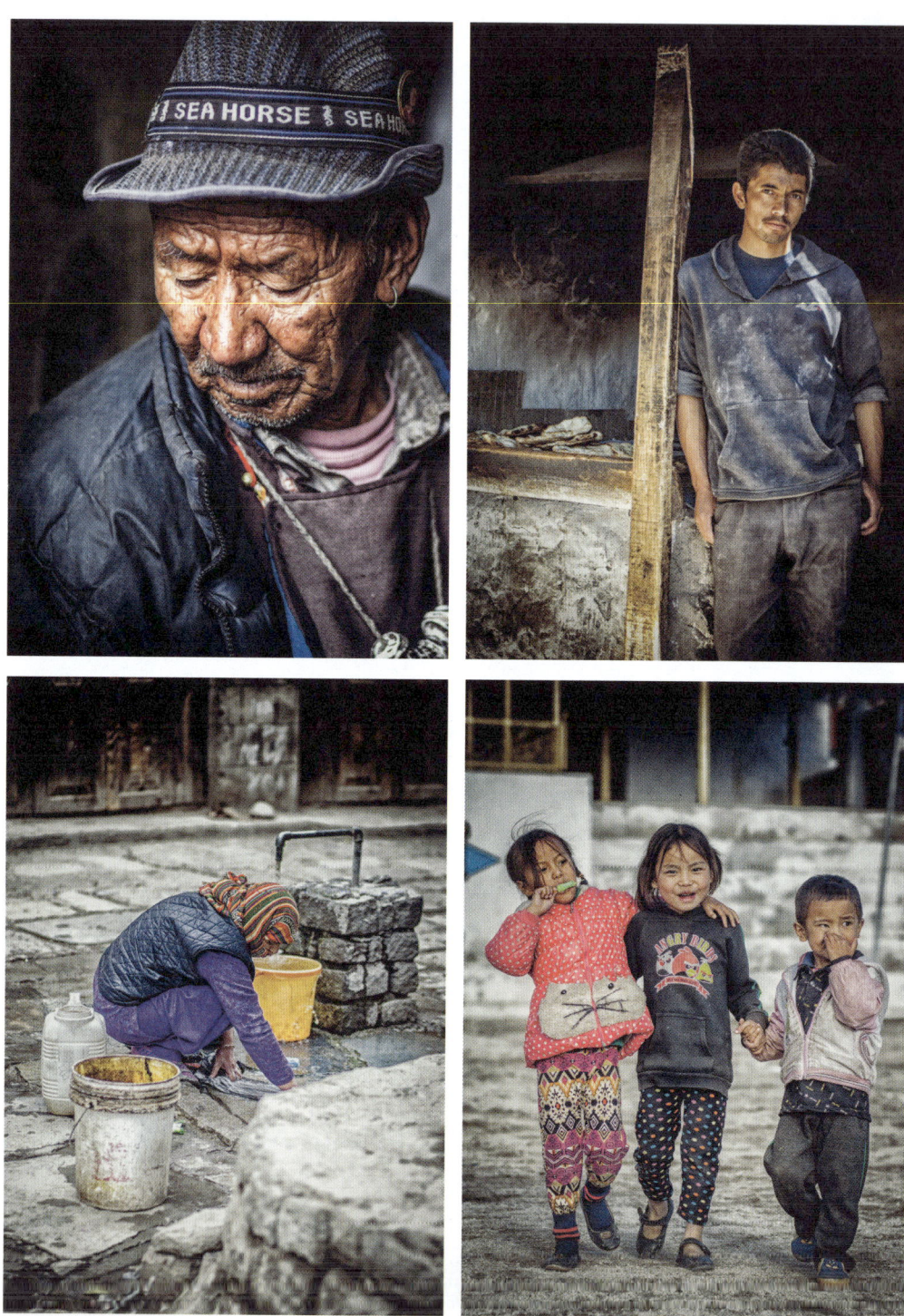

Clockwise from top left: A jeweller preparing to cast a ring; A baker in the Muslim quarter; Kids wandering the polo grounds; A woman cleaning clothes in Old Leh.

slicked-back hair and a big bling watch — assured me that he could get an experienced guide for me. But then he said that the guide would have his own 'pick thing and boot spikes'. I excused myself and walked out.

There was another company across the small stream, on the corner of Library and Fort Road. This one seemed legit; the office was filled with modern mountaineering equipment. I started talking to the guy behind the desk, who although young had a face that had been exposed to the elements. He was also wearing a mountain fleece with white chalk on it, suggesting that he was a rock climber. I felt confident that he knew what he was talking about, but I also got the feeling that he could not wait to get home, that he did not really want to be there. He told me that he would try to find someone, but I was not convinced that he would try very hard. I had visions of turning up at 8 a.m. only to find that he hadn't been able to get a guide, totally blowing my chances of reaching the summit before the storm came in. But then, it's India, I thought, and perhaps I should have a different, less Eurocentric expectation of professionalism. He would probably be fine.

Then there was Karma, an older gentleman who owned a company just down the street from Jigmet, in the small courtyard area on Upper Tukcha Road, just before the road starts weaving its way down the hill to the river. Karma was a strongly built man with a soft, jovial face, who seemed pleased to see me when I walked in, ready to take the time to talk.

The shop's small window was obscured by a large sign, and by a collection of antique gear, making it difficult to see inside. The office, a single room, was very small, dark, dirty and overflowing with loosely organised piles of ropes, crampons, heavy steel ice axes, army-surplus plastic mountaineering boots, helmets, cookers, tents, sleeping rolls and deflated rafts. The ceiling and upper walls were covered in soot from the kerosene lamps used during the frequent power outages.

Everything seemed old, well-worn and slightly neglected. Nevertheless, the gear was obviously tired because of use, and recent use too — the points on the steel crampons were shiny, not rusted — which reassured me that Karma had been out there, and knew what he was talking about.

'Tomorrow I will have a guide for you, I promise,' he said reassuringly. 'And he will be a good guide — many of the best guides have gone home, but I will find you a good guide. Just make sure you are here by eight o'clock in the morning. Then we will leave for the mountain.'

'OK, great,' I said, somewhat relieved — I still had to get home and pack, and I was feeling tired from all my running about, which worried me.

'Ah! On time! You must not be Ladakhi!' Karma laughed the next morning as he got up from behind his cluttered desk, putting down a screwdriver and a broken cooker to shake my hand. Stepping over the plastic boots on the floor, he placed his hand on my shoulder and led me outside.

'I like people who are on time — means it will be a good trip. It's good luck, you know.' Karma laughed again, and gave me a heavy pat on the back. 'Yes, good. Come, take a seat while we wait for Tashi, your guide.'

He gestured to the table and chairs in the courtyard, which was beginning to catch the morning sun. The eclectic collection of chairs was already crowded with people: guides, travel agents, bicycle-tour operators and proprietors, all wrapped in down jackets and drinking tea as they waited for either the sun or clients — whichever came first.

Karma turned and shouted, 'Tea! Padma! Bring us some tea!'

A young woman stuck her head through the door of the nearby tea stall and waved to acknowledge his request.

'How far away is Tashi, do you think?' I was anxious to get going.

'Hmm, five or ten minutes? But who knows — he is Ladakhi!' Karma laughed and slapped the table. Some of the other men at the table cracked a smile, as if bearers of some secret knowledge. I didn't want to be left out, so I smiled as well.

Now, seated and comfortable, Karma began an animated conversation in Ladakhi with some of the other men. Time passed slowly and I became occupied with my own thoughts. All my running around trying to find a guide, had left me exhausted. My body already felt tired, and it was only eight o'clock, I thought pessimistically. How can I cope with climbing up the mountain if I am already tired? How will I ever be able to make it to the top?

I began to feel nervous, particularly as I felt so much was riding on my ability to climb. Six months earlier, I had set up the Mastering Mountains Charitable Trust for the purpose of raising money to help people with MS get into the outdoors. The response had been incredibly exciting, with sponsors like Macpac, MitoQ and Petzl coming on board, and with interest in my trip from the media and organisations like Multiple Sclerosis New Zealand. Then there were all those people with MS or other disabilities who had read about me, talked to me or sent me emails, excited about Mastering Mountains, my trip and the hope they held out.

However, the involvement of all these entities meant that my successes — and failures — were going to be very public, out in the open for everyone to see in the blogs and vlogs that I posted. And that was frightening. It was hard enough to face my own failings and the impact of MS on my life, let alone have it all out there for the world to see. Not to summit would be totally humiliating.

I will summit, I told myself. I found myself clenching my jaw, angry at the disease. No way will I let it get the best of me, I said to myself, no way will I let it stop me. I simply will not allow myself to fail. I will prove that I am able.

'Ah! Here is your tea!' Karma said suddenly, startling me. Lost in my thoughts, I hadn't noticed Padma standing beside me with a teacup held out.

'Oh, sorry!' I said as she handed me a cup of milky chai tea. I smiled politely. I had forgotten to ask for black tea; I hate milky tea.

'You are very welcome,' Karma said, sitting forward in his seat with a warm yet expectant 'OK now drink it' smile. I took a small draught.

'Ah, that's good tea. Thank you,' I said. I'm sure it would have been good tea, had it been black, and I was grateful for the warmth of the cup in my hands. It was a cold morning.

Karma sat back in his seat and gave a satisfied smile to the other men at the table, seemingly proud of his happy client.

'Tashi shouldn't be far away now,' he said. He paused, then added, 'We were just discussing the rescue of a climber up on Stok Kangri. He slipped and fell 400 metres. He was very badly injured. Very sad.'

'But he survived the fall?'

'Yes, he did. But he was climbing without a guide. People think Stok Kangri is easy and they are not prepared. It is very bad, very dangerous. That is why you need a good guide — a guide like Tashi. People who go without guides take too many risks. Ah! And here is Tashi now!'

I turned and saw a flustered young man, a car pulling away behind him. He gave the impression either that he had just woken up or that he was in a bad mood — it was hard to tell which, but neither option inspired me with confidence. I must stop evaluating the situation according to Western expectations of professionalism, I reminded myself. Tashi joined us at the table in the sun, dumping his small pack on the ground and, pulling out a New York Yankees cap from under his arm, placing it over his messy hair.

'Nick, this is your guide Tashi. Tashi, this is Nick,' said Karma.

I reached out my hand. 'How's it going?'

'Good,' Tashi replied, somewhat apathetically. He gave a single, limp shake of my hand before sitting down abruptly. He picked some gunk out of his eyes, wiping it on his trackpants. Karma tapped him on the knee, said something, and pointed to the tea stall. Tashi stood up and hopped over, returning with a mugful of chai held close in a two-handed clutch.

Karma continued talking to his Ladakhi friends and Tashi sat silently, staring blankly into the shadows across the road.

'Should be a good day for the climb,' I said, trying to engage him in conversation.

Tashi looked up from his tea and gave a single nod. He pulled the hood of his jacket over his head, retreating into its shadows, shutting down the possibility of conversation. Karma had assured me that Tashi was fully qualified, had completed an Advanced Mountaineering Course and achieved full accreditation as a guide, but his lack of professionalism was making me uncomfortable.

Looking at Tashi, Karma and the other guides sitting around, there seemed to be a worrying absence of that sharp and authoritative engagement I had enjoyed in New Zealand and European guides. Just two months earlier I had been climbing with my good friend Nina in the Remarkables, near Queenstown. Nina, who is both an experienced climber and a doctor in Wellington, had invited me to join her on the climb as part of my preparation for the Himalayas. Together we'd hired a French climbing guide to give us a weekend of instruction. Thomas was highly experienced, and had lots of energy and an engaging decisiveness that inspired trust. The three of us climbed the classic route called Friday's Fool, a 200-metre climb on rock and ice, and took a fun route up the north-eastern ridge to the summit of Single Cone.

Friday's Fool was the first time that I had attempted a proper ice route, and although I was a bit nervous I was sure that, in Thomas's capable hands, everything would be OK. He led the route with ease, confidence and authority; Nina and I followed behind.

I love climbing with Nina, another person who is filled with grace, someone with whom I can be vulnerable and honest. In fact, Nina was the first climber or tramper to whom I had ever admitted the presence of MS. Climbing with a gracious person leads to enjoyable, restful exertion. I push myself not to prove anything, but only for the simple pleasure of climbing. This is the best, most satisfying type of climbing.

Tashi seemed slightly more lively after a second round of tea. This was a good sign, I thought. Karma stood up, announcing our departure.

'OK, you can carry your gear over to the car,' he said to me, pointing to the other side of the road. Tashi stood up quickly,

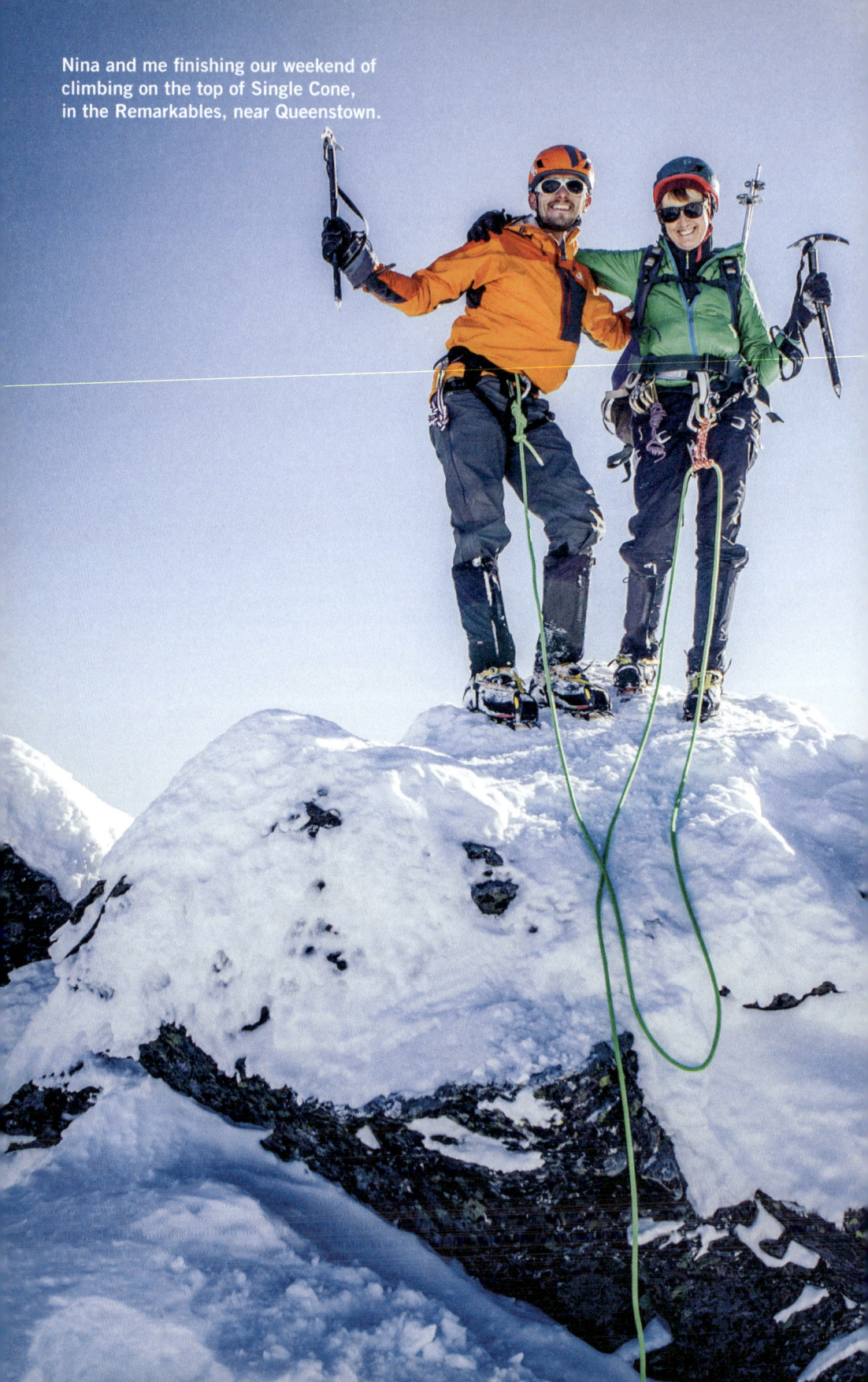

Nina and me finishing our weekend of climbing on the top of Single Cone, in the Remarkables, near Queenstown.

tapped Karma on the shoulder and whispered something. Karma was clearly taken aback, and his brow furrowed. I wondered what was wrong. The two of them went into Karma's office, emerging a few minutes later with an ice axe, a short length of well-worn rope, a sleeping bag and a pair of old blue leather mittens. Karma was clearly giving Tashi a bit of a telling-off. I wondered whether Tashi had forgotten his own gear.

Realising I was watching, Karma smiled. 'Ah!' he said. 'OK! Are you ready?' He rubbed his hands together enthusiastically.

'Which car is yours?' I asked. There were several parked across the road.

'Oh! The little grey one, the Tata Nano.'

I followed him across the road, carrying my 16-kilogram, 65-litre pack.

I was slightly miffed that Tashi was carrying only a small 30-litre pack, his sleeping bag tied haphazardly to the outside. I knew that I shouldn't judge a person by their gear, and that you can make incorrect assumptions about a person's climbing experience based on their appearance, however, it was hard not to wonder how much experience Tashi actually had — his casual cotton-based streetwear and lack of mountaineering equipment did not fill me with confidence. But I piled my stuff and myself into the compact car nevertheless, and kept telling myself that everything would be fine, and that I should stop being so Eurocentric in my expectations.

It took Karma several attempts to start the car — the key turned but nothing happened. He shifted in his seat, lowering his right shoulder and moving in closer to the key, allowing, it seemed, more subtle control. His tongue wiggled between his teeth, mirroring his efforts as he jimmied the key. I had a sinking feeling. I began to contemplate a morning of further delays. We were already more than 45 minutes behind schedule.

It was a relief when the car finally burst into life. Karma laughed, also relieved, I think, and patted the steering wheel affectionately. We pulled out into the chaos of Old Fort Road — the main drag through town — and the 600-cc engine struggled, the cadence of the sewing-

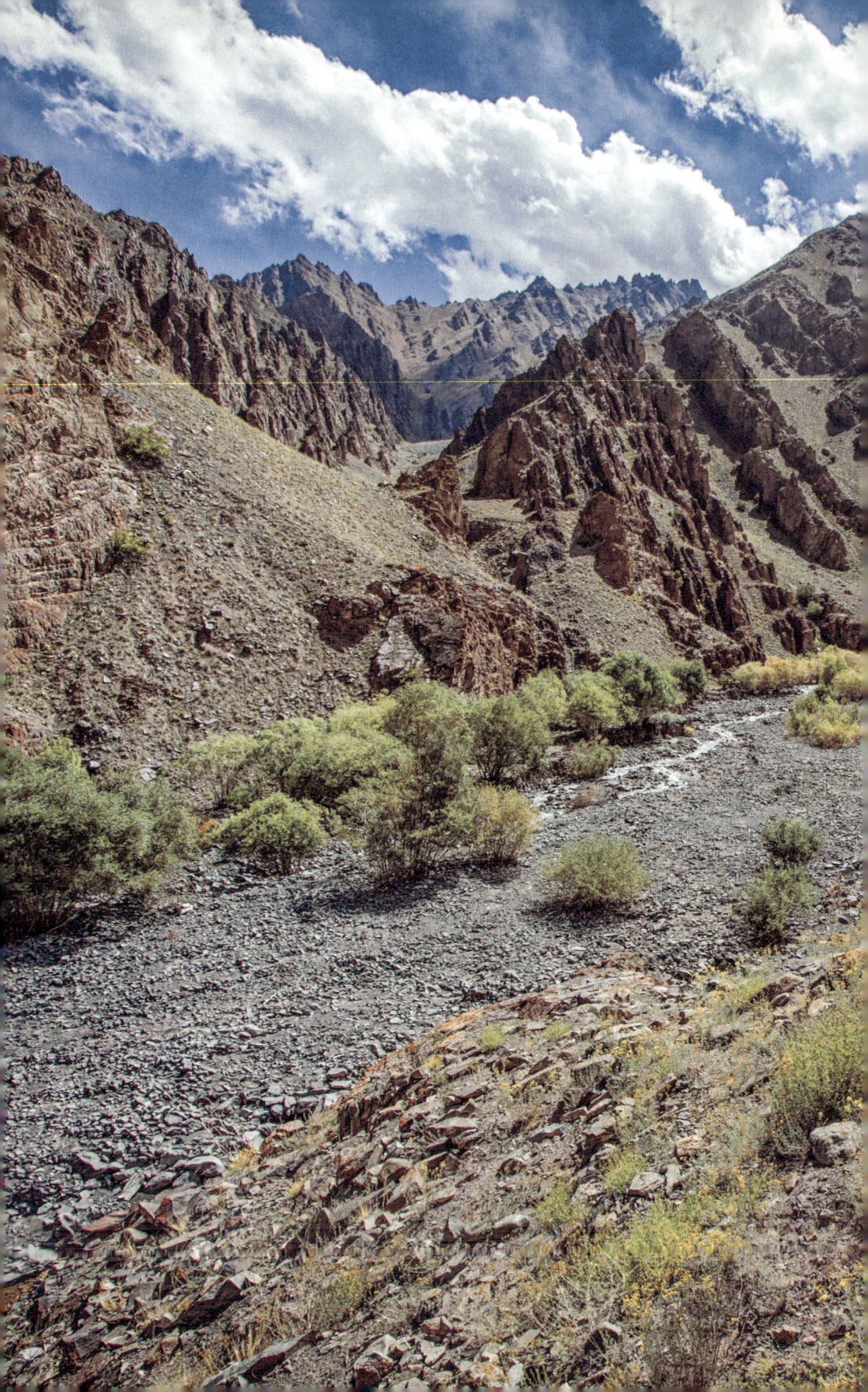

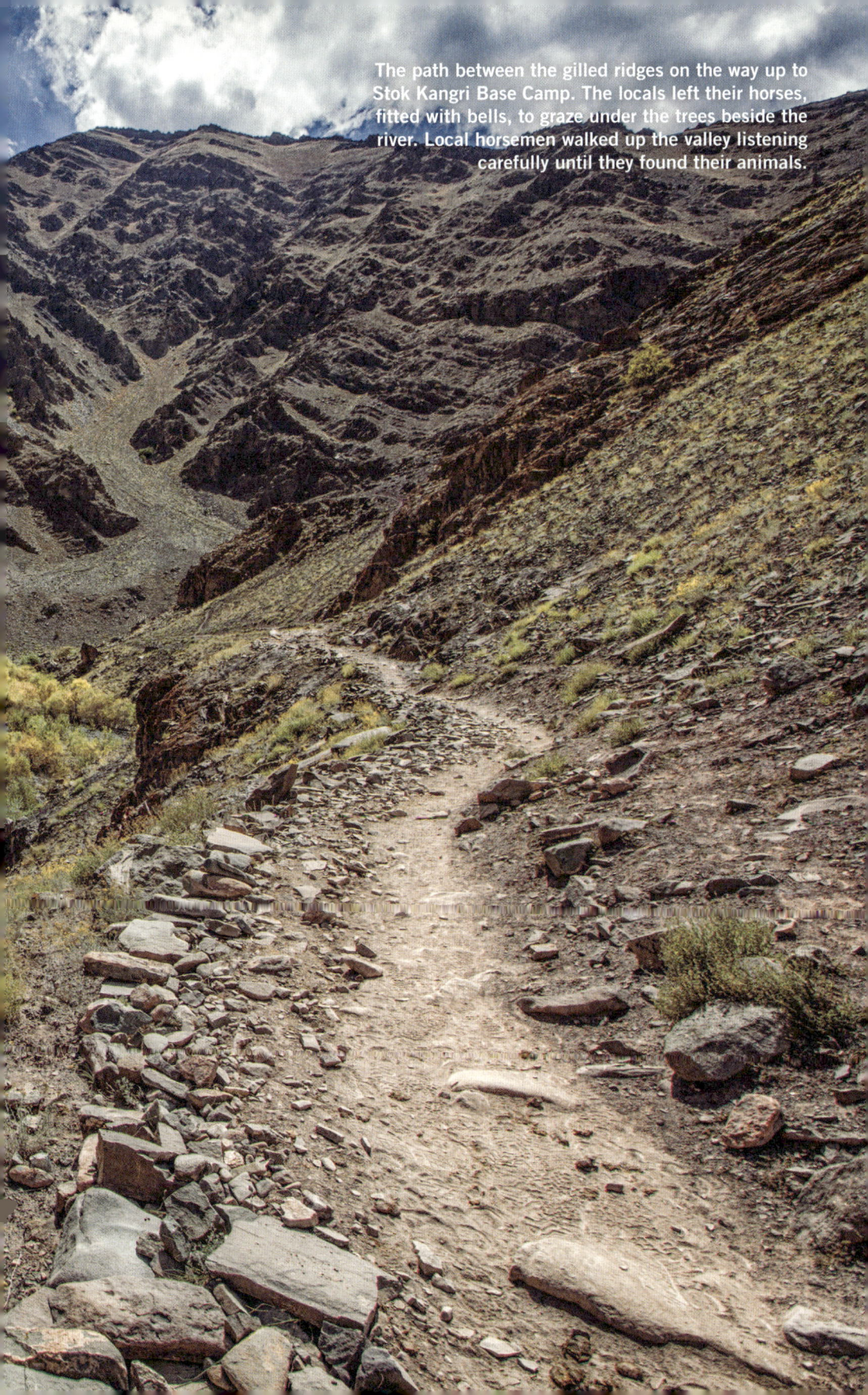

The path between the gilled ridges on the way up to Stok Kangri Base Camp. The locals left their horses, fitted with bells, to graze under the trees beside the river. Local horsemen walked up the valley listening carefully until they found their animals.

machine purr a bit sluggish under our weight.

'I own the only Nano in the whole of Leh,' Karma explained with pride. 'I flew to New Delhi, purchased it new from the Tata dealer and drove it all the way back.'

'Oh, wow! Good for you. How do you find it?' I remembered reading about the Tata Nano when it first came out.

'It is a very good car,' Karma replied. 'It uses the latest nano-technology in its two-cylinder engine, which makes it very powerful — that is why it is called the Nano. It is the best car of its type in the world. And it only cost two and a half thousand US dollars, brand new! Can you believe it? You can hardly pick up a motorbike for that much these days.'

The car rattled over the rough road, the little wheels dropping into potholes as we crossed the river and began to ascend past the old Stok Palace and into the foothills of the Stok Range. I was enjoying the drive, buoyed by Karma's positivity, and by the fact that we were finally progressing towards our goal.

Karma dropped Tashi and me off at an old bridge that spanned the river we would follow up to the Stok Kangri Base Camp. Beside the bridge was a small white marquee, shading a woman who sat behind a collapsible table, collecting fees from tourists hoping to climb the mountain. Tashi went over and dealt with her as I ran through all my gear in my mind, ensuring that I had everything I needed.

It was about 10.30 a.m. when Tashi and I finally geared up to start our trip. I felt positive: slipping on my pack is a bit like putting on my favourite gym shirt; it's comfortable, it smells like sweat and it means that a satisfying workout is ahead. We began walking up the edge of the valley, along walled country paths beside a small stream shaded by poplar trees, and past the farmhouses that lined the riverbed. The walking was pretty easy, time passed quickly, and I felt strong, which was reassuring.

I had certainly hoped that I would feel strong. Acclimatising to higher altitudes had been one of my focuses over the past six months. Back home I had been going to the gym three times a week, early in the morning, training for the trip, and I had completed numerous tramps with an altitude-training mask. This mask, which makes you look like Bane from *The Dark Knight* and sound like Darth Vader, simulates altitude by restricting the amount of oxygen you receive. I had been using the mask since February, steadily increasing the altitude, and building my tolerance through the hours spent at the gym each week.

For the month prior to my departure, I had been completing my hour-long cardio workouts with the mask set to 6000 metres: the highest it would go. I pushed it hard every time I went. Some mornings, when I was tired, it was so hard to breathe that my trainer thought I was going to pass out as I did my interval training on an exercycle or rowing machine. But I always kept going, even if I did feel as if I was going to pass out, hoping — choosing to believe — that my efforts would distance me from the possibility of failure. And it seemed that my hard work had paid off, given that I had not once experienced any altitude sickness.

After Gerwyn left, I had used my recovery time to acclimatise as well. Acclimatisation can also be achieved through short ascents to higher altitudes, and I had made two trips out of Leh for the high-altitude exposure. The first trip took me to the top of Khardung La, which at 5359 metres is the highest motorable road in the world. I hired a taxi to get there, the rough road being far too long and arduous to walk. It was an impressive drive, as the road took us to the edge of huge cliffs, beneath massive, crumbling granite faces, topped with towering, needle-sharp spires. It seemed an impossible location for a road.

Arriving at the crest of the hill, the driver parked his taxi beside the teahouse and took a break, while I climbed up to the top of a small knob just above the pass. I fell into a slow, steady pace as I climbed the short distance. Slow and steady meant less huffing and puffing, and less exhaustion in the legs. The air was cool and snow lay on the ground around the pass, but the sun was intense and quickly warmed me as I climbed, particularly given the absence of a breeze. It was very pleasant.

Two days later, and feeling somewhat stronger, I made a second acclimatisation trip. Wanting to do a bit of exploring, I decided to camp for a few nights at Pangong Lake, which was at 4349 metres, and reached via the 5330-metre Chang La. To give myself maximum flexibility as I travelled through this sparsely populated border region of India, I decided to hire a motorbike for four days. In Leh, there were two choices when it came to hiring a motorbike: either the modern 220-cc Bajaj Avenger or the much larger 500-cc Royal Enfield Bullet, with its old-school Harley-Davidson styling and thumping engine. I decided to go with the Avenger as it gave better economy — an important consideration when heading out into an area devoid of petrol stations — and was lighter to handle, which would be beneficial should I come off.

Coming off the bike was a continual concern for me. Not only were the roads rough, often either potholed or covered with sand and stones washed down off the mountains, but also other drivers seemed to know no rules. People overtook on corners, sped through the small towns, and would not necessarily stay in their lane. Winding up the narrow road towards Chang La, round all those blind corners, I lived with my finger on the horn, tooting for all I was worth in the hope of warning any unsuspecting locals that I was coming.

Despite the terrifying experience of joining the chaotic flow of traffic, the best part of the trip was travelling the road from Chang La to Lake Pangong. Down off the pass, large icefields terminated on or just above the road and supplied a stream that supported the bright-green valley floor, herds of yaks and a small lake. Above towered bone-dry mountains. Without any vegetation, all the variations in their geology and the colours of the rocks were in plain view: the naked faces of massive mottled blocks of reddish-brown, zebra stripes of light on dark and dark on light, and swirling earth tones similar to the stormy cloud bands of Jupiter, all bleeding into the water-coloured valleys of tumbling scree.

I spent two nights at the lake, perched on a spit of land, away from any other people. A few kilometres back down the road were a series of temporary campsites, set up for summer guests. The campgrounds, with their tents already in place, did not appeal, not least because I

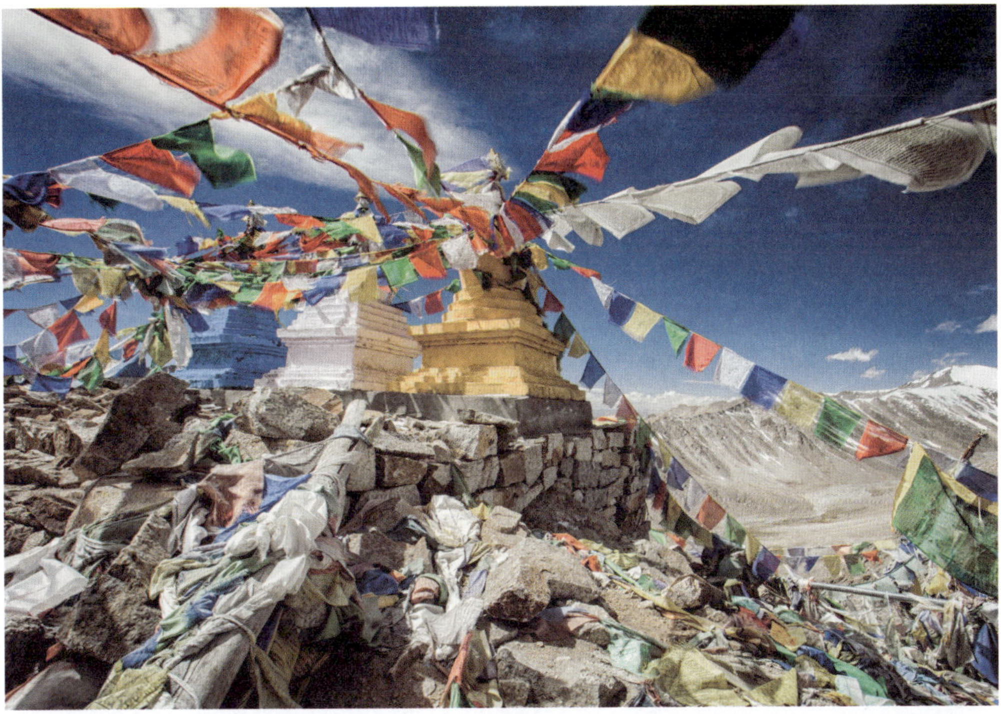

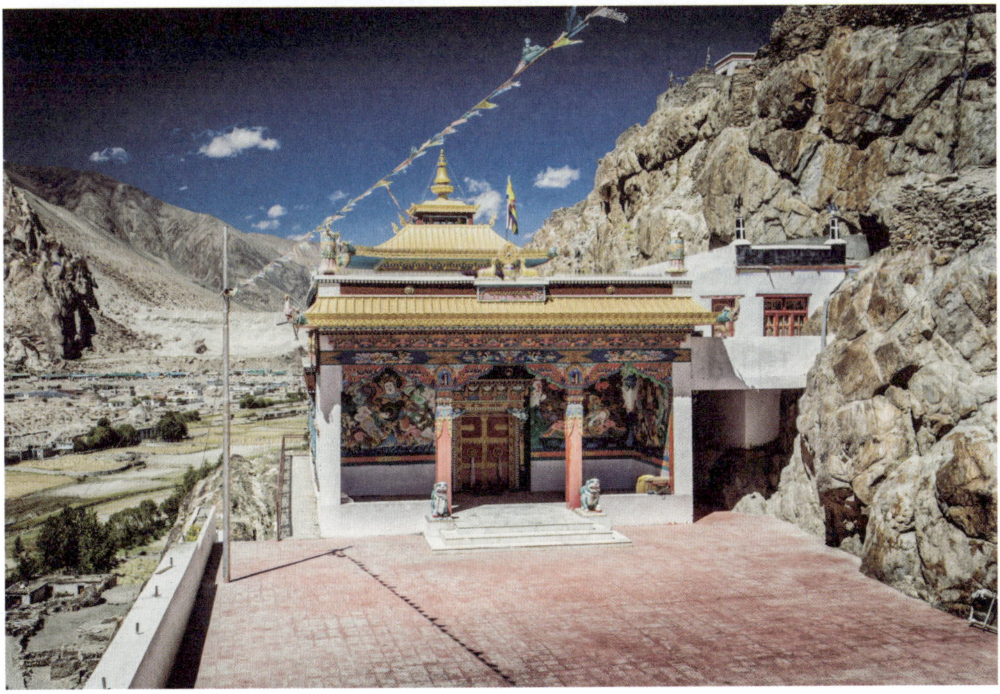

Top to bottom: The prayer flags marking the top of the Khadung La Pass made it difficult to walk around without getting in a tangle; The monastery at Tangtse, where I stopped on my way back from Lake Pangong.

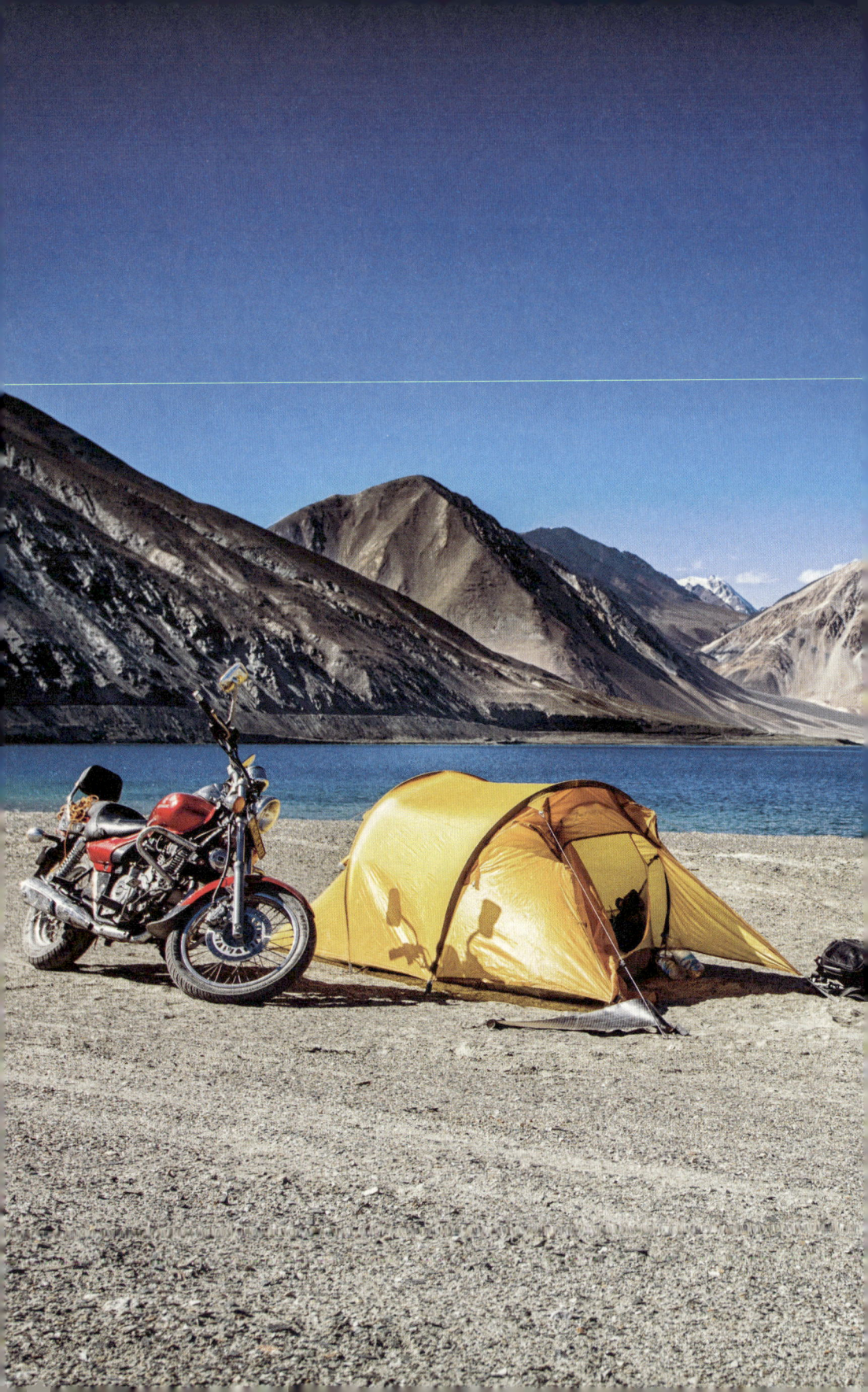

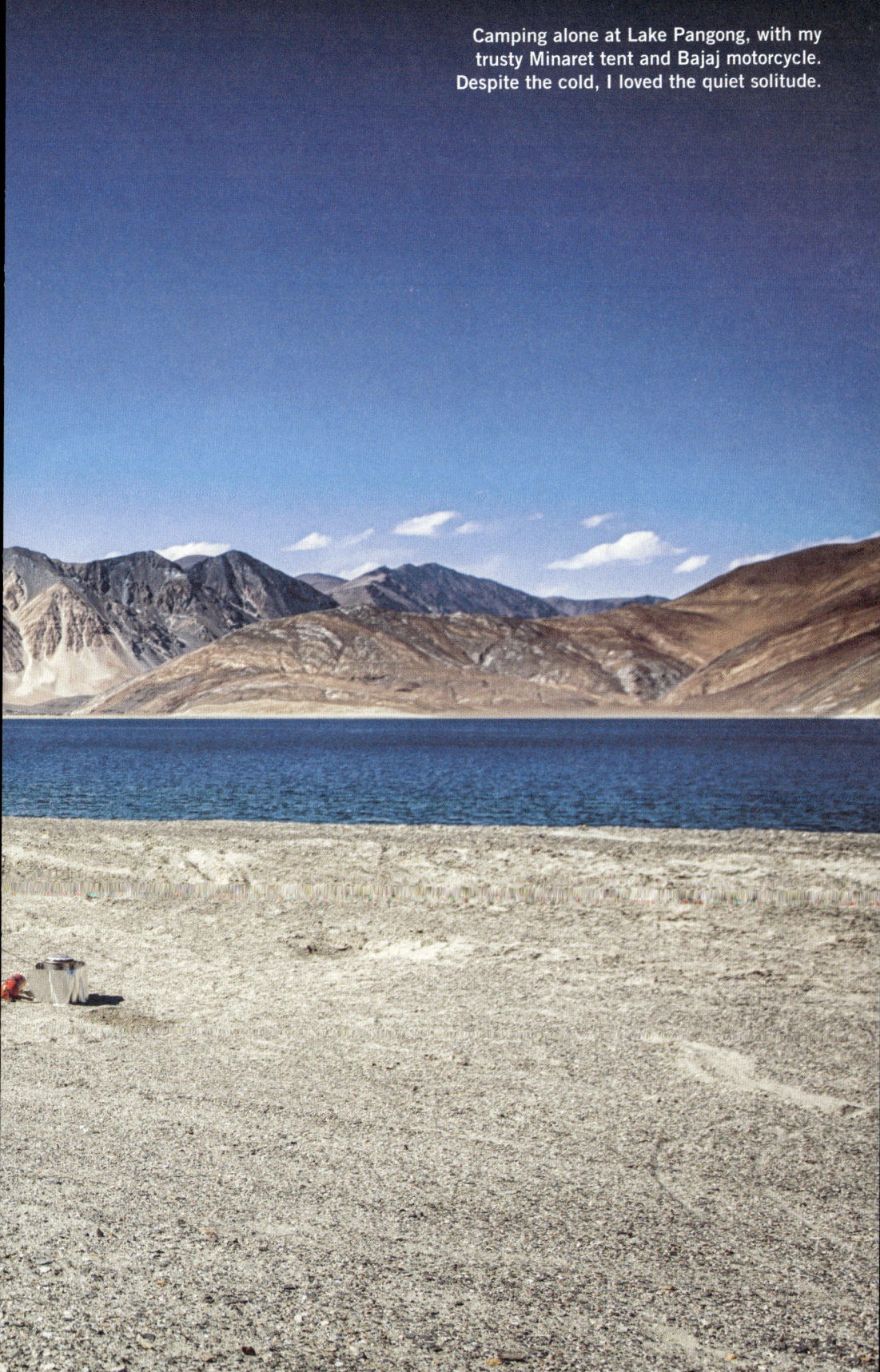

Camping alone at Lake Pangong, with my trusty Minaret tent and Bajaj motorcycle. Despite the cold, I loved the quiet solitude.

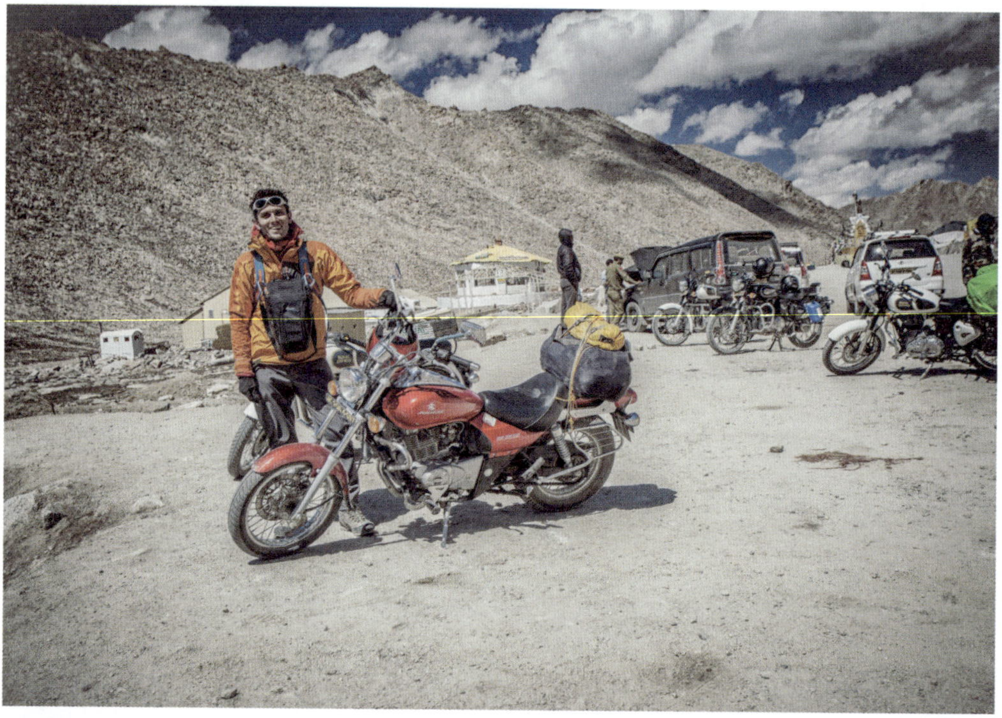

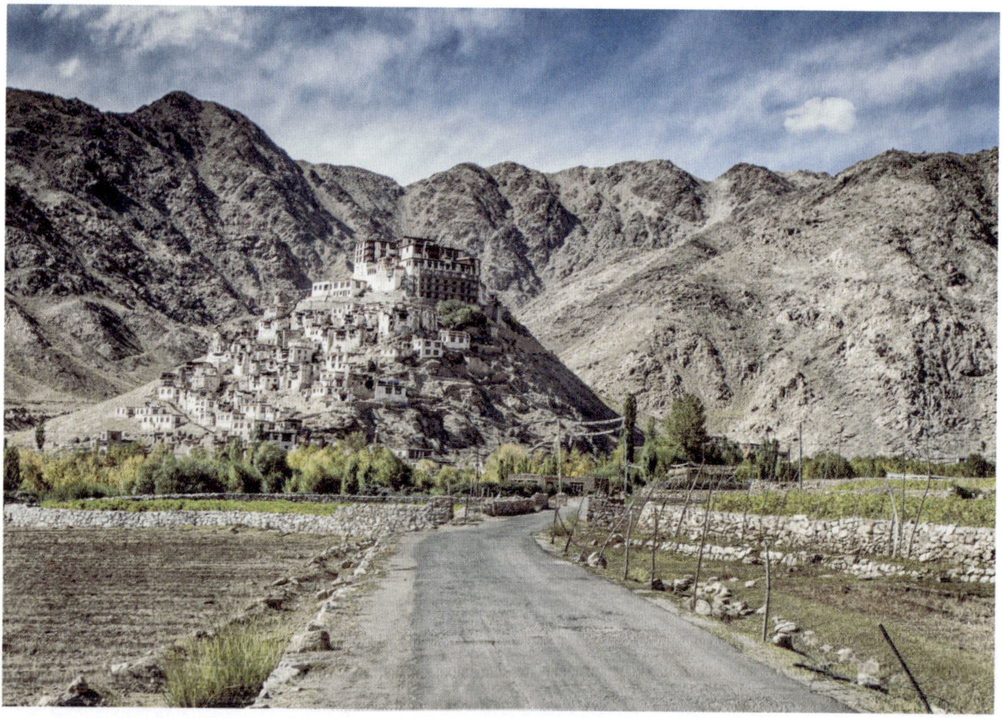

Top to bottom: At the top of Changla Pass;
The monastery at Chemrey on the way back from Lake Pangong.

would be able to hear everything that went on in the neighbouring tent 30 centimetres away — which could have been particularly awkward, given the number of amorous young couples there for the weekend. I was not sure what the rules around free-camping were exactly, but I had been told that you could camp anywhere, so I continued on past the campgrounds and down a rough gravel road, to arrive at my solitary spot on the spit of land.

During the day I would sit and watch the lake as it changed colour, starting in the morning as a deep royal blue, turning to turquoise around the middle of the day, then returning to its former blue. The landscape also changed with the light: the colours of the hills and the 6000-metre peaks that surrounded me would alter, intensifying then fading, and individual features would become more or less clear. I became mesmerised by the scene as I sat there, reading and watching, watching and reading.

I was reading Robert McFarlane's history of mountain-eering, *Mountains of the Mind: A History of Fascination*, and I came across a quote from Rousseau: 'In short, there is a kind of supernatural beauty in these mountainous prospects which charms both the senses and the minds into a forgetfulness of oneself and of everything in the world.' This was it exactly, I thought as I basked in the near-perfect beauty of the scene. I say 'near perfect' because the Indian Army always seemed to have a boat on the water, patrolling the border with China, a reminder of the hostilities that made this beauty so fragile.

Nevertheless, I found myself enjoying the process of 'forgetting oneself'. It was incredibly freeing to let go of the catalogue of accomplishments that I used to establish my identity, forgetting the facade of strength and the need to pursue physical achievement, choosing not to be defined by multiple sclerosis. Instead, I found myself choosing to let my self-worth be carried by the knowledge of God's unconditional acceptance, enjoying a deep sense of rest, a state of grace. When it was time to leave my spot on that narrow spit of land it was with regret but also a feeling of being at peace with whatever the trip ahead might hold. I felt a profound sense of joy, a satisfaction that was far greater and more nourishing than anything my pursuit of physical achievement could provide.

Tashi and I had just entered the wide, rocky gully that was the entrance to the heart of the Stok Range and were walking up the riverbed. Rocks and debris lay strewn everywhere and the washed-out banks, still raw from the massive floods that had devastated the area back in 2010, made walking on the edge of the river difficult. We were now at around 4000 metres; confined to the uneven surfaces of the riverbed, carrying a 16-kilogram pack, I felt utterly exhausted. On top of that, my legs were beginning to feel like jelly, which was distressing. I considered asking Tashi if we could swap packs. In fact, I thought about it quite a lot.

I began to regret my decision to not hire a porter — not that it had been entirely my decision. I had always intended to have someone to help me carry my pack, as a key part of my plan to manage fatigue. Gerwyn had encouraged me to carry my own pack up Stok Kangri, saying it would give me a greater sense of achievement, and I must admit that the idea of accomplishing the peak under my own strength, carrying my own gear, did appeal to my ego. However, the prospect of failing to complete the climb was deeply frightening, and I was worried about the added physical pressure of carrying a pack. That was why I had wanted a porter.

However, during our negotiations, Karma had insisted that there were no porters available for hire. When I asked if my guide would be able to carry some of my equipment, Karma smiled, leant forward, and told me that the guide had enough of his own gear and could not possibly carry any of mine. That's why I was slightly miffed when I noticed that Tashi was carrying only a 30-litre pack.

There was only one reason why I did not call out to Tashi and ask him to swap packs: I did not want to shatter the illusion that I was a strong, capable climber. I liked the fact that Tashi was impressed by my nice new Macpac gear. When I had mentioned Macpac's

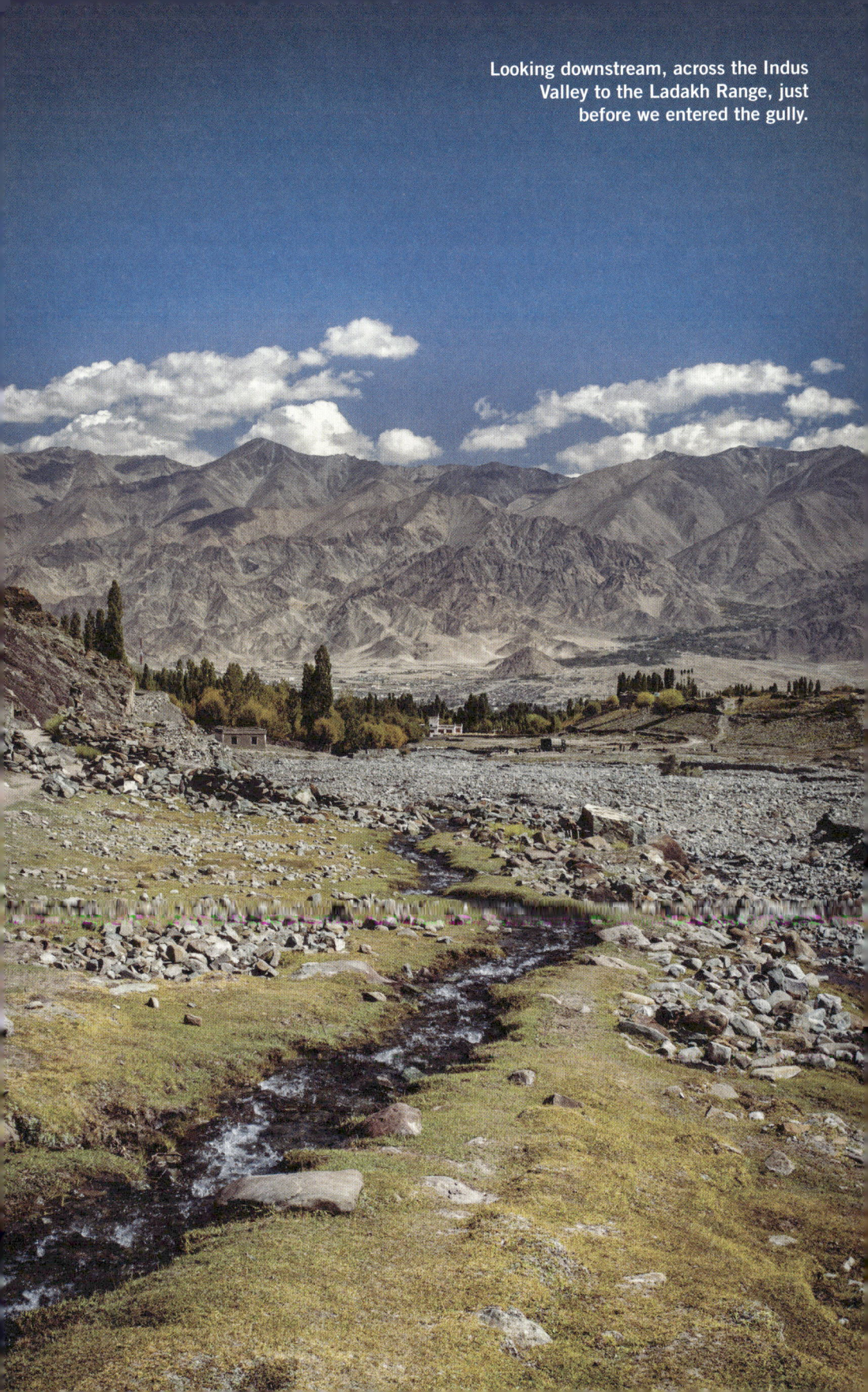

Looking downstream, across the Indus Valley to the Ladakh Range, just before we entered the gully.

sponsorship to him, it seemed as if I was suddenly somebody, worth something, momentarily free from the dark grip of MS. I did not want to break this fragile spell, so I soldiered on, refusing to ask for help. Grace can be quickly forgotten.

Tashi, who was able to handle the altitude and negotiate the streambed much faster than I was, maintained a substantial lead throughout most of this time. I did my best to keep up with him, pushing myself as hard as I could. Again, I found myself on the losing side of that pursuit of rest — each time I caught up with Tashi he would immediately stand up and move on. I tried to engage him in conversation, to create small breaks without appearing weak, but the language barrier made these conversations difficult to maintain.

Perhaps it goes without saying that I was delighted when we began to encounter tourists who were heading down the mountain. Stopping to chat provided a moment of reprieve in which to catch my breath, and also gain some insight into conditions on the mountain. Most of the people I spoke to had made an attempt on the summit a day or two earlier, but everyone had a tale to tell and I was eager to listen.

'Hey!' I waved to a fit-looking guy in his mid twenties who was on horseback.

'Hey, man, what's up?' he answered in an American drawl.

'Just heading up to Mankarmo for the night, then to Base Camp and the summit tomorrow. How about you? Did you make it?'

'Dude, I made it to the top yesterday morning — talk about a fuckin' buzz! The view was totally awesome. I was, like, totally tripping out. I mean, like, totally tripping out.' He emphasised the last few syllables, pausing between each for added effect. The pleasure of recalling the memory was written all over his face. It was exciting, infectious. 'And then, to top it off, I swear I saw K2, all the way in fuckin' Pakistan! It was so incredibly clear. Fuck.'

'It was unbelievable.'

He ran his fingers through his hair and stared off into the distance.

'Wow! That's sweet, man! K2? That is unbelievable. What time did you summit?'

'Around eight, dude — it took us seven and a half hours to get to the top and I was stoked. But, dude, it was so fuckin' cold. Unbelievable. Down around minus four or minus five degrees Fahrenheit. So what's that in Celsius, around minus fifteen or twenty or something?'

'Yeah, that sounds about right. But wow, that is cold! You were OK? Had enough gear?'

'Bro, I have an awesome down jacket and some good boots, so I was totally fine with the cold. You really need good mountaineering boots, though, and a good jacket. Do you have some solid four-season boots and a good jacket?'

My heart sank just a bit. Karma had assured me that my three-season tramping boots would be fine up the mountain. I had been going to hire some proper mountaineering plastics, but he had dissuaded me, offering to purchase my boots when I returned.

'Yeah, man, I have an awesome expedition-weight down jacket, so I'm all sorted there. And I have these boots —' I lifted my foot to show him — 'which are three-season. My guide reckons they should be OK.'

The American laughed. 'Yeah, I would probably wear a couple of layers of socks with those boots, if I were you. But, if your guide thinks you'll be OK, I'm sure you will be fine. At least . . .' He paused. 'Well, just wear lots of socks, that's all.'

'OK.' I chuckled. 'I have a few pairs of thick socks, so I'll be sure to chuck them on. Thanks for that.'

'All cool, dude. Also, make sure you use poles on the way down the mountain. I didn't and I totally smashed my knees coming down. It's pretty steep and, I mean, they are totally fucked. I barely made it back to Base Camp. I spent the rest of yesterday recovering, but they are still screwed. Fortunately this guy had a spare horse that I could use, otherwise I would still be up there.'

Next, I encountered a group, some of whom were also on horses. Some of them had made it to Base Camp but then experienced acute altitude sickness, necessitating their retreat and explaining why they looked so ill and miserable.

After them, also on horseback, came a European climber. I

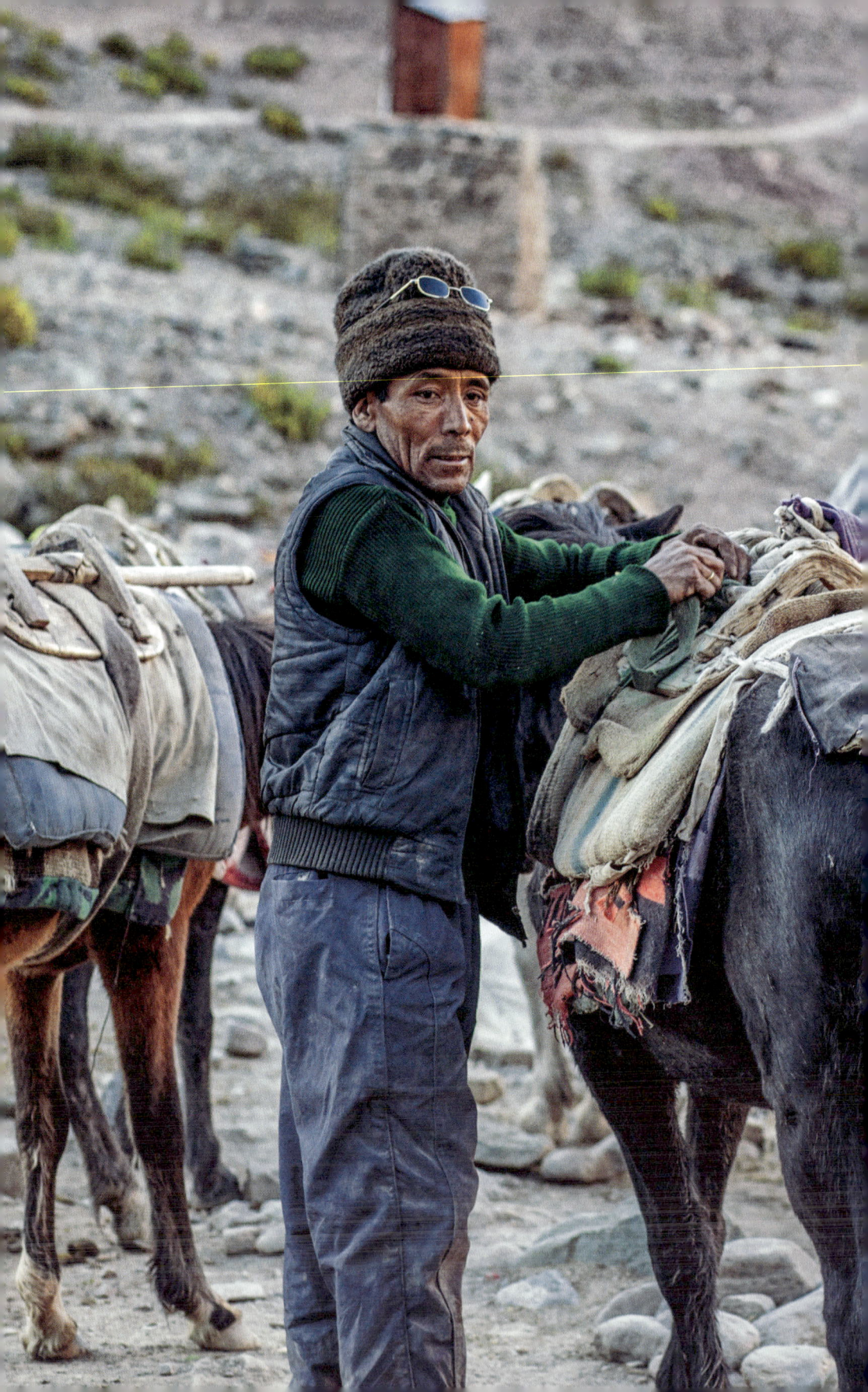

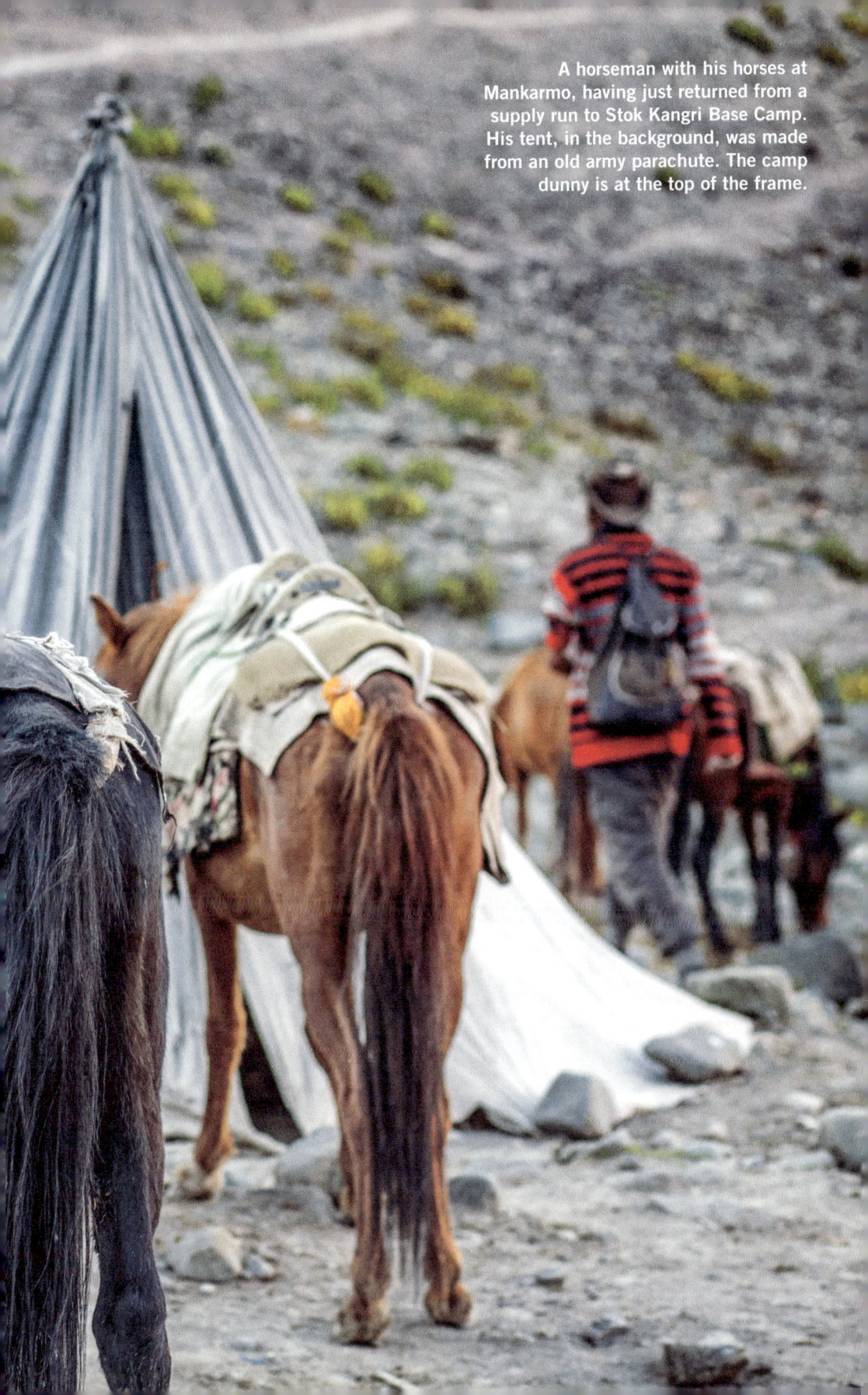

A horseman with his horses at Mankarmo, having just returned from a supply run to Stok Kangri Base Camp. His tent, in the background, was made from an old army parachute. The camp dunny is at the top of the frame.

could tell he was experienced. It often shows in a person's face. Or perhaps it was the particular combination of technical garments he was wearing — the black-and-yellow pro shell-wear and well-used technical climbing boots. He looked as if he had just come off a summit attempt.

I gave him a wave and walked over. A horseman was holding the reins, and he stopped the horse.

'Hey, man, how did you go?'

'All right.' The climber was friendly, but obviously tired.

'Where are you from?'

'Switzerland. You?'

'New Zealand. Did you climb this morning?' I asked carefully.

'Yar.' His shoulders slumped a little.

'What was it like? Did you make it to the top?'

'Yes. I left at twelve thirty a.m., just like everyone recommends, but I summited at five. I couldn't see anything up there because it was still dark. And I didn't want to go all that way and come down again without seeing the sunrise, so I sat and waited.'

'Bummer. But well done on such a fast ascent. Were you cold?'

'Not to begin with — I had been moving fast. But I didn't have any insulation to sit on while I was waiting and it was so cold, and windy, perhaps minus twenty or minus thirty. My feet and hands went numb. Then I got back to Base Camp and realised that I have four or five frostbitten toes — a couple on each foot — and then a few toes and fingers with frostnip too.' He spoke very matter-of-factly.

'Damn. Were they able to treat you at Base Camp?'

'No. That is why I am heading down today. I should be able to get treated at the hospital in Leh tonight.'

'Good call. Hey, but was the sunrise worth it?'

The Swiss climber smiled. 'Yes, it was worth it. All the peaks around were orange, like fire. It was wonderful. There was a bit of cloud this morning — I think that front is on its way — but it was still beautiful. I just wish I realised how cold I had got. Frostbite is . . .' He paused. 'Well, it's not ideal.'

'Yeah, I bet. But well done on making it down.' I smiled at him, then

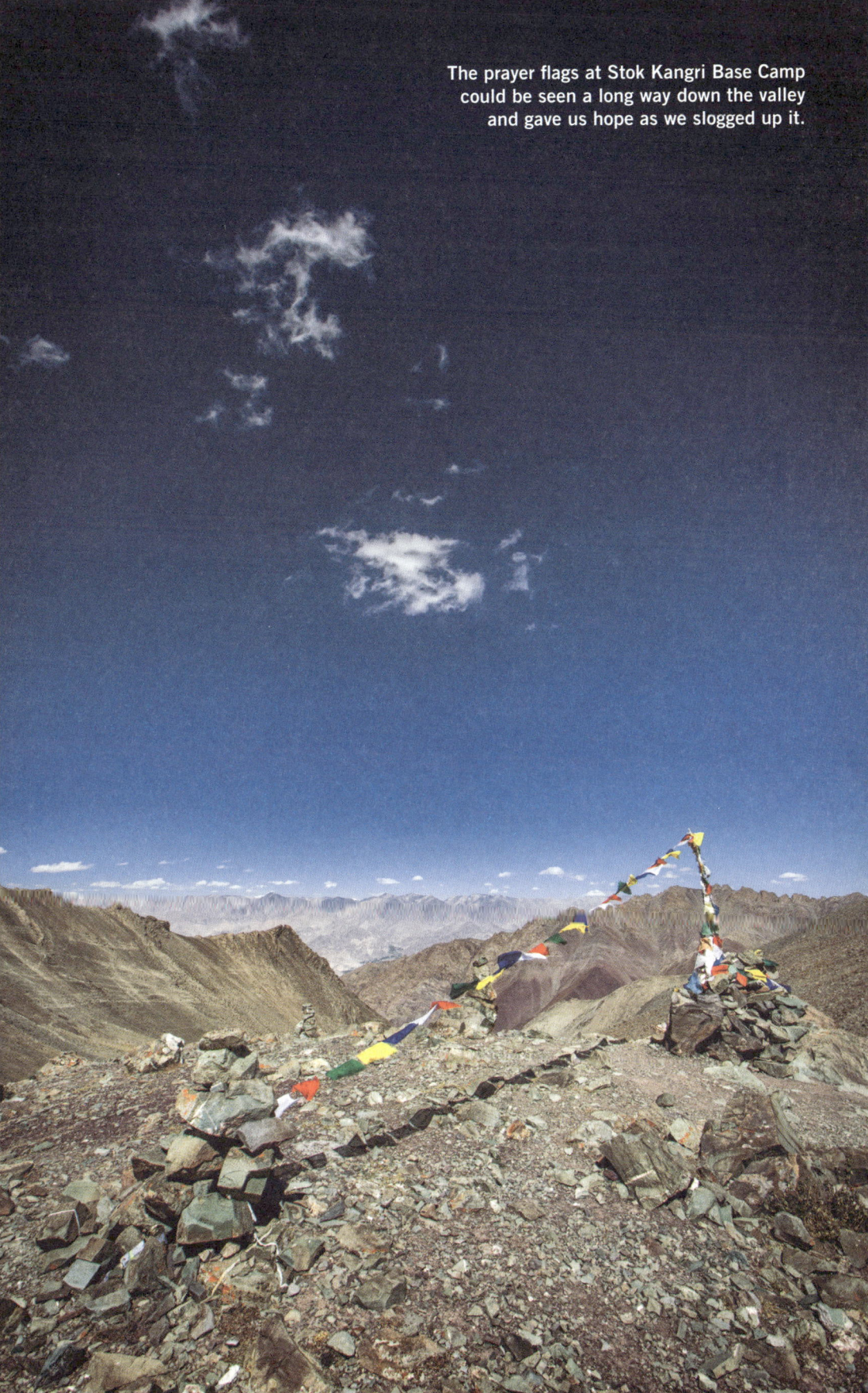
The prayer flags at Stok Kangri Base Camp could be seen a long way down the valley and gave us hope as we slogged up it.

looked at my boots, slightly worried.

Ill health, exhaustion and cold became recurrent themes among those we encountered as Tashi and I pressed on. What was particularly alarming was the fact that most of them had been unsuccessful in their summit bids. This surprised me. I had assumed that Stok Kangri was a pretty straightforward climb — an assumption that was steadily eroded by the stream of injured and would-be summiteers. Clearly many had underestimated the seriousness of the climb and the difficulties posed by the onset of winter. But I would not be one of these casualties. I would make it to the top.

The only climbers I met who had made it to the top unscathed were a group of gargantuan, bearish Polish climbers, complete with leather-trimmed glacier glasses, big climbing boots and white-zinc noses. I am not exactly a big guy — I'm more lanky than anything — and if the correlation between size and success meant anything then I was pretty screwed. And that wasn't taking into account of my boots. But I am a New Zealander, I thought. Our mountains make us tough. I will make it.

The dreaded descending triad of my watch's alarm — 'Da-de-do, da-de-do' — woke me at 12.45 a.m., just three hours after I had fallen asleep. Though I did not feel ready to wake, I sat bolt upright as a wave of adrenaline hit me — this morning was the morning. My stomach clenched as I raised my eyes towards the peak that I could not yet see, and thought of the hours ahead: a 1200-metre ascent towards one lonely peak. This was no small task.

It was cold outside and I had difficulty lighting my stove for breakfast, the lack of oxygen at 4930 metres and a steady breeze complicating things considerably. Normally, petrol is very volatile and it lights easily when I use my flint to throw a spray of sparks into the little priming dish on my MSR Whisperlite. But this morning it was more difficult.

I took off my gloves so that I could hold the flint closer to the fuel and threw another spray. This time it caught, but the flame was lazy and blown by the wind. I moved my body to shield the struggling fire, and placed the aluminium guard around the stove. Then I turned off my headlamp as I waited for the stove to heat enough to vaporise the fuel. It was a clear night, and the stars were mesmerising. But I felt tired.

I had not slept well, filled with anxiety about the climb, worried by the prospect of not being able to complete it — a fear compounded by the fact that I did not feel confident about Tashi's ability to lead and support me. I had climbed into my tent a bit before seven o'clock, with the hope of sleeping a good six hours. But sleep did not come easily, and I lay there tossing and turning as I ran through my gear and the day ahead, creating contingency plans for various situations that might arise. What will I do if I run out of energy? Do I have enough food for a 12-hour day? Tashi had not brought a medical kit, so how would I use my basic medical equipment to fix a sprained ankle? What about a broken leg? These thoughts came thick and fast as I tried to gain a sense of control and preparedness in a situation where the only acceptable outcome — a successful bid on the summit — seemed so elusive.

I put on my headphones and listened to Morten Lauridsen's *Lux Aeterna*, the most beautiful and peaceful piece of choral music I have ever heard. I love choral music and the deeply immersive experience of being surrounded by voices in harmony. Perhaps this love comes from my experience as a young soprano in a choir, or perhaps it has something to do with the fact of being caught up in a creative act so much greater than yourself, giving a sense of transcendence — I am not entirely sure. Whatever the case, it is the music that always grants me peace when I am anxious or sad, reminding me of that transcendent reality.

The piece opens with the words 'Requiem aeternam dona eis' ('Grant them eternal rest'). I love the tension built through the dissonance of the opening chords, the tangle of voices resolved in a closing repetition of the word 'requiem', which means rest.

I tried to focus on this sense of resolution as I battled with my

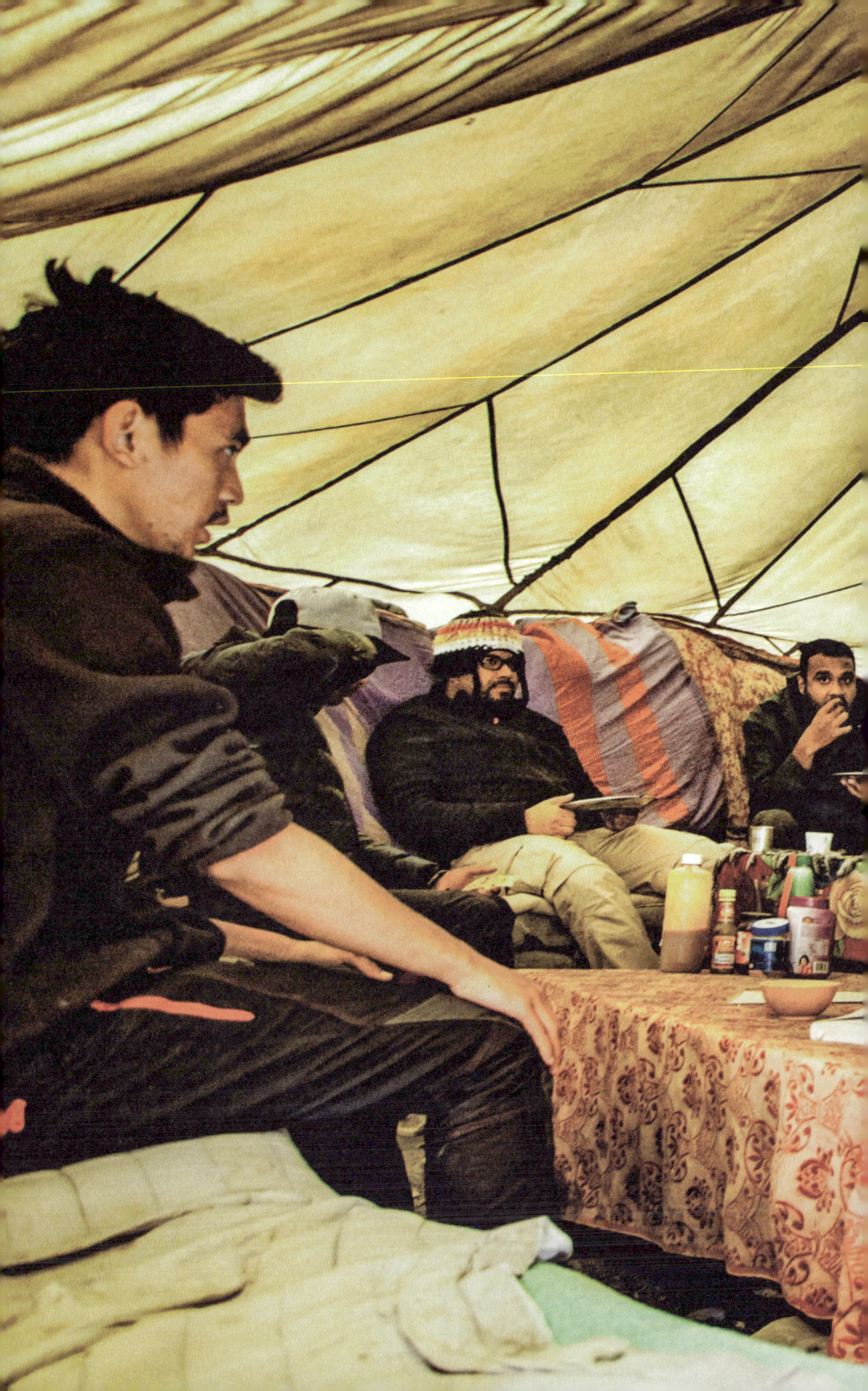

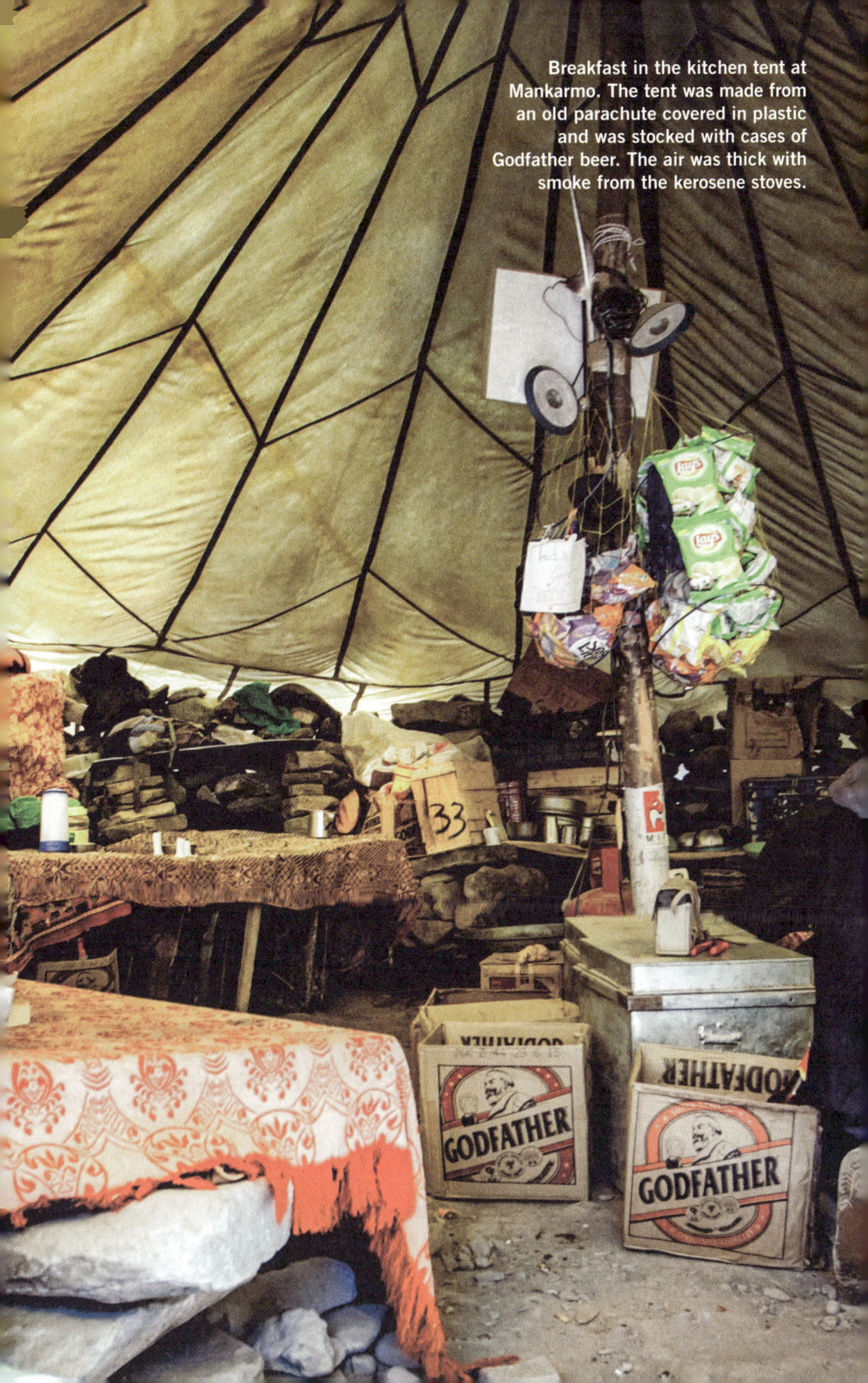

Breakfast in the kitchen tent at Mankarmo. The tent was made from an old parachute covered in plastic and was stocked with cases of Godfather beer. The air was thick with smoke from the kerosene stoves.

mind, in an effort to let myself be carried through the music into a state of rest. But my mind would not be so easily controlled and it kept returning to think about situations that might derail my attempt on the summit, and ways to deal with those situations. I was going to reach the top — I was going to make it, come hell or high water.

The last time I looked at my watch it was a bit after 9.30. I dozed fitfully after that, only to be woken by my alarm three hours later.

I placed my pot on the stove to boil water for coffee and breakfast. It was beautiful under the stars in the fresh, cool breeze. It was now 1.10, and the plan was to leave at 1.30, but I had not seen any sign of Tashi.

I got up and walked down to the large kitchen tent that sat on the edge of Base Camp, and to the guides' tents beside it. I peeked inside the kitchen tent, hoping to see the flash of a headlamp or hear the roar of a burner. The cook and his aide were asleep on the floor, but there was no sign of Tashi.

I walked past the guides' tents slowly, although I didn't know which tent Tashi was sleeping in. There was not so much as the rustle of a sleeping bag or zipping of a jacket.

I'm sure it will be fine, I told myself. Tashi has it all under control. He's a qualified guide; he knows what he's doing.

I walked back to my pot of water, now boiling, poured myself a coffee and made my breakfast. I had created my breakfast very carefully, trying to pack in the highest calorific content per gram. I stirred the hot water into my packet of gluten-free porridge, complete with raisins, a good serving of cacao powder and a big dollop of coconut oil. Just as I was finishing the packet, around 1.30, I saw Tashi's headlamp emerge from one of the tents. He threw me a quick wave as he wandered towards the kitchen tent. I quickly chucked my spoon and empty breakfast packet into the tent, picked up my bag and walked down to join him.

We set out around 1.45, climbing up out of the camp and around the ridge that stood between us and Stok Kangri. We made solid progress for the first hour as we traversed the scree slopes beneath the ridge and made our way towards the Stok Glacier. I was reassured by a feeling of strength as the time slipped by within my bubble of light, the rhythm and the blur of the edges and shadows lulling me into a trance-like plod that moved me steadily along the path.

The first thing to disturb this rhythmic pace was a growing sense of discomfort in my stomach. Perhaps my breakfast had been too rich, I thought as I pressed on, trying to ward off the feeling of nausea. It would pass, I told myself. I would not let a bit of an upset stomach deter me.

The next disturbance came from Tashi, who suddenly stopped, placed his hand on his stomach, and bent over as if he was about to throw up. I stood there frozen, unsure what to do, as I watched Tashi retch and hold himself. He stood like that for a few minutes, fighting the urge to vomit, then sat down in obvious discomfort.

'We should rest, so food can digest,' he said, oblivious to the unconscious rhyme.

Sound advice, I thought, as we sat for a while.

I looked at my watch: 3.21 a.m., 5494 metres. Good progress, I thought. Approximately 500 vertical metres in roughly an hour and a half — not bad, given our breaks. We were standing at the edge of the glacier that forms something of a highway up the mountain. Tashi stepped on to the glacier.

'Hey, Tashi, shouldn't we put on crampons?' I asked. The glacier was topped with a heavy layer of glassy-smooth ice.

'No. The glacier not that steep. You be fine with no crampons.'

I looked up and down the glacier, grateful for the 100-metre reach of my headlamp. He was right, the glacier was not particularly steep at this point, but looking down it I could see a large crevasse and, beyond that, boulders. Tashi was already walking.

'Um, Tashi, can you wait for a moment? I don't feel comfortable going on to this without crampons. I'm going to put them on.'

Tashi came back to me and stomped around, trying to keep warm, while I attached my crampons and pulled out my ice axe. It was starting to get cold.

'OK?' he asked when I had finished.

'Yip, let's do it,' I replied. 'Hey, how are you feeling?'

'Bit sick. But I am OK.'

If he had asked me how I was feeling, I would have told him that I was feeling increasingly nauseous.

I stepped on to the glacier, the sharp points of my crampons biting into the ice. It was on my third or fourth step that I heard a loud crack, sharp like a rifle shot. I froze, startled, wondering what was happening as the glassy layer of morning freeze strained, popped and shifted under my weight. I looked up at Tashi, wide-eyed.

'It's OK, not bad. Keep walking,' he said.

'Why does it not happen for you?'

'No crampons,' he shouted, pointing to his feet.

Half a dozen steps later, it happened again.

We continued up the gently sloping ice, round a few crevasses, and then began to ascend an increasingly steep slope, still on the glassy-smooth surface.

'Tashi!' I shouted. 'Shouldn't you put on crampons? It's pretty steep.'

'No, don't need them. I know how to walk on glacier well. Special technique,' he said, smiling proudly.

I felt that Tashi was being a bit cavalier walking without crampons, but reasoned that he had grown up around ice and snow and knew what he was doing — surely. Once again I told myself to be open to new ways of doing things.

Tashi was now 10 or 12 metres ahead of me, ascending a steeper section of ice. I was watching him carefully, worried, as he climbed what was easily a slope of 15 to 20 degrees. He put one foot forward, and as he began to transfer his weight on to it the foot slipped, ever so slightly. But it was enough to make him freeze mid-stride, with both feet planted on the ground.

Holding his ice axe — one hand on the adze and the other on the pick — he reached out his arms and plunged the spike into the ice, to get a more secure bite, I assumed. He then leant forward, placing

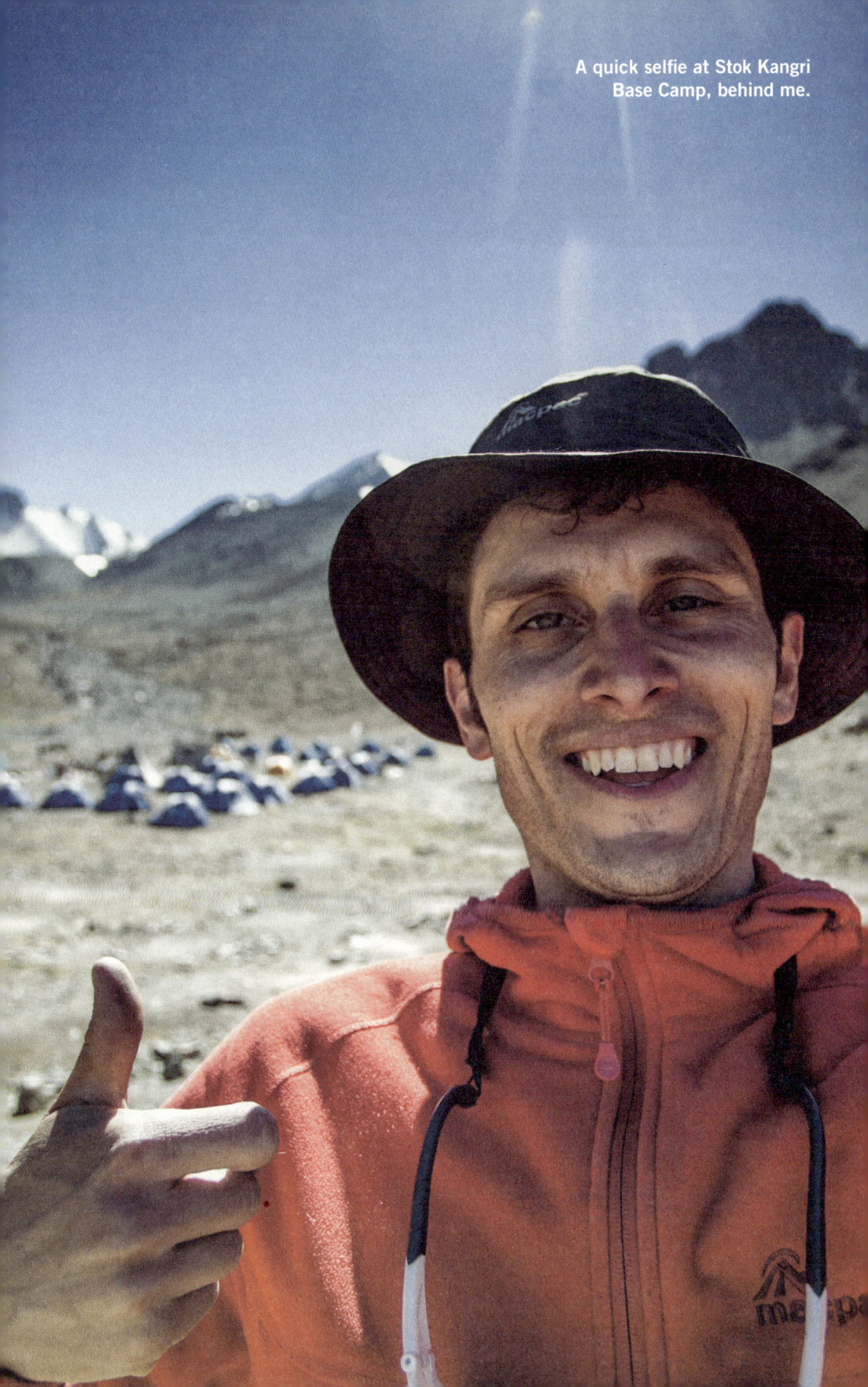
A quick selfie at Stok Kangri Base Camp, behind me.

his weight over the axe, causing both his feet to slide out from under him. He fell, face first, and started sliding towards me. He made a quick attempt to arrest his slide, but he wasn't holding the ice axe properly and it blew out of his hands and was left behind.

I didn't know what to do. As a result of his unsuccessful attempt to self-arrest, Tashi had rolled over on to his back and was now coming down head first — he was sliding straight towards me, and at an increasing speed. I thought of the crevasses beneath us. I knew that if I did not stop him he would end up in one, severely injured or worse. But he was coming at me fast, and I was afraid that he would knock me over and sweep me down with him. I had an ice axe and I knew I could self-arrest. Nevertheless, sliding down an icy slope towards a crevasse is never a good situation to be in.

I quickly stomped my feet into the ice as hard as I could, widening my stance slightly. I braced myself for impact. I made hand contact with his left shoulder before he hit me. I pushed him out, away from me, while also trying to get a hold of him, to stop him. But I couldn't. I couldn't hold his shoulder and he continued to slide past me. Not wanting to move my feet, I twisted round and reached out. I just managed to grab his ankle. Tashi came to a stop but I stood there, frozen, my heart racing, afraid to move.

'That was close,' I said tersely, as I offered him my other hand to help him up.

'Sorry, sorry, very sorry,' he muttered frantically.

I held his arm, lest he slip, as we carefully walked over to a more level area. He immediately plonked himself down, pulled out his crampons, and attempted to attach them. I walked over and retrieved his ice axe, which had come to a stop on a rock a short distance away.

'Sorry, sorry,' Tashi kept mumbling.

I then discovered the reason he hadn't attached his crampons in the first place. His crampons did not fit his boots: they were too big. This annoyed me. I had asked him if he had fitted his crampons to his boots when we did our gear check at Base Camp, and he had assured me that they fitted. Next time, I'll ask to see it, I thought.

'Sorry, sorry, sorry,' he continued to mutter.

'It's OK, Tashi,' I said, trying to be gracious. 'No one was hurt this time, so it's OK. But I'm worried about your crampons. Are they going to be OK, or shall we turn back?'

'OK, OK,' he said, standing up. 'We continue. Not far, then we take them off.'

'Are you sure?'

'Yes. We continue.' He put on his backpack.

'How are you feeling?'

'Hmm, sick. But we continue. You?'

'I'm actually feeling pretty sick too, nauseated.'

'Continue?'

'Yes, let's continue. We can do it.'

'Good, good.' Tashi turned to the slope and started walking.

▲▲▲

I paused for a moment. My stomach felt strange. This can't be happening, I thought, as I took a few more steps.

Then I had it — the urge — and this time there was no mistaking it: it was a stomach cramp, signalling the onset of diarrhoea. When you've got to go, you've got to go, as they say. 'Crap,' I muttered to myself.

'Tashi! Wait up!' I yelled as I frantically looked for a place to relieve myself. I don't know what I was looking for exactly — somewhere to hide, perhaps. I was surrounded by the sterile white surface of the glacier. To defecate here seemed a crime.

Another stomach cramp.

'Crap!' I muttered again, more loudly. I *had* to go, and anywhere would do. I turned off my headlamp, dropped my pants, crouched and let it rip, right there on the glacier.

It took a while for the diarrhoea to clear my system. Just when I thought it was over and stood up, I'd get another cramp, squat again and go another round. Exposed to the cold, I realised how freezing it was, as my nether regions slowly turned numb.

Fortunately, I was facing away from the mountain, overlooking the

Indus Valley and the city of Leh. Watching the shimmer of the city lights beneath the starry sky was like being on the top of the Ararimu hills again, near the old macrocarpa tree, overlooking Auckland, only more beautiful. Seeing this spectacular view was some small consolation during this time of cold misery — a consolation followed closely by the fact that nothing had landed in my pants.

Finally confident that I had sufficiently evacuated my bowels, I stood up carefully, legs still apart, and turned round to waddle over to my pack. But there was Tashi.

'You OK?' he asked, holding out a roll of toilet paper.

'Thanks, man.' I laughed. He may not have brought a medical kit, but at least he had loo paper ready in my time of need. 'My roll's at the bottom of my pack.'

'OK, OK.'

'I think I feel a bit better after that,' I said, relieved in more ways than one.

'Good, good. Take your time.'

I looked at my watch: 4.06 a.m., 5623 metres.

My relief from the sense of nausea was short-lived, however. I felt increasingly sick and my breakfast began to creep its way back up my throat.

'Tashi, can we take a break?' I asked, sitting down on a rock.

'OK, OK. Take your time.'

I felt absolutely miserable. I was starting to feel tired, my hands and feet were freezing, and I had an overwhelming desire to throw up. I could not think of anything else, much less enjoy the climb. I was tired of trying to subdue the urge to vomit. Stuff it, I thought. I'm not afraid of a good chunder. So I stood up and let it go.

'No, no. This is bad, very very bad.' Tashi sounded distressed.

I watched the vomit splash up off the glacier on to my pants and freeze. I wiped my mouth and nose on my glove, the orange leftovers freezing immediately. It was cold.

'This bad. Very bad.' Tashi was concerned, but I felt better.

'Is this altitude sickness, do you think?'

'No, not altitude sickness. Maybe some bad water, because we both have.' Tashi rubbed his stomach. I had wondered about the water too. Base Camp had been running out of water as the streams froze over. We had both drunk some tea with our dinner. I had been hesitant about drinking it at the time, as I suspected that the water hadn't been boiled properly, but I was desperate for some liquid and took it in, hoping for the best.

'You want to go down?' Tashi asked.

'Actually, I feel a lot better after that. The nausea has gone. How about we continue?'

'You sure?'

'Yeah, man, only another five hundred metres to go.'

I was not going to let a stomach bug stop me.

I looked at my watch yet again: 5.35 a.m., 5769 metres.

'Tashi, I need to stop. I need a break.'

'OK, OK,' Tashi replied, and we sat down.

We were about 350 metres below the summit — so close, it seemed. The sky was just beginning to fill with light, separating it from the mountain. Above us we could see two headlamps painstakingly moving up the ridge to the summit. Above them the clouds were racing. It looked as if the climbers were having a hard time up there, those last few hundred metres exceptionally tough work. Tashi estimated it was about −20°C, even though we were reasonably sheltered from the wind. I could not imagine how cold it must be higher up. My hands were numb, buried in my armpits beneath the warmth of my massive down jacket. I was struggling to cope with this.

I was needing to break more and more often. I felt annihilated. Without food in my stomach, I was quickly running out of energy. My diaphragm was exhausted, made worse by the bouts of vomiting and the odd dry-heave along the way, making it difficult to breathe deeply. Shallow breathing did not provide enough oxygen and I felt as if I was being smothered. Exhausted and starved of air, my limbs —

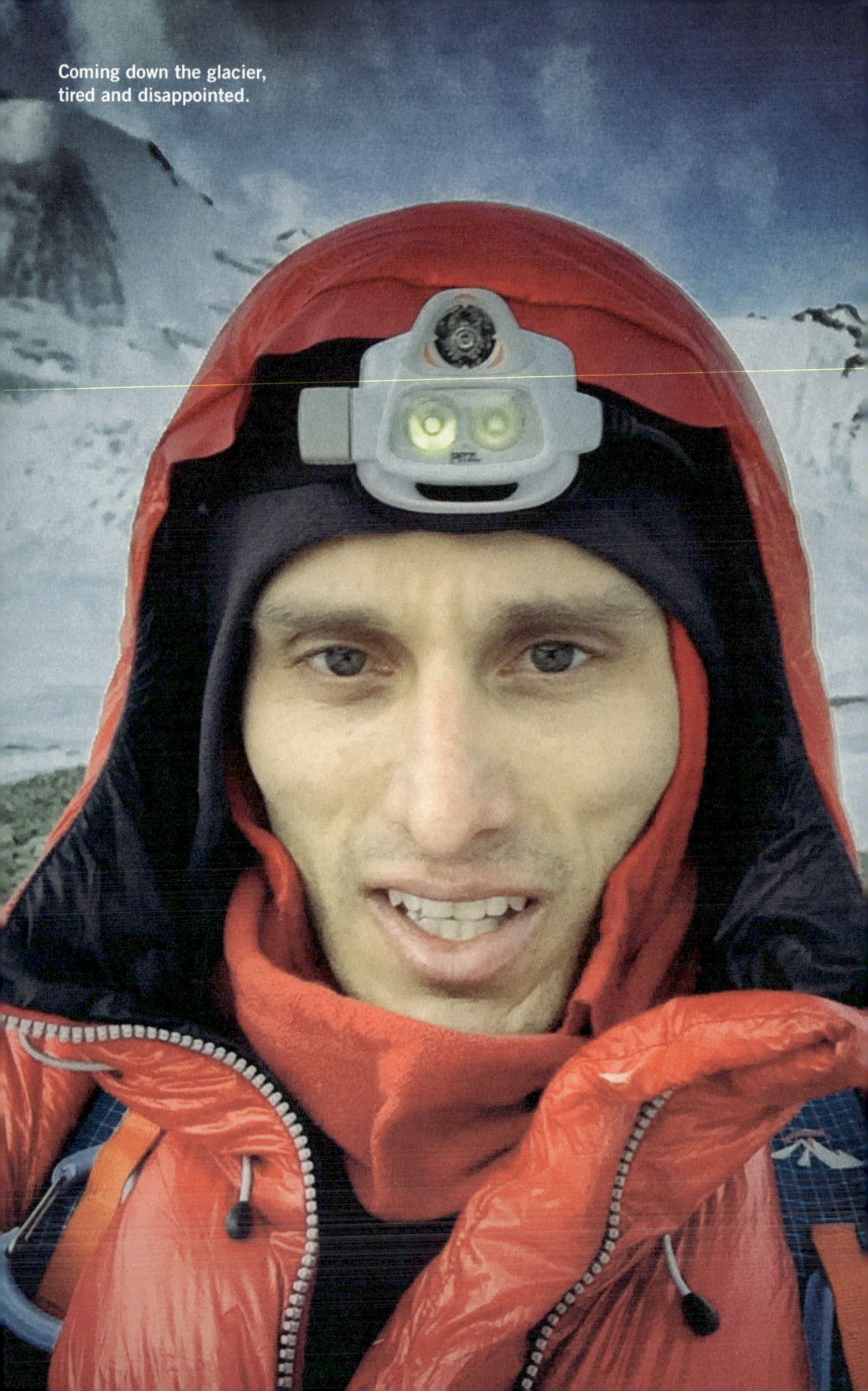

Coming down the glacier, tired and disappointed.

particularly my feet — had fallen prey to the intense cold that came with the slower pace. I couldn't feel my toes at all and the question of frostbite haunted my thoughts.

'What do you think?' I asked Tashi, nodding in the direction of the ridge.

'Up high is very cold and very hard — strong winds.'

We sat and watched as another pair of climbers turned round. It was Johann, a man I had become friendly with at Base Camp, and his guide.

'I think we should turn back as well,' I said, in a moment of clarity. Tashi looked at me.

'I think I could make it to the top, but I won't have enough energy to get back. I'm too exhausted and I'm finding it too hard to breathe. I will have nothing in reserve if we go on. And my feet are numb, and I don't want to get frostbite. What do you think?'

'Yes, we go back to Base Camp,' Tashi replied. 'These clouds will bring snow soon. It is good to go back.'

We got back to Base Camp around 8.30 a.m., just as the snow flurries began to set in. The last hour had been exceptionally difficult. I had felt defeated and totally exhausted, without either the strength or the will to go on. I was on the brink of collapse, especially when Tashi suddenly walked off, leaving me to walk the last 30 minutes to Base Camp alone. That happened just after I had asked him to carry my pack — a huge admission of failure as far as I was concerned. In despair I had gone straight to my tent, where I had fallen asleep.

Tashi woke me at ten o'clock.

'Hello, Nick? Are you awake? Nick?'

'Hi, Tashi,' I replied through the tent fly.

'OK, OK. They are closing camp — too cold and there is not enough water. The weather is turning bad too: we need to get down the mountain today. We can't stay tonight.'

I unzipped the door of the tent so that we could talk. I had not even thought about the weather's impact on our ability to stay the night at Base Camp.

'What are we going to do?'

'You think you can walk back out today?'

'Not a chance. I feel absolutely knackered and still really nauseous. My legs will give out under me if I try to walk down the stream to the road. There's just no way I'll make it. Sorry.'

'OK,' Tashi responded. 'Well, there is a horseman who can put you and your pack on a horse all the way to Stok, but we have to leave now.'

This was a godsend.

'Oh, wow. How much?'

'Two thousand five hundred rupees,' Tashi replied.

I let out a low whistle — it was a lot of money — but then, I didn't have much of a choice.

'OK, let's do it.'

▲▲▲

It was around 5 p.m. by the time Karma dropped me back at the guest house in Leh. I immediately crashed into bed, devastated and numbed by the sense of defeat. My mind was in turmoil as I thought about what had happened, and about the future.

Still nauseated, and choking back tears, I thought about how I had come down off the mountain. It was humiliating: I had joined the ranks of abortive summiteers as I rode down through the valleys, parading my weakness. I chose to believe that MS was the problem, that if I had been an ordinary person I would have had the strength and stamina to push through and accomplish my goal.

Choosing to think this way had a massive impact on my view of the future. I felt as if my desire to climb was nothing more than a self-inflicted pipe dream, the vain hope of a weakling. I despised myself for being so stupid, for being so ambitious. Since when does anyone make a comeback from MS? I asked myself, choosing to ignore the huge number of stories I had read and heard to the contrary. What a wanker — what a vainglorious wanker, I thought, trying to climb a mountain with MS.

I thought about my plans to climb in Nepal, to continue climbing in New Zealand. Under the overwhelming pessimism, those dreams were crumbling, slipping like sand through my fingers, leaving me with nothing but a fistful of gravel. If I couldn't climb Stok Kangri because of the MS, how could I hope to climb anything else?

I was an utter failure, I told myself, and all those people who had supported me would know that — I would be a laughing stock.

Approaching Island Peak Base Camp, nestled on the left between the moraine, beneath the massive vertical faces of Kali Himal that rise to the peak on the right.

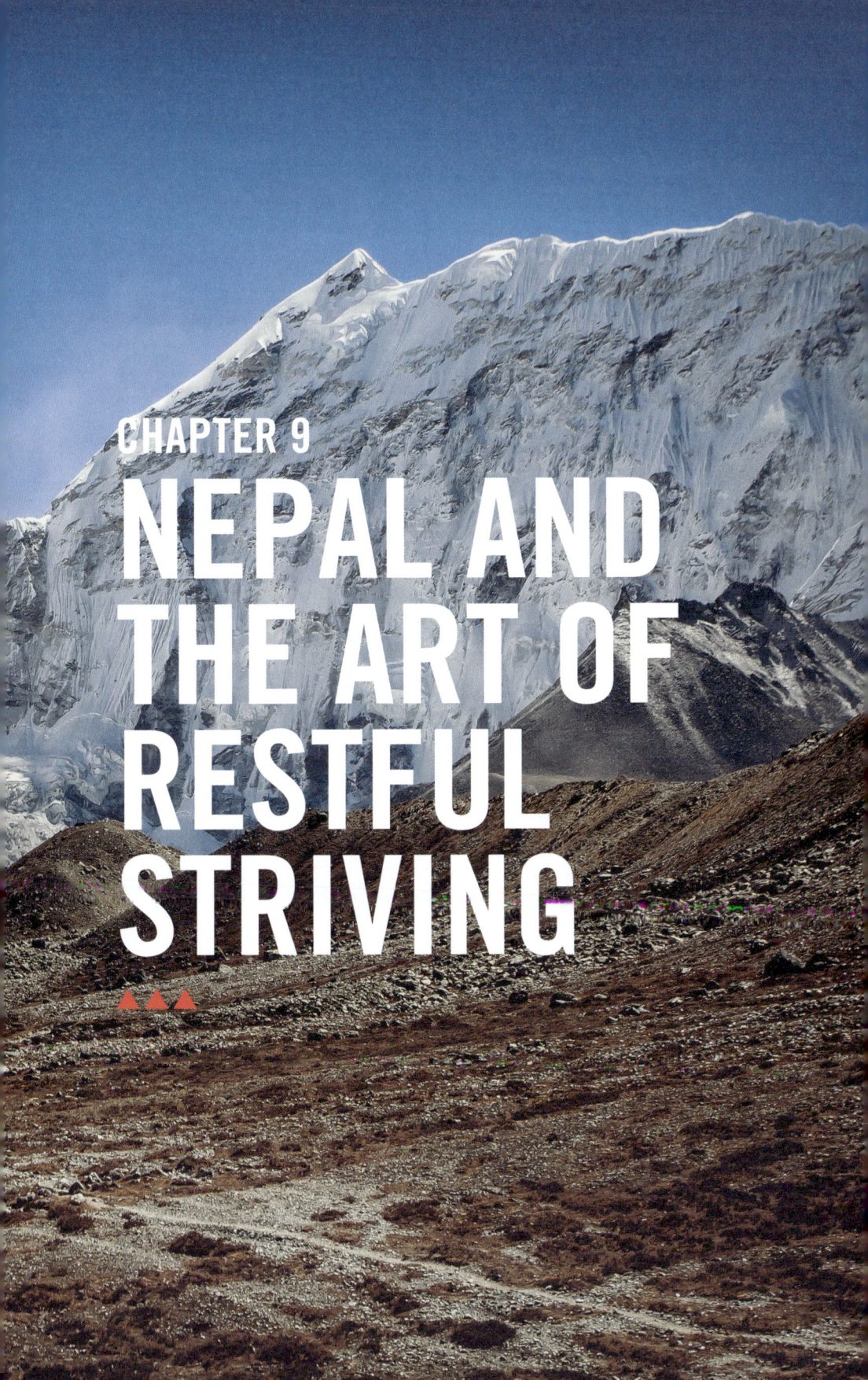

CHAPTER 9

NEPAL AND THE ART OF RESTFUL STRIVING

October 2015
Everest Region, Nepal

It was just before midday when Pasang and I arrived at Island Peak Base Camp. It had been a beautiful morning as we walked up through the glacial valley to the camp, positioned at 4975 metres. It was hard to walk and hold a conversation at that altitude, so I had a lot of time to think.

I was completely blown away by the enormity of the mountains around me. A few days earlier I had met a geologist whose special area of knowledge was the formation of the Himalayas. We'd had a long conversation, and I kept returning to his descriptions of the geological processes involved in the creation of these mountains. He had explained that the Himalayas provided one of the most dramatic examples of the effects of plate tectonics. The plates, floating on a global pool of magma, had collided, pushing the Himalayas up from the seabed faster than they could be eroded. As I looked up at the mountains around me — Lhotse on the left, Island Peak in front — it was almost impossible to comprehend the timespans involved in the life of a Himalayan mountain. These mountains had weathered millennia of frightful storms, jet-stream winds, ice ages, earthquakes, torrents and glaciation. In the span of their life, my life was but a hiccup.

Even more astounding, perhaps, was the fact that through all of

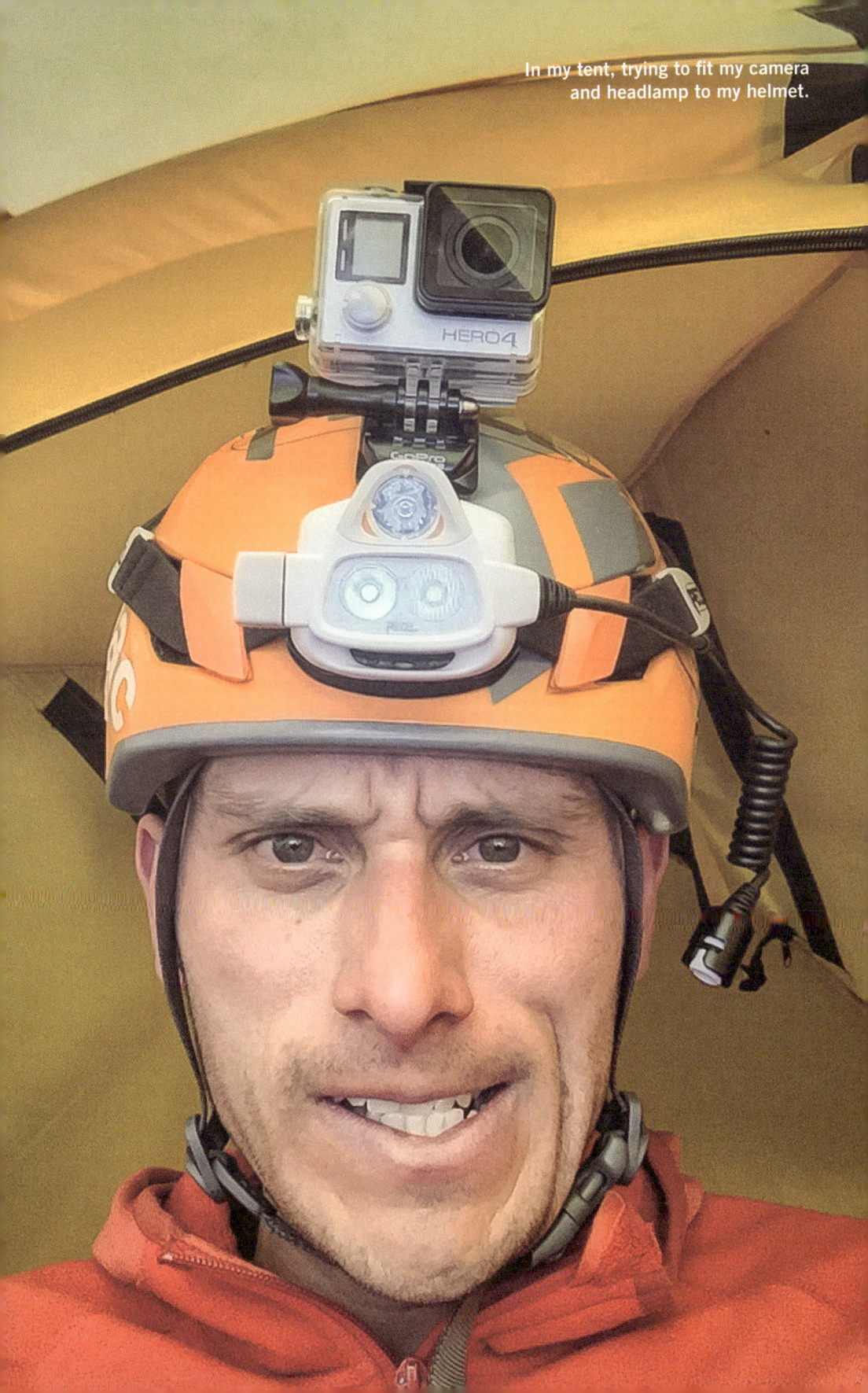
In my tent, trying to fit my camera and headlamp to my helmet.

this the mountains remain so incredibly beautiful. Their faces were huge, reaching up for kilometres above me, and magnificent in detail. Looking at them was like watching the night sky in the early-morning clarity of Poihipi Road. Just as it was possible to get lost in the detail of the Milky Way, so it was possible to be held spellbound by these mountain faces. The scale of this alpine beauty was overwhelming: the delicate fluting of the snow above a rocky bluff, the cauliflower face of an icefall, the swirling bands of granite, the unblemished swathes of snow, and the calligraphic sweep of crevasses. I was surrounded by this breathtaking beauty — a beauty created through the violence of tectonic collisions and the unrelenting assault of the weather.

While it was deeply humbling that my 30 years of life paled to nothing in comparison to their span, and my 1.8-metre frame was dwarfed beneath their 8000-metre stature, I found comfort in this confrontation of my attempts at self-definition. In fact, it was almost laughable, the ridiculousness of trying to define my value through something as small and fleeting as my body and its abilities. I needed to accept a definition that was based on something outside of myself and my abilities. It seemed so obvious. That's when I turned to prayer, moving my concerns about identity and my desire for a stable sense of self away from my capacity to perform and anchoring them in the beauty of the Eternal, of which these mountains are but an echo. I realised it was only when I did this that I would have an identity as unmoving as the mountains; that I would have peace and rest, a moment in grace.

Base Camp was all set up for us when we arrived. Pasang and I each had our own private tent, and we also had a dining tent, complete with chairs, a table and a red-and-white chequered tablecloth. In the midst of such apparent extravagance I felt like royalty as we sat down and had a cup of tea. I had not been much of a tea drinker prior to this trip — coffee has always been my drink of choice — but here in the mountains masala black tea was a highlight of my day, a purveyor of happiness and joy.

Like many things in Nepal, whether an ornately decorated temple or air thick with the smoky-sweet musk of incense, masala black tea was a rich sensory experience. Its particular intensity is said to be the result of being grown at altitude. It's often infused with cinnamon, ginger, pepper and other spices, and the complex flavours simultaneously deliver an invigorating boost and a restful sense of calm. It was the perfect drink after a day in the mountains. The morning's walk had left me a bit tired, partly from the altitude, but mostly from the beating heat of the sun, so it was good to rest and drink the tea in the shade.

After our tea break Pasang and I went through our gear once more, setting up the safety lines for our jumars, the devices that enable a climber to ascend a rope, and checking the fit of our crampons.

Pasang cursed suddenly. 'What's wrong?' I asked.

'My crampons do not fit — I brought wrong crampons,' he said, holding out a boot and crampon for me to see. The crampon's front bale, the part that attaches to the toe of the boot — was designed for high-altitude mountaineering boots, like those Pasang would wear up Mt Everest, not for the standard four-season boots we were both planning to wear for this climb. I could not believe my luck: two guides, both with sets of misfitting crampons. This time, however, no amount of persuasion would convince me to go up the mountain with someone who did not have fitting crampons. I felt a sinking feeling, a ruffle in my sense of calm.

'These are new boots,' Pasang explained, 'and these are my favourite crampons. I forgot to try them at home when I picked up my equipment.'

An easy mistake, I told myself.

'What are you going to do? Because we're not going to go up if you don't have proper crampons.'

'Hmmm. I will go talk to the guide over there and see if I can borrow his,' Pasang replied, pointing to a cluster of tents close by. 'He is Sherpa from Khumjung — we went to school together.'

As Pasang wandered over to the tents I finished packing my gear, stowing it in my bag in the order in which I would need it the following morning. I found myself trying to think through possible solutions to Pasang's misfitting crampons. Perhaps he could run back to Chukhung and get another pair from the teahouse we were staying at. I felt a bit annoyed, but kept reminding myself that this was about the journey, not the destination.

A few minutes later Pasang was back. 'The other guide, he has very nice pair — very new,' he said, smiling and holding up a pair of crampons.

I felt a sense of relief: the trip was still on.

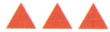

On his 1924 expedition to Everest, George Mallory reputedly carried with him 60 tins of quail in foie gras, 48 bottles of vintage Montebello Champagne, plus all those wardrobe items that were essential for fine dining: bow ties, Norfolk jackets and knickerbockers.

I think my dinner was probably better than any of Mallory's, not least because it was so unexpectedly good. Pasang and I had settled down to eat just before 5 p.m. so that we could get an early night. Our cook had created a beautiful egg and garlic soup for the entree, followed by dal bhat with a stunning vegetable curry. Dal bhat, which consists of rice (bhat) and lentils (dal), is a staple meal for many Nepali people. It was about the only food that I could afford at the teahouses we had stayed in as we made our way up from Lukla to Namche and Khumjung. The higher we got, the more expensive the food had become.

Supplies of fuel and food for all of the teahouses were flown in to Lukla then carried by yak or dzo (a cross between a cattle beast and a yak), taking days to arrive in the upper reaches of the valleys. Not only that, but the higher you go, the greater the volume of fuel consumed in cooking. Understandably, the cost of food climbs significantly at altitude, nearly doubling as we approached Island Peak.

Nevertheless, teahouses are pretty cool places. They are often

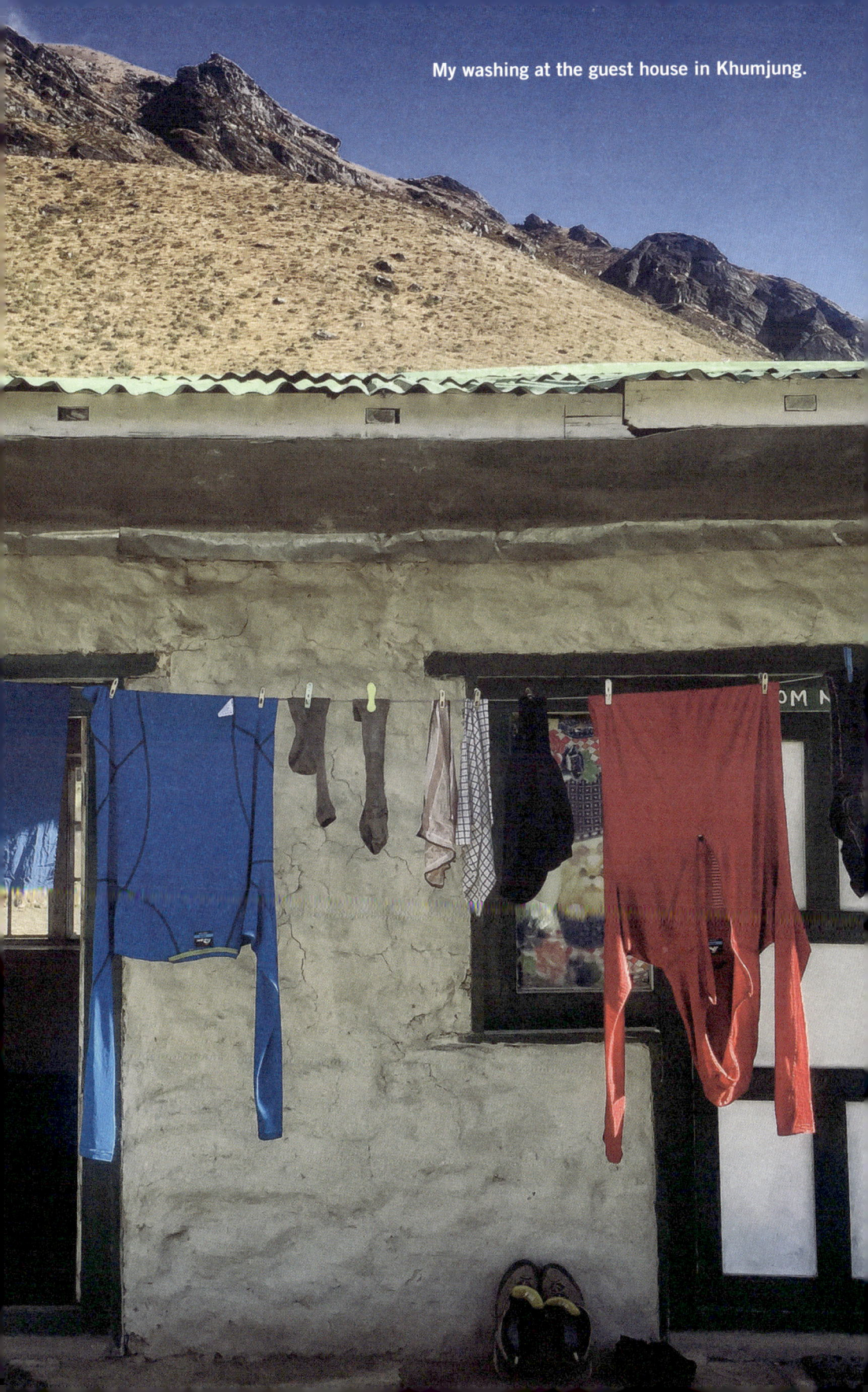
My washing at the guest house in Khumjung.

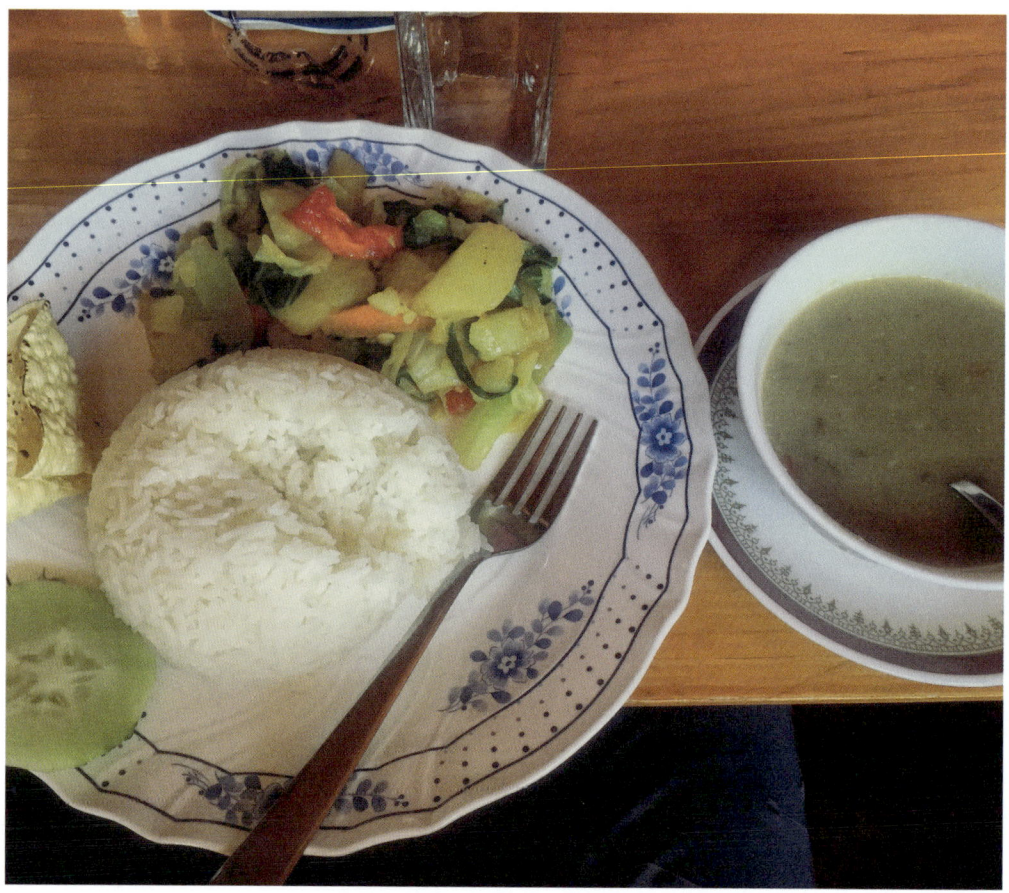

My plate of bhat (rice) and vegetable curry, served with a papadum, next to my bowl of dal (lentils). When you order dal bhat, you get an unlimited supply of rice and lentils: great for filling up at the end of a long day.

run by a family and connected to their home, with a large living area and many small guest rooms. In the centre of the living area is a potbelly stove that comes to life in the morning and early evening. The guest rooms are not heated, so at night everyone comes out, sits around the fire and drinks tea. I really enjoyed these times, seated on the comfortable, cushioned benches that run around the walls of the room, talking to the other trekkers, climbers and Sherpas. I loved the stories of the disparate lives intersecting in the room, hearing about other people's hopes and dreams, summits and defeats. The wood-panelled walls are decorated with flags and photos of climbers, and often there are pictures of family members who have accompanied major expeditions and summited big mountains. Sometimes, these are the same people who are serving you food or working on the earthquake-damaged house down the road.

All of the teahouses have fairly standard menus with a good number of options, but most of the main courses are pretty expensive. Often I didn't find them filling enough for dinner and I could never afford a dessert. That's why dal bhat was so good. Not only was it one of the cheaper options, but the cook would also make a big pot of dal bhat for the family, the Sherpa guides and any other visiting locals. The Sherpa people are very generous, and they would always keep my plate full of rice and lentils, meaning that I could eat as much as I wanted.

But a full stomach was not the only reason I liked eating dal bhat. Sharing the same dish as another person naturally creates a point of connection, something I really valued with people such as Pasang and some of the other guides. They would often eat tiny raw chillies with their dinner, and they would offer me some as well. I found the chillies excruciatingly hot, and general hilarity inevitably erupted as I scoffed down mouthfuls of rice in an attempt to cool my mouth. 'If you eat chillies, then you will need to eat too much food and won't have any money to buy more,' Pasang would quip.

'You eat whole chilli today, before Island Peak,' Pasang told me now, grinning. 'It will be good luck.'

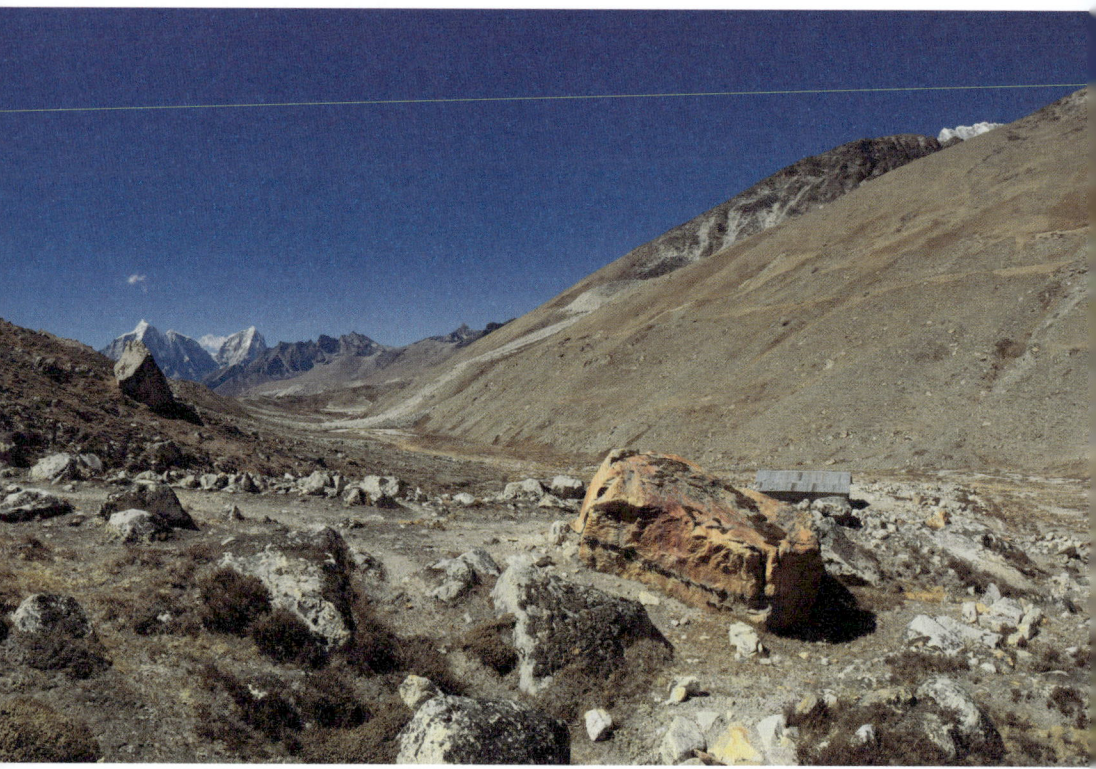

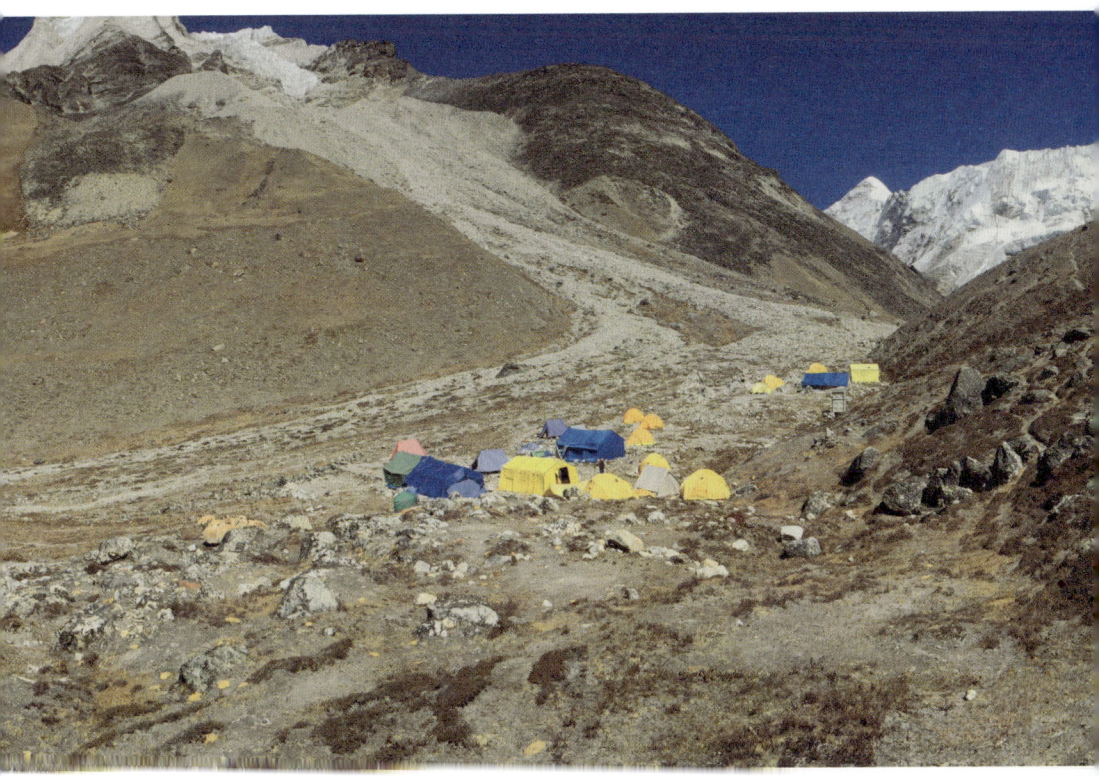
Island Peak Base Camp.

I laughed as I picked a round chilli — the hottest sort — off the plate.

'Ooh, I don't know,' I laughed. 'I don't think I'll be able to sleep if I eat one of these.'

I took a small bite; a bit of chilli does spice up the dal bhat and add some variety. As the familiar burning set in I pulled my handkerchief out of my pocket, ready to mop up the sweat and tears. I had learned that one should never touch or rub one's eyes while eating a chilli.

Having survived the chilli, with the aid of a couple more helpings of dal bhat, I was full and ready for a snooze. Then the cook walked in with dessert: huge, hot mango slices, accompanied by hot mango juice. I was not expecting this at all, but I secretly relished the opportunity for a bit of high-altitude gluttony.

'This is amazing!' I told Pasang.

'You get good food at Base Camp,' he laughed. 'It makes you strong. You'll be like Sherpa.'

It was without doubt the best meal I had eaten in Nepal, and I had enjoyed every mouthful. I was entirely satisfied, notwithstanding the absence of genteel dining attire like Mallory's. I was sure I stank: I had been wearing the same shirt for the last 11 days and during that time I had washed it once — if you could call it washing. My hair, greasy and unwashed for the same length of time, stood on end in a manic mushroom-meets-David-Bowie kind of style. Bow ties and Norfolk jackets would have been wasted on us — down puffers and warm mountaineering pants were the way to go.

Pasang and I migrated to our tents at around 6.30. As I lay down I felt profoundly at peace. I didn't feel as if I had anything to prove. I didn't even need music to help me fall sleep: the rumbling boom of ice falling off the faces of the unshakeable mountains was music enough.

As I closed my eyes, I thought of Psalmist's words 'He will not let you stumble; the one who watches over you will not slumber', and fell asleep.

My alarm went off at 12 a.m. and I was instantly awake.

'Nick,' Pasang called through the fly of my tent. 'Are you awake?'

'Yip,' I replied. 'I'll get dressed and I'll be out.'

'OK, breakfast will be ready in a few minutes.'

It was a relief not having to worry about whether or not my guide was going to wake up, I thought, as I pulled on the clothes I had carefully laid out beside me. I felt good — confident and strong.

I came out of my tent and entered a world sparkling with ice. A heavy frost had fallen during the night, covering everything with a thick layer that glistened brightly under the light of my headlamp.

'You sleep OK?' Pasang asked.

'Yeah, I slept like a log — those mattresses are so comfortable. I feel really good. How about you?'

'I am good. We are going to smash this today!' Pasang laughed and raised a hand in the air, inviting a high-five.

'Sure are.' I chuckled.

We had some warm soup and tea for breakfast, then Pasang asked for my drink bottle, which he filled with boiling water.

'Here, put this in the pocket inside your jacket. It will keep you warm,' he said. 'And, remember, tell me always how you feel. If you are cold, we stop and you put on more clothes; if you are hot, we slow down; if you are tired, we turn round. You tell me how you are and nothing will go bad. Communication is good. OK?'

'Yes,' I smiled. 'Communication is good.'

'And, remember, no shame in turning round. If you don't feel good, we turn round — good decisions keep us safe.' He placed a hand on my shoulder. 'You ready?'

'Yes, I'm ready,' I replied. It was 1.10 a.m.

I was incredibly excited. This was not the bolshie hype I sometimes feel before doing something risky. This was an excitement in which there was nothing to prove, and therefore nothing to lose. I felt unburdened by concerns about what might happen in the future or how I would address any problems that may arise. It almost felt like being a child again, about to journey up Ruapehu, towards the icy summits, completely present in the moment.

This confidence arose in part from my total trust in Pasang's ability to lead me. But more deeply, perhaps, it originated in an amazing sense of being buoyed or carried. Feeling completely at rest in my identity, I was entirely free to enjoy the moment and delight in the simple pleasure of walking in the dark, up a mountain, towards a summit.

And there was much to delight in. Below, the ground and all the rocks were still covered by the glistening carpet of ice fractals, shimmering like glitter. Above, the stars were amazing, so clear and so sharp — they seemed closer, more intense. Around us, there was a boom of avalanches and a crack of glacial movement. Beside us, we saw a nocturnal animal, perhaps a lynx, slinking away into the night, its eyes flashing as it watched us.

Sometimes I would look at my feet and the narrow ledge we were following, then cast my gaze off the ledge, down the mountain and into nothing but inky-black space. Wrapped in my down jacket it felt as if I was journeying to a different world, floating free of the earth.

▲▲▲

'Three fifty-one,' Pasang called out. 'So good time. Very good speed.'

'Yes!' I quickly looked at my watch. 'And just over three hundred metres to go!'

We had just arrived at Crampon Point, as it is called, at 5825 metres, where we would take a quick break, put on our crampons, and join the glacier on our way to the summit.

'How you feeling?' Pasang asked.

'I feel fantastic. You set a perfect pace up the hill. I feel really good, not tired at all. Hey, and this is the highest I have ever been.' I laughed.

We had cruised up the hill — hardly pushing it, I thought — and I felt confident, strong, and, reassuringly, I was not feeling any negative effects of altitude.

'Good job.' Pasang laughed too, imitating an often-used phrase of mine.

'How are your hands and feet? Not cold?' he asked.

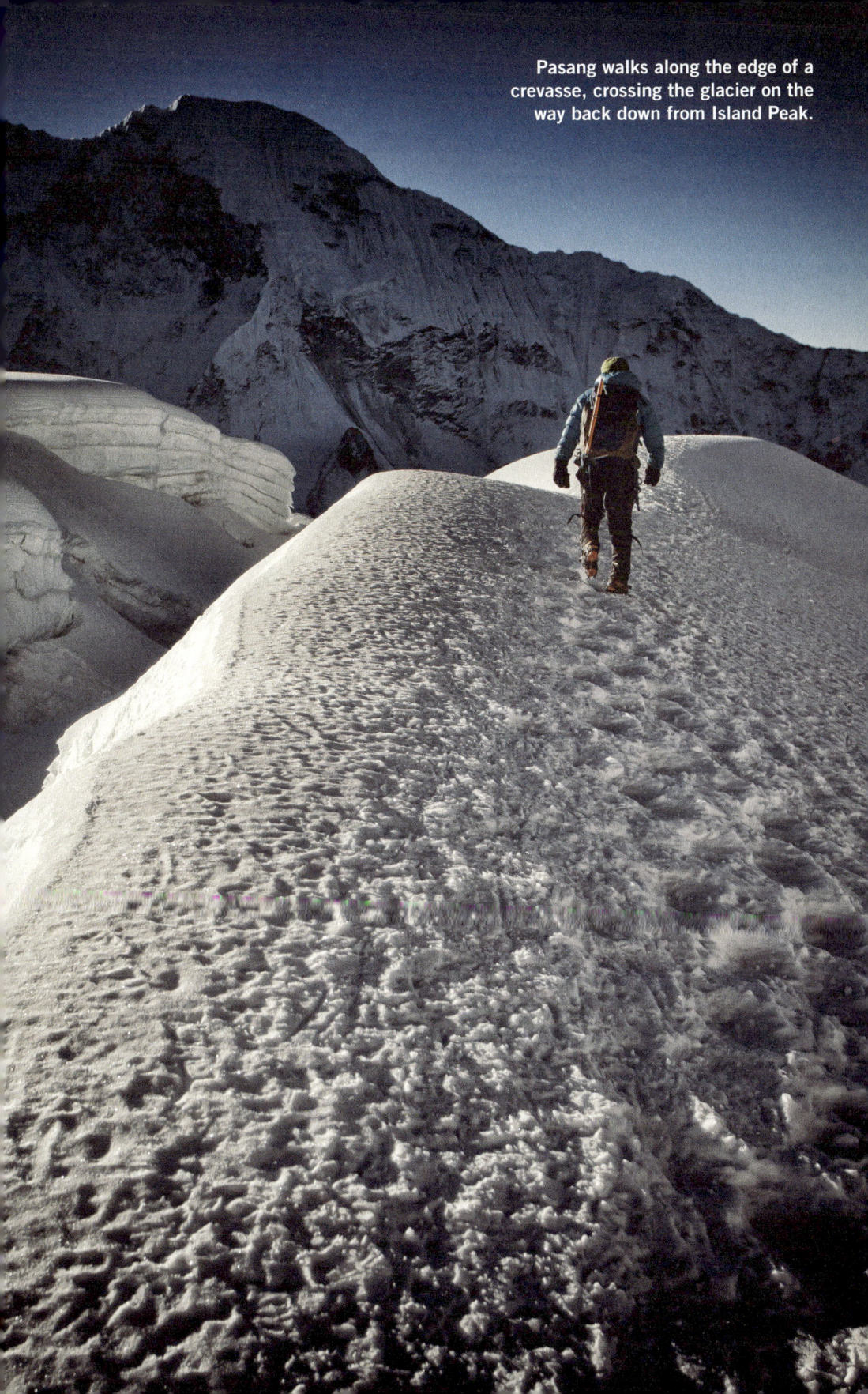
Pasang walks along the edge of a crevasse, crossing the glacier on the way back down from Island Peak.

'Yeah, great. The feet are a little bit cold, but not too bad.' I sat down and started digging out my gear for the next leg of the climb: my harness, ice axe and crampons.

The crampons were hard to put on in the cold, and difficult to attach with gloved hands. I ditched the gloves, and the tips of my fingers stuck momentarily to the frozen steel points, chilling my hands. I quickly laced the nylon webbing through the rings as tightly as I could, my hands becoming less deft by the moment as numbness set in.

We started up the steep ice ramp that led on to the glacier. My crampons squeaked as they shifted on the ice — the surface of the glacier was hard, frozen solid. As we walked from Crampon Point, up towards the large ice plateau that feeds the glacier, we first had to cross a large area of crevasses that had opened as this river of ice slid over an edge, fracturing under tension as it entered an icefall. The track, which followed slithers of ice between the crevasses, often came very close to the edge.

At one point I peered in, approaching the edge as close as I could without leaving the security of the well-formed footbed. Under the light from my headlamp the sides of the crevasse were an icy blue that faded into darkness, the bottom of the crevasse beyond the reach of my lamp. I suddenly got a sense of the precariousness of my position, gasped, looked straight ahead, and quickly walked on, using my ice axe with perfect plunge-step-step technique. The crevasses looked amazing as we zigzagged between them. There were often huge icicles round the edges, which made them appear like massive fanged mouths, hungry for a climber.

It was after we had crossed the crevasses and reached the ice plateau, at around 5900 metres, that I found myself feeling slightly dizzy and disconnected from my surroundings. I found it difficult to judge depth — something that happens only when I am extremely fatigued, or oxygen deprived. A flicker of fear rippled through my mind as I realised the potential implications.

I had experienced this feeling before, when I had traversed the ridge from Mt Robert to Angelus Hut in Nelson Lakes National Park earlier in the year. Dad and I were on our way to climb Mt Hopeless and I had used my altitude-training mask, set to +4000 metres, for the traverse of the Robert Ridge. I lasted for quite a number of hours, cruising along at a simulated altitude of about 5500 metres. At Julius Peak the nausea and dizziness really kicked in. The next one and a half hours were incredibly hard. I slogged my way along the ridge, feeling increasingly unwell but determined not to give in to the urge to remove the mask and take a deep breath. You won't be able to steal a breath of oxygen-rich air on Island Peak, so get used to it, I kept telling myself that day.

The rocky terrain of the ridge took on that sense of flatness that comes with the struggle to judge depth. I found it hard to walk over the loose rocks that form the path, and began to trip and stumble. Then, as we crossed the ridge above Fourth Basin, not far from the hut, I kept experiencing waves of exhaustion. My head was beginning to throb. Part of me still did not want to take the mask off. I was determined to complete the day's tramp with it on — which, given my physical condition, was entirely irrational. But when I looked down the scree slopes towards the hut I knew there was no way I could safely descend them and complete the tramp with the mask on.

I also knew that I would not have the energy, so I removed the mask, and somewhat begrudgingly took in lungfuls of oxygenated air. As I slowly made my way down to the hut my faculties gradually returned. While I was disappointed at not being able to complete the day's walk with the mask on, I was shocked at how strongly the lack of oxygen had impacted on my rational processes, and how quickly I had developed a form of altitude sickness.

That's why I was frightened when I started to feel dizzy and dazed on Island Peak. It was the first time I had experienced these effects on this trip. Was this altitude sickness? I wondered. What if it suddenly gets worse, like before? Once again I felt swamped by the fear of not being able to complete the climb.

Communication is good, I reminded myself. Don't be stupid about this, like last time.

'Hey, Pasang,' I called. 'I'm feeling a little bit dizzy and slightly dazed. It's not too bad, but I'm just letting you know.'

'OK,' Pasang responded. 'Take deep breaths and we go a bit slower. Tell me if it get worse.'

'OK,' I said, focusing on my breathing. It's OK if I have to turn back, I reminded myself. It's not the end of the world.

I looked at the stars, so bright above us. I stopped and covered my headlamp with my hand, allowing my eyes to adjust to the darkness. It was an astoundingly beautiful sky; the stars were so incredibly sharp. At altitude you don't necessarily see more stars, but you do see them with much greater clarity. I stood enveloped in the blackness, unable to see anything but the mass of detail above me, and felt a glimmer of peace.

I thought about the morning so far: it had been a truly beautiful experience, this journey into another world. Throughout the morning I had felt that sense of restful striving — the same as when I had climbed with Nina in the Remarkables. 'Restful' and 'striving' are not two feelings that often come together, but they are the words that captured the way I felt. I felt rested in the belief that my value was extrinsic to my person, undiminished by my failings. I had nothing to prove and there was nothing that I could lose. I took in a few deep breaths, enjoying the cool, fresh air. I looked at the stars for a while longer. The short break and deep breaths helped, and I felt the dizziness slowly subsiding.

'Nick!' shouted Pasang, now a fair distance ahead of me, his headlamp washing me in light. 'You OK?'

'All good,' I told him as I resumed the slow march onward. 'Just taking a quick breather.'

Kick, breathe; kick, breathe, stand. Pause and breathe. Plunge, breathe; zip, breathe, brace. I looked at my watch: 5.04 a.m., 6121 metres. We had crossed the plateau and had begun climbing the 200-metre, near-vertical ice ramp that would take us on to the summit ridge. I had been going at it for roughly 30 minutes: kicking my crampons into the ice, standing up on the front points, plunging my axe into the face, then zipping my jumar up the fixed rope, bracing for a moment in preparation to bring my feet up, repeating the process. The top had just come within view of my headlamp. I was close. This had been one of the hardest parts of the morning for me. The ascent up the ice ramp was tiring and it seemed to go on and on, becoming increasingly steep, until it was now near-vertical.

I paused, breathing as deeply as I could. It's amazing how altitude affects your body's ability to operate. You have so little energy, and a single step or action will require all you can muster from a single breath. I was not particularly exhausted, but energy production requires oxygen, and I was struggling to generate the energy I needed. The breaks were becoming more frequent — the air was getting thinner and I found myself huffing and puffing for longer. Making it more difficult was the hacking cough that I had developed. The air at altitude is so cold and so lacking humidity that it dries out the lining of your lungs, causing a dry, irritating cough that is difficult to suppress. But that's not to say I wasn't enjoying the experience — I was loving it.

I climbed up on to the summit ridge at 5.11 a.m. Pasang was coming up behind me. The ridge was knife-sharp and I grinned. There is something particularly thrilling about a knife-sharp ridge leading upward into the cloud or the darkness. The anatomy of the ridge was profoundly alluring as its curves and lines converged at a point ahead of me — a point still hidden from sight, promising the pleasure of breathtaking beauty. I could hardly wait for Pasang to reach the ridge and transfer us on to the set of safety lines that had been set up at the beginning of the season.

In 1997, when I was 12, Grandma and Papa had given me Colin Monteath's book *Hall and Ball: Kiwi Mountaineers* for Christmas. It was a large, full-colour book with pictures on every page, and I was completely enthralled by it. I had memorised the captions of the most significant photographs, and had read and reread the story as it recounted the highs and lows of the climbing careers of these two mountaineering giants, Rob Hall and Gary Ball.

The pictures that held my attention the most were those that showed sharp ridges leading to peaks. I would imagine myself as one of those people toiling upward towards the summit, moments away from seeing the view from the top and soaking in the splendour of a mountain panorama. One image I returned to over and over was a small photograph in the margin, at the bottom of a page. This was of Jan Arnold, her arms thrown into the air in pure elation, as she returned to Base Camp after successfully summiting Mt Everest. I loved this photo because of the joy it communicated, the thrill of completing a climb, and in time it came to symbolise all that I hoped mountaineering and the mountain experience would deliver.

And here I was, standing on a razor ridge moments away from the summit. I was enormously excited. Adding to the excitement was the precariousness of this final stage of the ascent. The ridge was only wide enough to support a single trail of footprints. On my left there was a 900-metre drop down into the Lhotse Glacier, and on my right the 200-metre drop down into the ice plateau we had just crossed. I already knew those drops were there, because I had studied the map, but when I looked the beam of my headlamp merely dissolved into the blackness below.

Pasang led the way along the ridge, checking the anchors that attached our safety line to the mountain. When we came to the last section of the line, however, he stepped aside to let me pass, so that I might reach the summit first. I was a little taken aback by this — it was not something I had expected. I did not feel my enjoyment would have been diminished if he had led the way and reached the summit before me, but nevertheless I felt humbled by his generosity and thoughtfulness in allowing me to experience the thrill of summiting first.

'Are you warm?' Pasang asked as I walked by.

'Yes, all good,' I said, smiling.

'Feet and hands OK?'

'Hands are fine, but my toes are a bit numb.'

'OK. It is very important you stay warm on the summit. Keep wiggling your toes, don't stop. And move your body if you start getting cold. Then you get no frostbite. OK?'

'OK, will do.'

'After you,' he said, gesturing with his ice axe.

Roughly half an hour had passed since we had first joined the ridge, and now the sky was just beginning to lighten with that pre-morning cast of blue, providing just enough light so that we could make out the ridges, faces and valleys around us. I looked up towards the summit. The light from the sky was beginning to find its reflection in the scalloped surface of the summit icecap, and now only the brightest stars were visible.

I felt a twinge of nervousness as I began moving, huffing and puffing, towards the summit. I kept coughing, trying to dislodge the tickle that wouldn't quite go away. Until this point I had not considered the act of summiting to be guaranteed, and I had refused the impulse to regard the summit as my destination. Realising that I was actually about to summit, I felt unready and slightly frightened, as if I was about to lose some sort of virginity. My childhood dream of summiting a Himalayan peak was about to be realised.

As I neared the top, the summits beyond Island Peak began to appear in my field of view. I felt a rush of excitement and I tried to pick up my pace. Step, pause, step, breathe; plunge, zip, breathe. Micro-pause and pull. Repeat. The last little bit was steep. Equipped with my jumar, I pulled hard on the safety line, dragging myself up, before zipping it along the line again. Step, pause, step, breathe; plunge, zip, breathe. Micro-pause and pull. The ice glistened with the gentle swaying of my headlamp. I looked up again. Now it was not just the distant peaks that I could see, but also the faces and heads of the valleys. Step, step, breathe; plunge, zip, pull, breathe. My breathing became shallow as I pushed up the last few metres and the view began to unfold. My rapid breaths were burning in my chest as I fought the urge to cough. Step, step, plunge, breathe; zip, pull, step, freeze.

As I stepped up on to the small ice platform on the summit I was enveloped in the most intense wave of excitement that I had ever experienced.

It felt as if the world had fallen away around me. Sheer faces and enormous peaks surrounded me. Never had I felt so alive, never had I been so astounded by a view. The sense of height and the scale of the mountains was absolutely exhilarating.

'Woohoo!' I screamed. There were no other words to describe the moment.

'We made it, Pasang!' I shouted, both my arms in the air. 'Wow! Well done!'

I looked around, at the stunning tooth-like peak of Ama Dablam, to Baruntse, and then to distant Makalu. I turned, and there was the gentle pyramid of Lhotse Shar, and then the overwhelming mass of Lhotse and Nuptse, rising like a cresting wave above us.

'Woohoo!' I screamed again. 'This is amazing!'

'Five forty-five, which means it takes —' Pasang started to count on his fingers — 'two, three, four, five. Four hours and half. Quite fast, we are.'

'Wow!' Normally it takes climbers between seven and nine hours to summit.

'This is amazing!' I laughed, blown away by our speed, and the fact that I had made it. I had so enjoyed the morning that summiting seemed like an unexpected bonus, a surprise. I just could not get over it. Words failed me.

'Unbelievable,' I said under my breath, then I just stood in dumbfounded silence, admiring the view.

The sun began to light the edges of Lhotse, lacing it with gold. I turned round again and watched the light catch the top of Ama Dablam, warm rays working their way down the face.

'Gosh, Ama Dablam is a magnificent mountain. It's hard to take your eyes off it, isn't it?'

'Yeah. So beautiful,' Pasang replied.

The light hit the next row of peaks — Cholatse and Tabuche among them — and then the next, and the next. One by one, peaks on the distant horizon were aflame, welcomed into the new day. There was an amazing sense of the earth revolving under the sun, of a new day in progress, of time in relation to distance.

'Such clear weather,' Pasang finally said, breaking the silence.

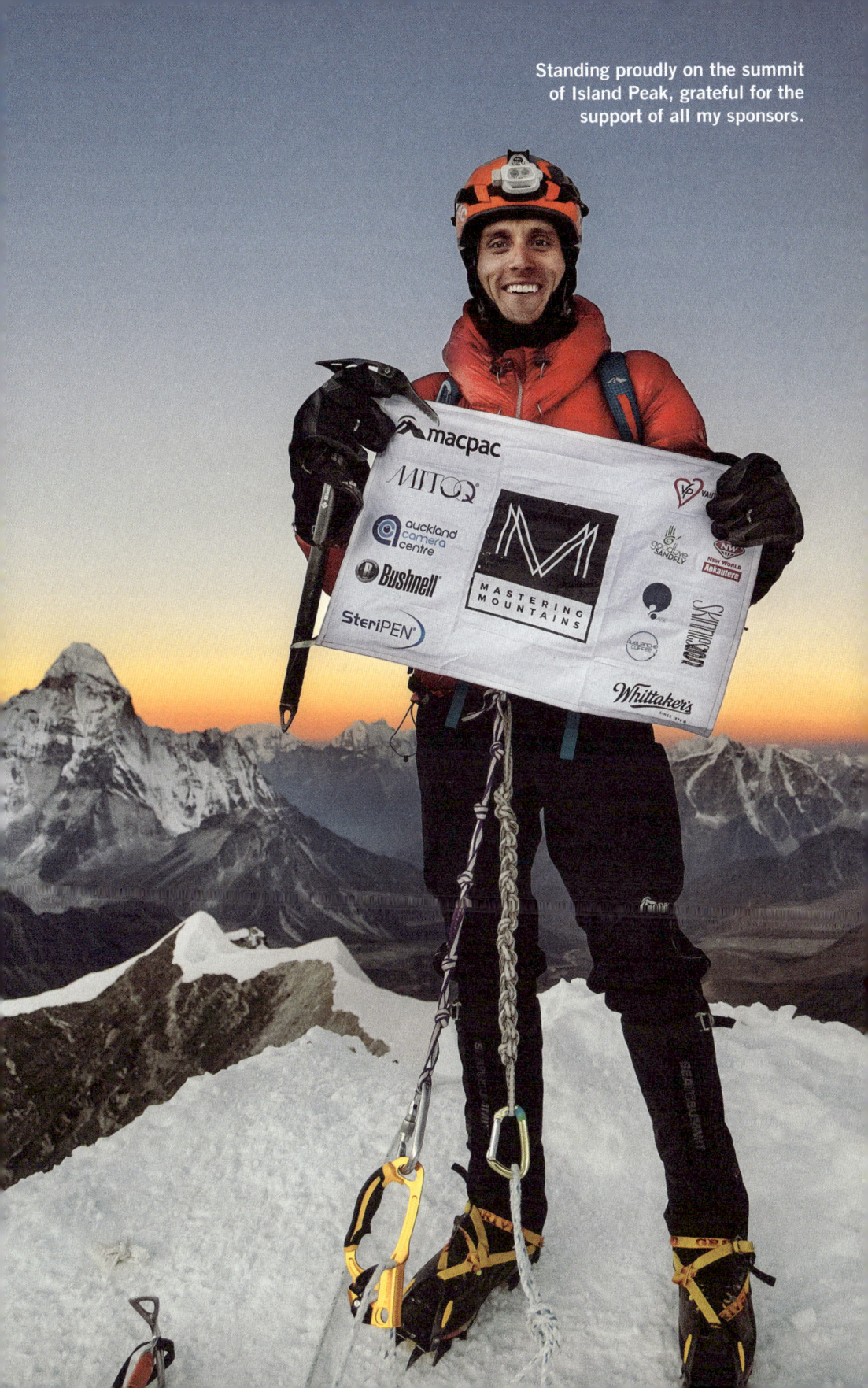
Standing proudly on the summit of Island Peak, grateful for the support of all my sponsors.

282 TO THE SUMMIT

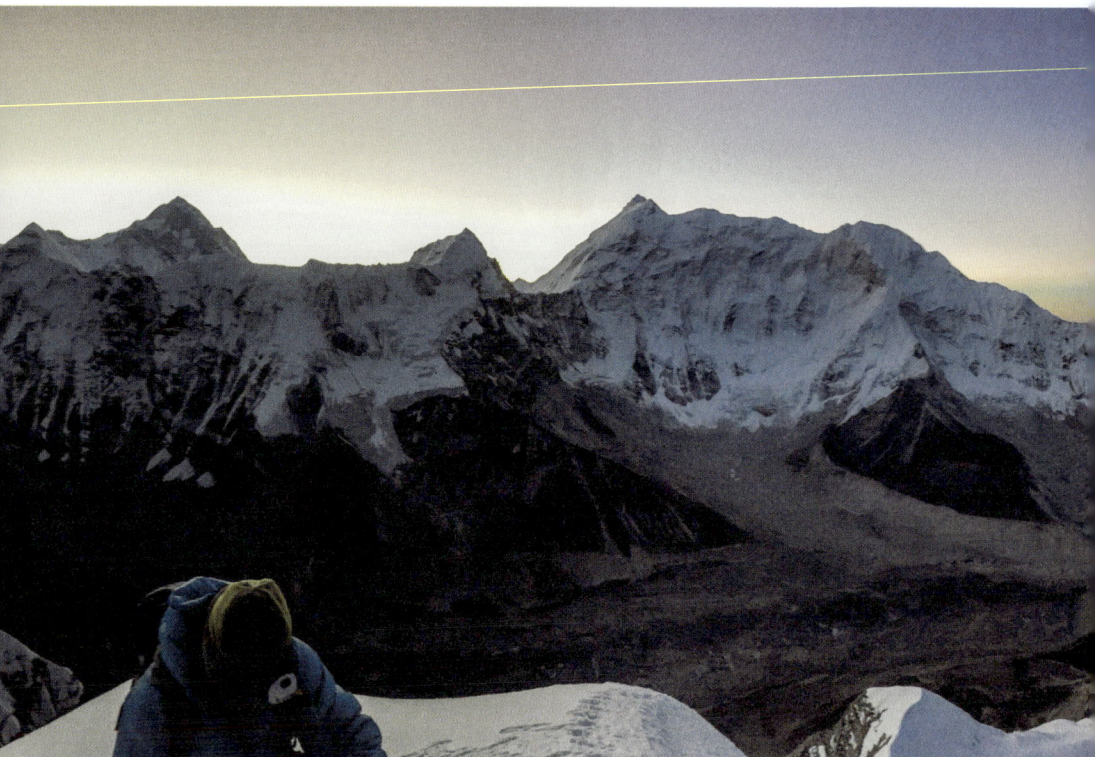

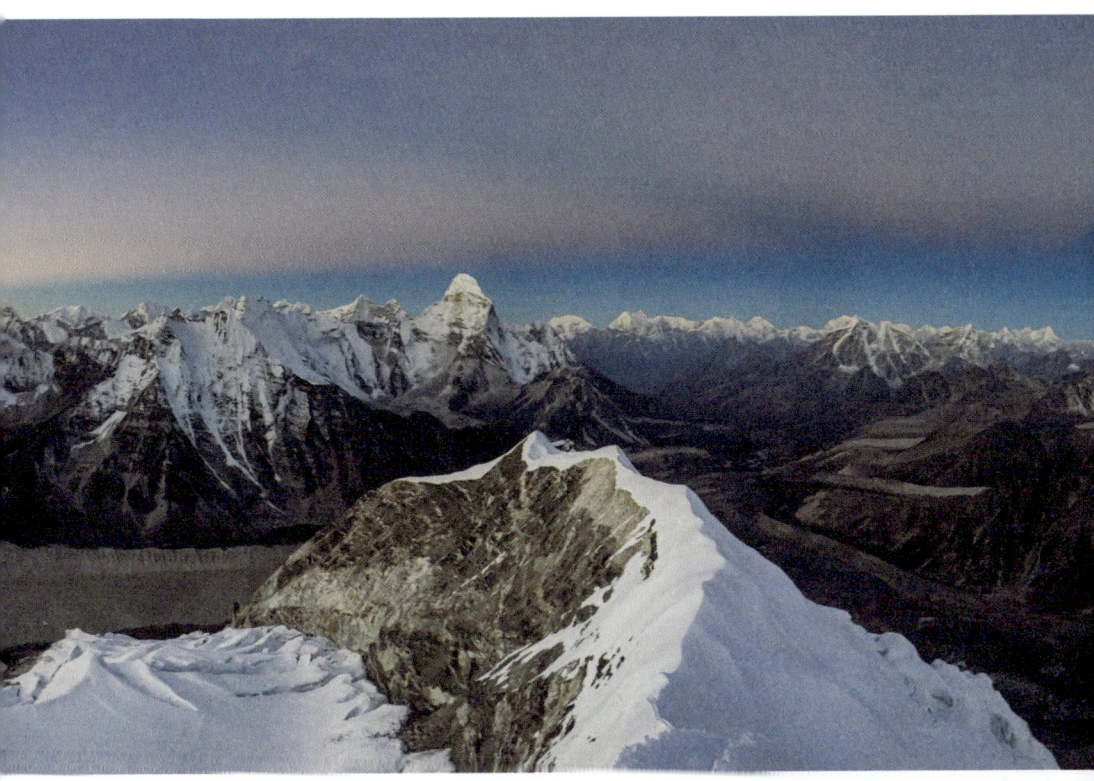

The sky erupting in colour with the rising sun. The summit ridge and glacier is beneath us, Ama Dablam rises sharply on the right, while Kali Himal and Makalu dominate the skyline on the left.

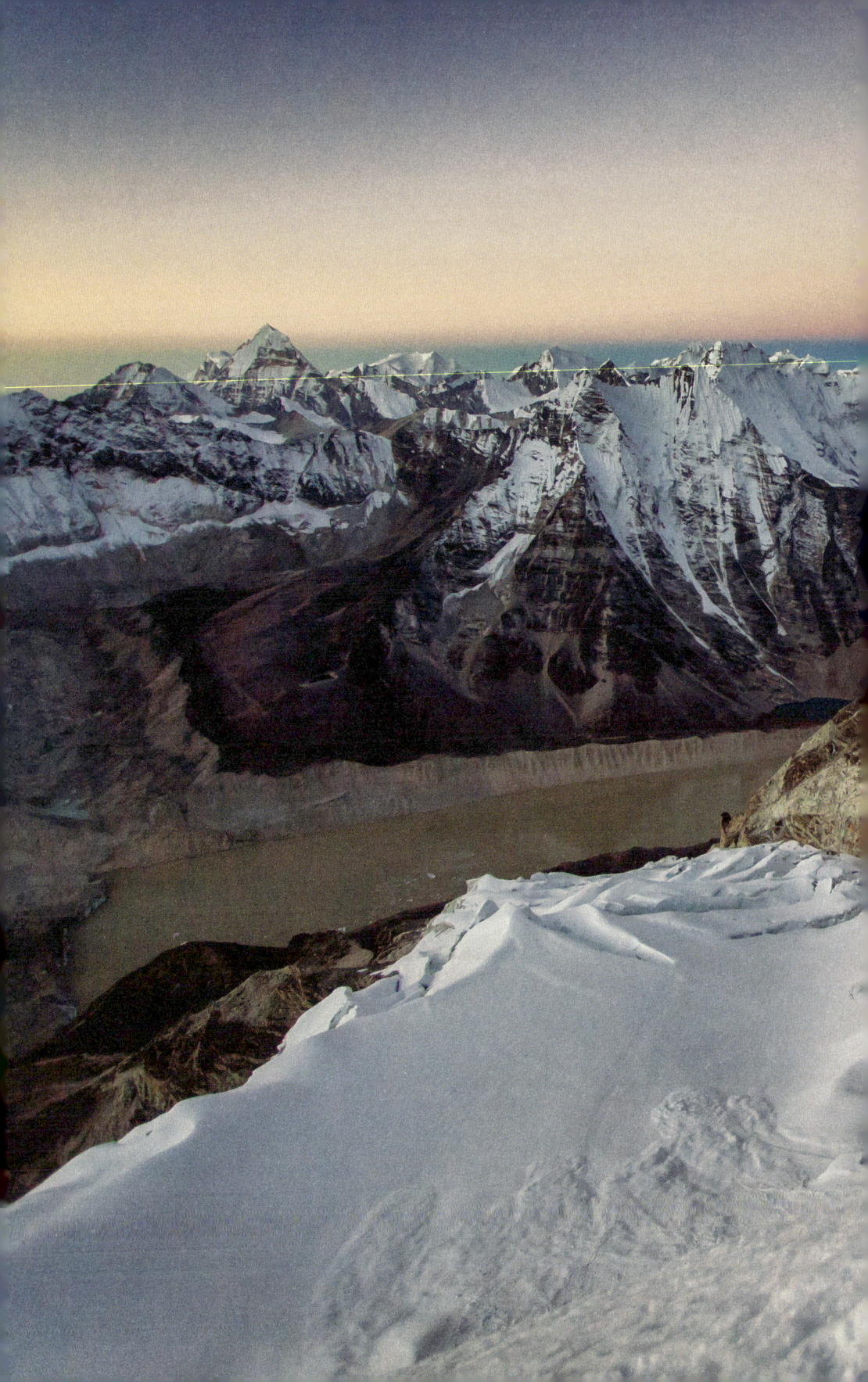

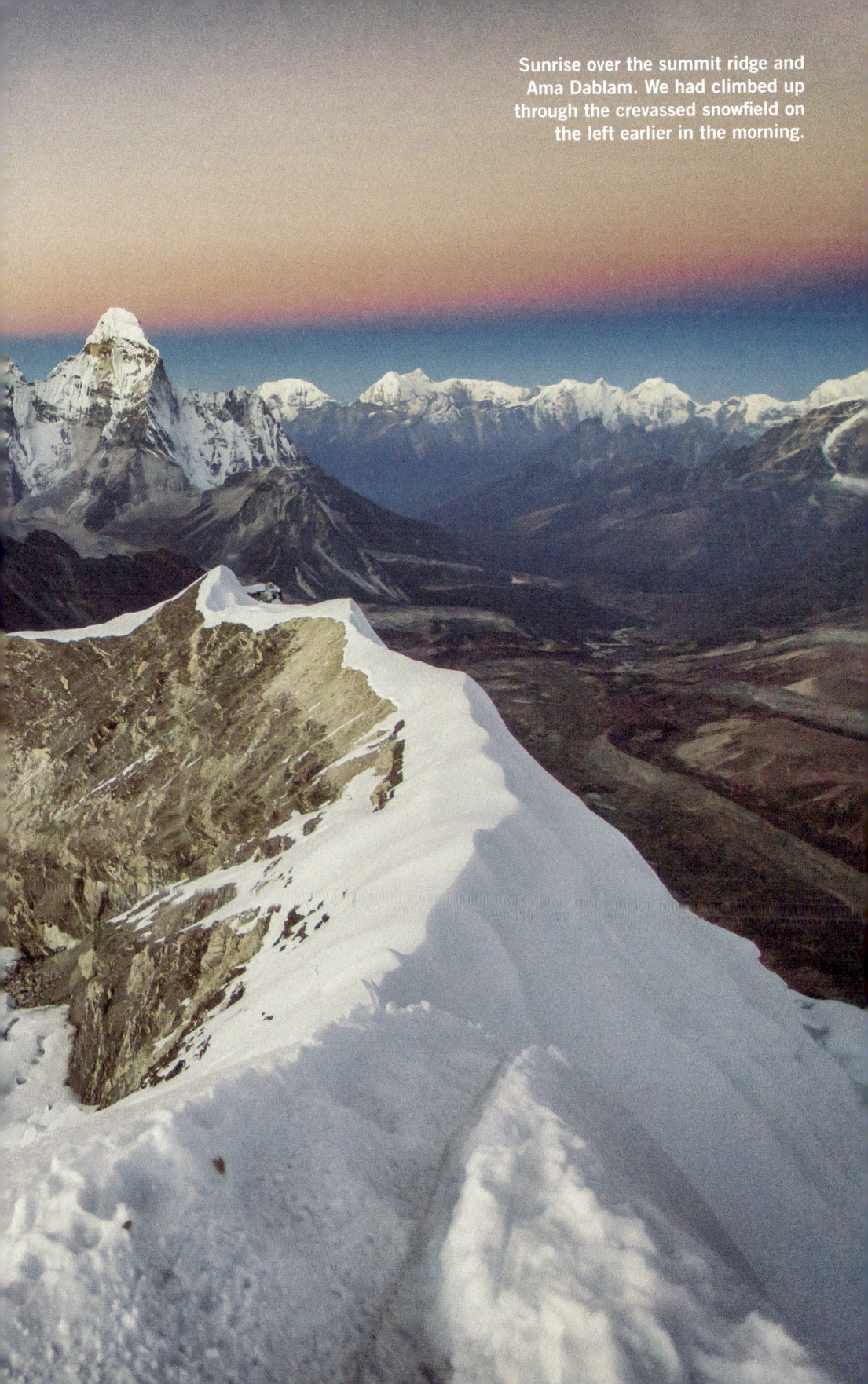

Sunrise over the summit ridge and Ama Dablam. We had climbed up through the crevassed snowfield on the left earlier in the morning.

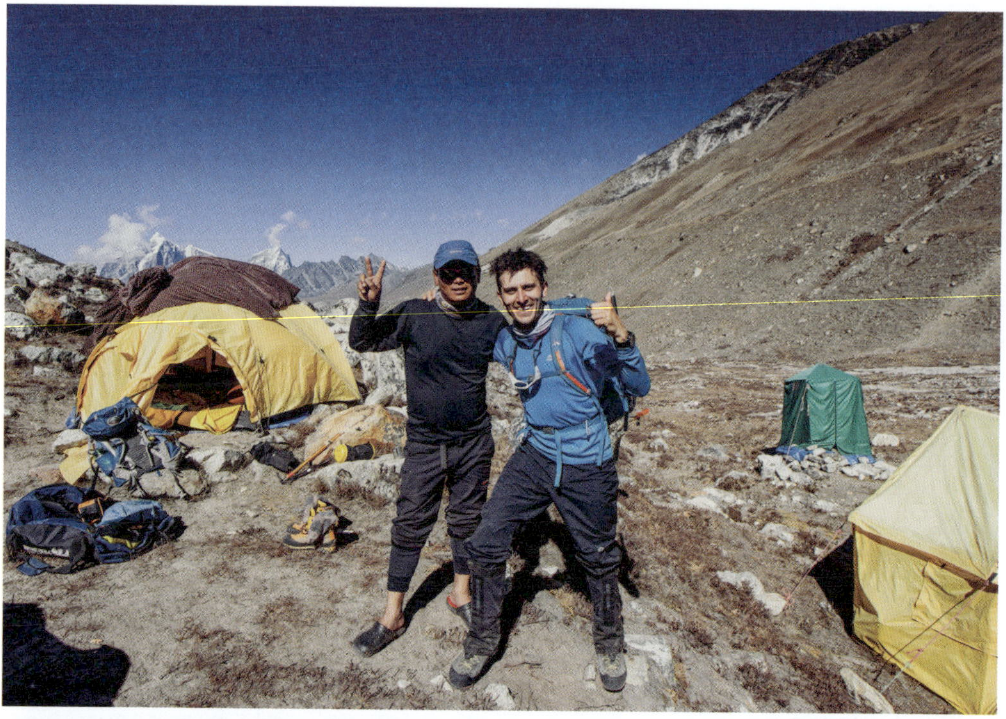

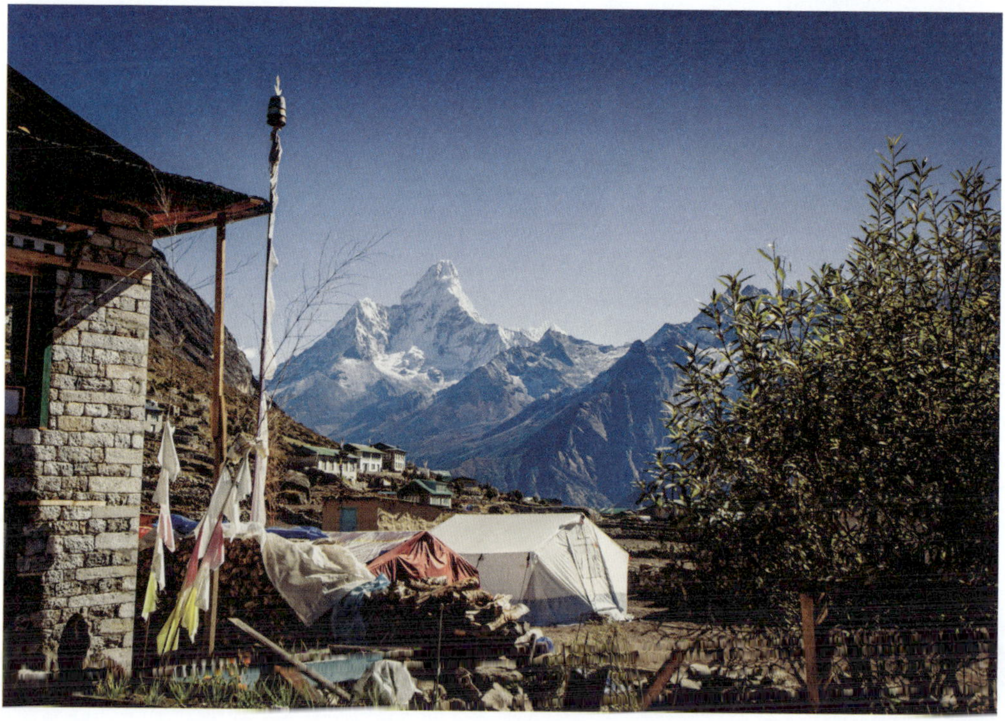

Top to bottom: Back at Island Peak Base Camp;
The view of Ama Dablam from the Khumjung teahouse.

There was not a breath of wind, nor even a cloud in the sky.

The mountains were more beautiful than I could describe. Looking down into the valleys, across and into the cols, I again felt an incredible sense of opportunity and potential. As I had at Ball Pass, I felt as if the sky posed no limit, and that there was incredible beauty out there, waiting to be known.

'We made it, man,' Pasang said with a grin.

'We made it!' I screamed, fist pumping the air. I was once again filled with a sense of exhilaration. I could hardly believe it.

Pasang laughed.

'This is your first step,' he said, smiling. 'Next Ama Dablam.'

'You reckon?' I asked, grinning, giddy at the thought.

'Yeah, you do it no problem.'

I smiled and turned my face towards the rising sun.

'Remember this?' I asked Pasang. I'd had my GoPro camera on my helmet during the climb, and I showed Pasang the video of the two of us summiting. I had been watching it over and over all morning. That moment when I had reached the top, had summited, still sent chills down my spine. I could hardly believe that we had done it. I felt profoundly grateful.

Pasang smiled.

'That was very good morning.'

'Man, it sure was,' I said, shaking my head.

Seven days had passed since then, and now we were sitting in the sun outside our guest house in Khumjung. I was enjoying feeling the warmth soaking into my bones.

'How you feeling?' Pasang asked.

'Pretty terrible, eh, just shattered. It's still just so hard to breathe.'

After summiting Island Peak we had returned to Chukhung for a rest day, then headed over Kongma La Pass towards Everest Base Camp. I had developed a case of what's known as the Khumbu Cough, which occurs when the inside of your lungs crack from the cold,

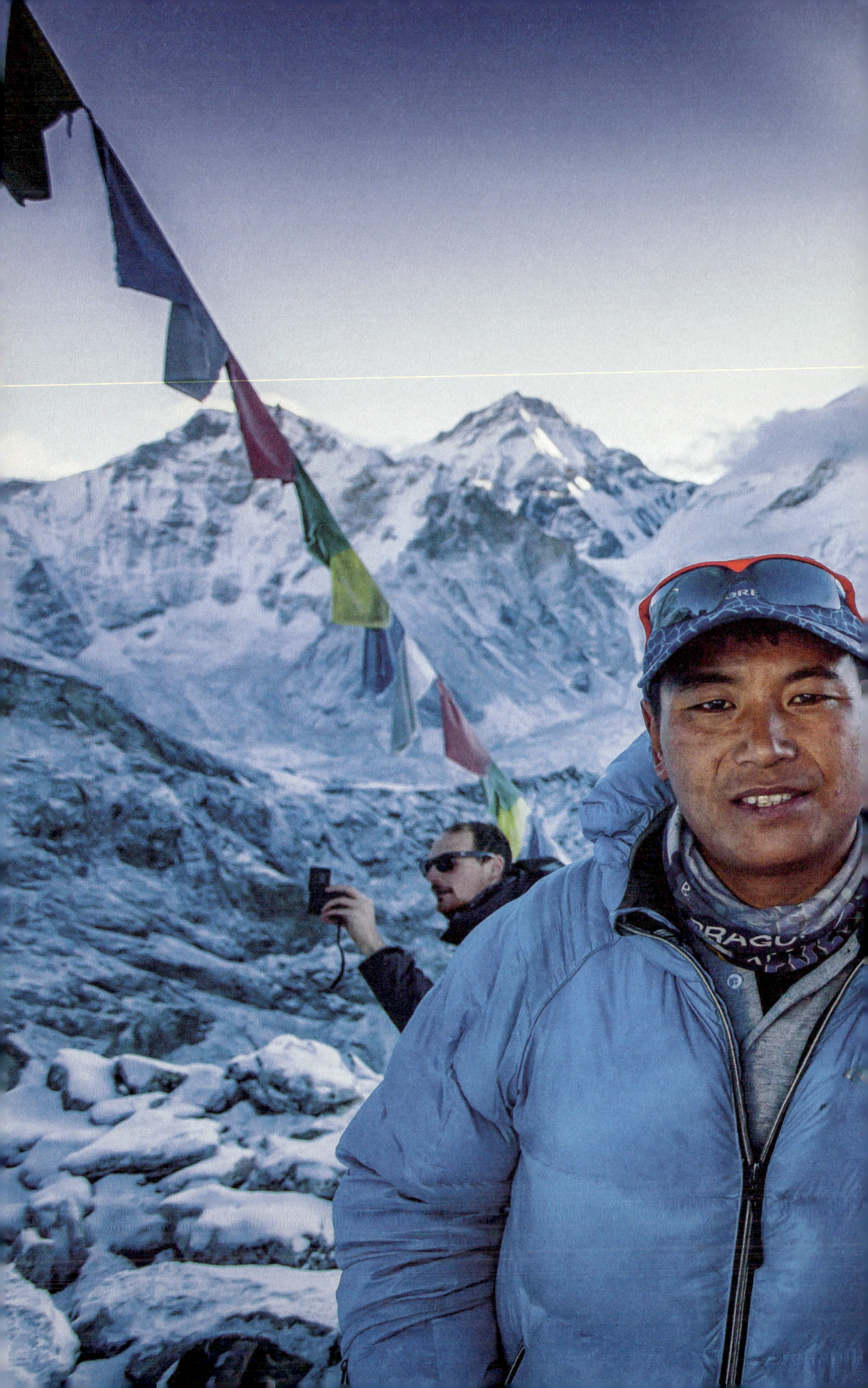

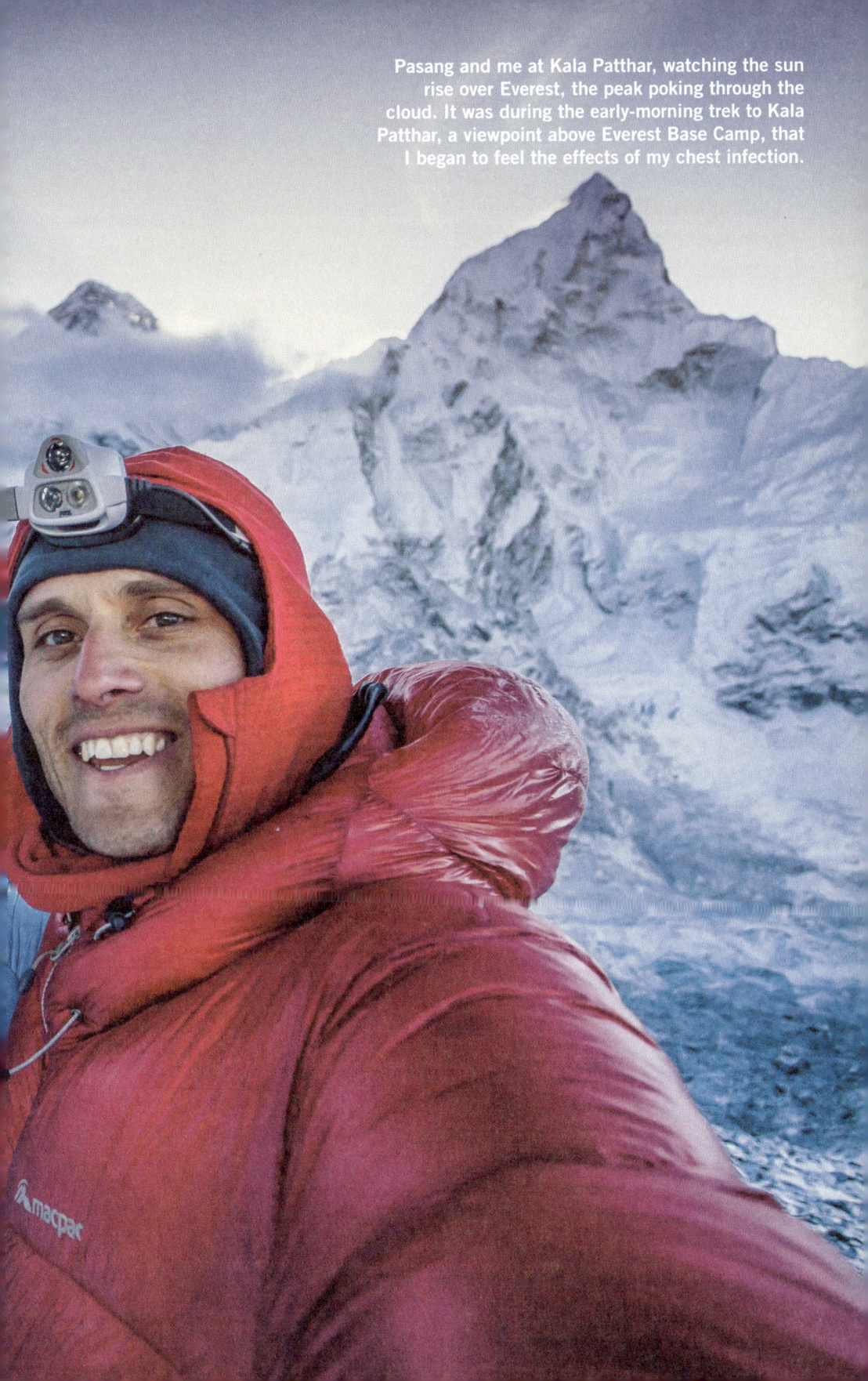

Pasang and me at Kala Patthar, watching the sun rise over Everest, the peak poking through the cloud. It was during the early-morning trek to Kala Patthar, a viewpoint above Everest Base Camp, that I began to feel the effects of my chest infection.

dry air. Although we'd made it to Everest Base Camp, and had gone on to climb Kala Patthar and watch the sun rise over Everest, I had struggled. My chest had burned all the way up and I felt exhausted coming down.

We had decided to return to the lower altitude of Khumjung so that I could recover, but my cough had developed into a full-blown chest infection, and now I felt absolutely exhausted. I was also worried about the MS playing up. I had begun to experience a few balance problems and I felt extremely lethargic, so we had decided to cut the trip short by a week.

'I think it good to get you back to Kathmandu — the doctors are better there. You look very, very sick — like a ghost,' Pasang said. 'Next time, I think we make more rest days. And we take canned tuna for you. You have lost too much weight — you are too thin and too weak.'

'Oh, cheers, bro.' I smiled and winked. 'Yes, I agree. More rest and more fish and protein will definitely be the way to go. I don't think dal bhat is enough all on its own — not enough protein.'

'What, dal-bhat power don't last twenty-four hour?'

We both laughed. I coughed.

'And I think you're right, more rest days would be good next time. But I also think I need to learn how to rest better. I was too worried about writing my blog post when we got back from Island Peak and I didn't rest properly. Resting is an art, I reckon — and a jolly hard one too.'

Pasang smiled.

I closed my eyes and returned to my enjoyment of the sun. I wondered briefly what Gerwyn was up to. After I'd left Leh and flown back to meet him in Delhi we'd flown to Kathmandu together, then he'd gone off to see a friend whose house had been destroyed in the April earthquake while I was climbing. He was due to arrive back in Kathmandu a few days after me. It would be good to see him again.

'It's been an absolutely amazing trip, Pasang. Thank you so much for your help. You've been incredible.'

'Thank you,' Pasang replied 'We have been very blessed.'

'Yes, very blessed.' I nodded. 'I'm going to be super-sad leaving, I must say. I just love it up here. It is so beautiful. I'm going to miss it a lot. But, at the same time, I feel at peace — I don't have anything to prove, and I have nothing to lose. It's all good. Island Peak was amazing. I feel very grateful.'

'You be back soon,' Pasang said, nodding towards Ama Dablam.

'I think you're right.' I grinned. 'You still reckon I would make it?'

'Yeah, no problem. Just next time we get you some tuna.'

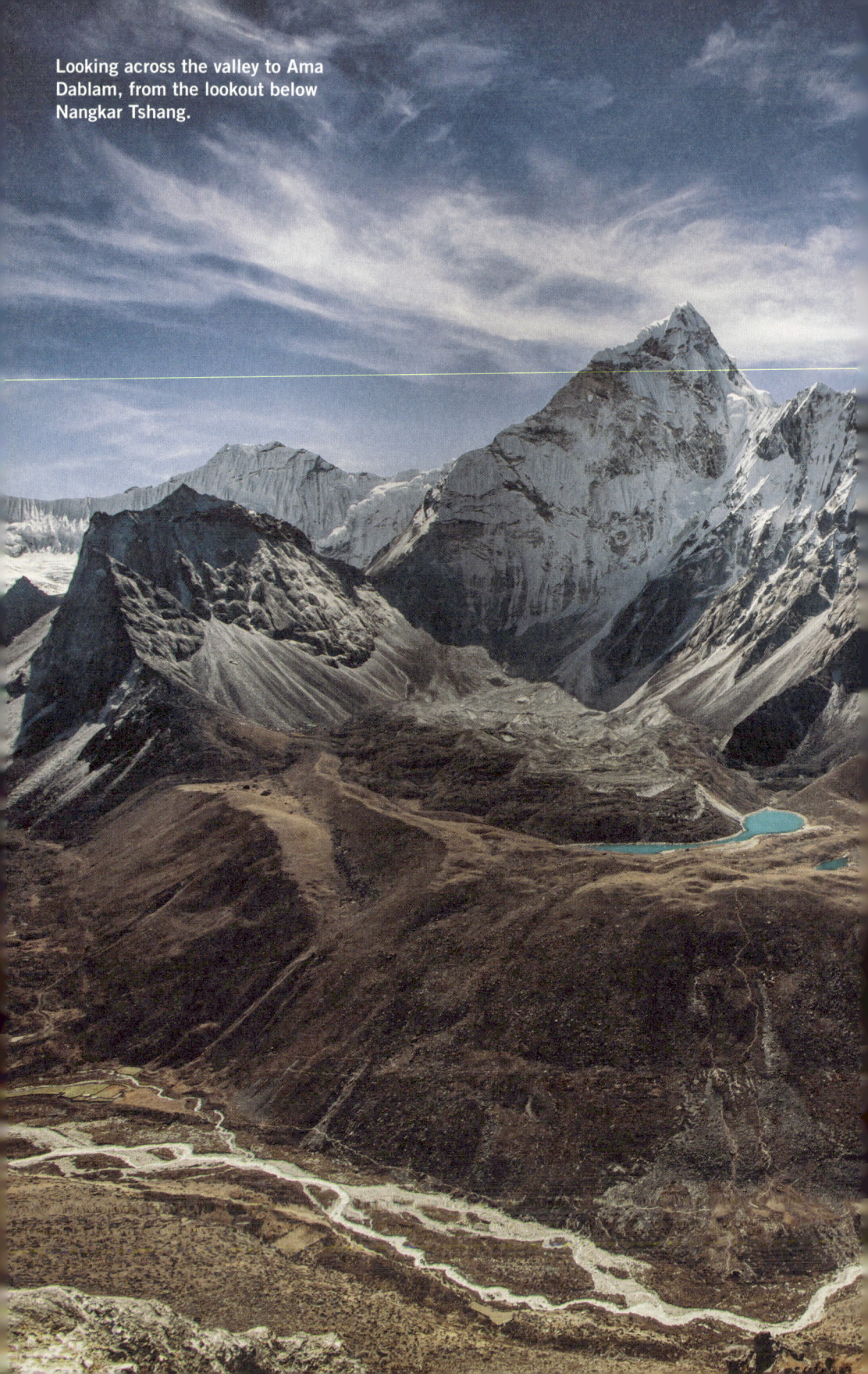
Looking across the valley to Ama Dablam, from the lookout below Nangkar Tshang.

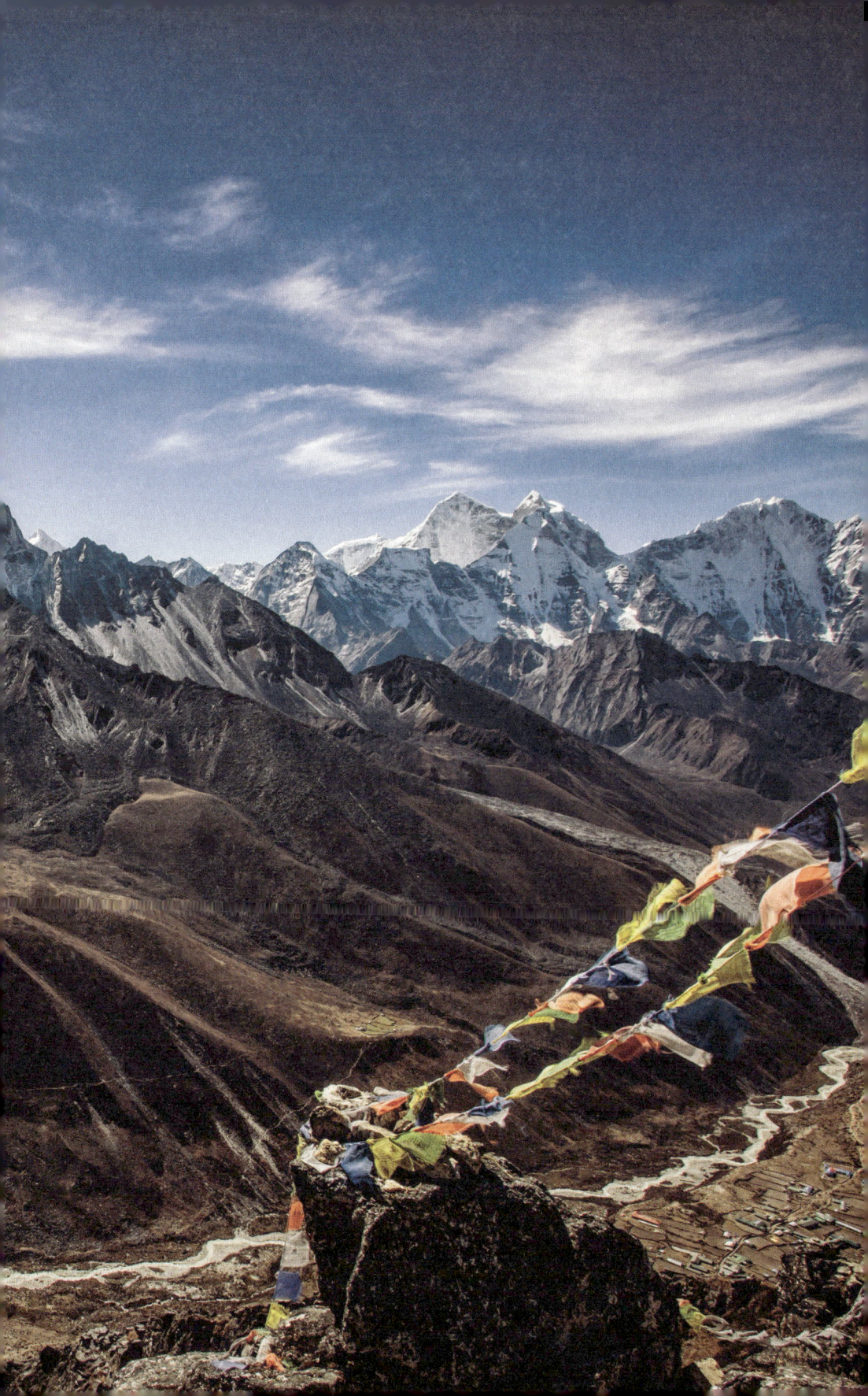

AFTERWORD: MASTERING MOUNTAINS

Writing this book has been the hardest single thing I have done in my life — much harder than climbing Island Peak. I knew it was going to be hard work, trying to bring all this together in three short months. What I was not prepared for was the emotional and physical response to revisiting many of these points in my life.

I realise now that there were many periods of my life — most of them the most difficult times — when I wanted to grieve, but I had refused to engage in that process. Writing this book and revisiting those tough times that I had tried to forget was very confronting and, at moments, left me overwhelmed by grief. Although it was not pleasant, I am incredibly grateful for this process, as it has made me more grateful for grace.

Physically, writing this book has been tough as well. The MS has been playing up quite significantly, the consequence of not resting after my return to New Zealand from Nepal. Nevertheless, it has also been a joy to write and incredibly cathartic.

Coming back from my trip to India and Nepal, I felt excited about the Mastering Mountains Charitable Trust and its goals. When I first created the trust in 2015, its purpose was to establish and support a scholarship programme that would enable people with MS to get into the outdoors again. However, the purpose of the trust has evolved with time, and it has become more clear to me as I have talked to other people and travelled overseas.

When I reflect on all the factors that carried me to the summit of Island Peak several stand out, and these form the core of Mastering Mountains' goals. First, the importance of gracious community. The trust aims to support people with MS as they make changes by providing an environment in which they can be vulnerable and weak, yet accepted.

Second, the realisation that I could take control of my MS, and that it did not have to mean the end of a rich life, was pivotal in my decision to resume climbing. Again, the trust hopes to help change perceptions around MS, making people aware that, while it brings change to a person's life, it does not necessarily have to bring an end to the pursuit of their passions. Closely related to this, Mastering Mountains also hopes to highlight the importance of correct nutrition, lifestyle choices and exercise as a means of remaining healthy with MS.

Finally, the need for financial support. During many of my lowest times my parents have been a support to me in many ways, including financially. I could not have got this far without them. For this reason, the Mastering Mountains Charitable Trust, working together with Multiple Sclerosis New Zealand, will sponsor people so that they can get out and enjoy nature or pursue their own passion.

You can find out more about the trust at masteringmountains.org.

September 2016
Palmerston North, New Zealand

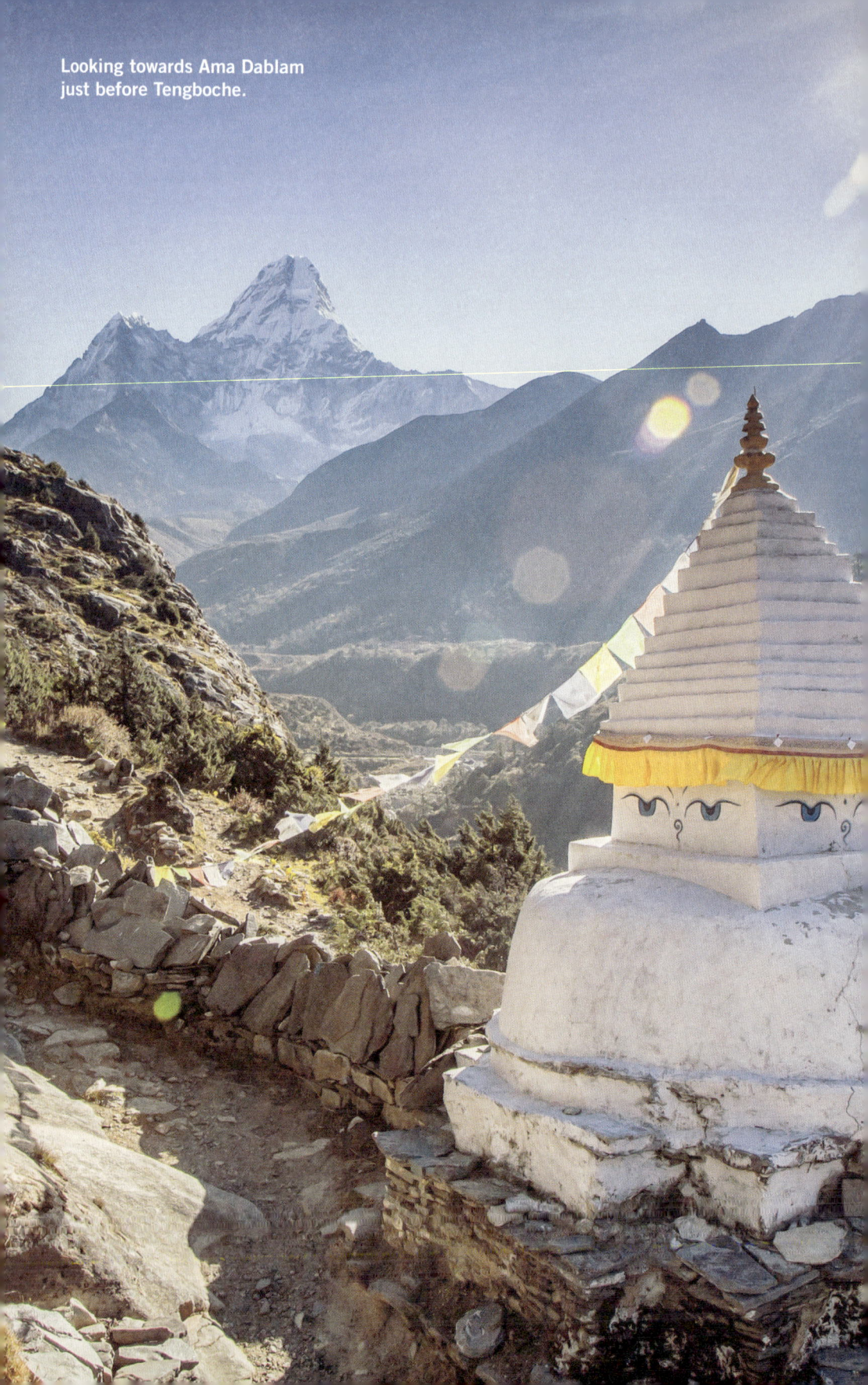
Looking towards Ama Dablam just before Tengboche.

ACKNOWLEDGEMENTS

There are so many people I should thank for getting me to this point. So many people have had an impact on my life — more than I could list. Nevertheless, those who have been the greatest help and support are my family. My parents, Peter and Alex, have always been there for me, ready to help and support me. Mum has been amazing in her tenacity as she has figured out a diet that works for me, and for being a shoulder to cry on. Dad has been an amazing support as well, going with me to doctors' appointments, taking me tramping and carrying most of my gear, and massaging my legs when they tighten up with spasticity. A big thanks go to my siblings — Fleur, Jonathan and Charles — for being patient with me.

My grandparents have also had a huge impact on my life. Grandma and Papa, Grummy and Jimpo, all fuelled my love for mountaineering and tramping by giving me books, boots and climbing gear for various birthday and Christmas presents. Mopsy and Popsy, in my frequent trips with them out on the Waitemata, developed my love of the wind, the sea and desolate places — a love that still finds expression in my love of the mountains. All of them have been an amazing support, and I love them dearly.

A big thank you also goes to my extended family, to my aunts and uncles, and in particular to Aunty Kate, for teaching me how to use a camera, and to Uncle John, for being a great friend.

A number of people in the USA deserve my thanks. First among them, Joey and David Brame, who had an amazing influence on my understanding of grace, for which I will be forever grateful. Thanks also to Jonathan Brown for being a true brother, helping me to work through many of the complex issues I faced in the US, and to Bert and Marie Walker, and Marc and Helen Chetta, for their incredible hospitality and generosity to me, and for their medical support during my times of struggle. I would also like to thank Julie and Mel Lacock for their friendship and generosity in supporting me in healthy eating.

I have found great encouragement and support in several communities in New Zealand. To Nina, Mark and Helen, thank you for providing a gracious climbing community, allowing me to join in despite my limitations. Nina and her husband Peter have also been huge and active supporters of Mastering Mountains. I would also like to thank Nina for her care and concern, for checking up on me, and for reading the medical sections of this book.

Thank you to my church family for their gracious support and regular encouragement.

In my opinion, Macpac Palmerston North is the best store in the country, largely as a result of the awesome management by Jody and Lana. As all these ideas started formulating in my mind, Jody encouraged me to pursue my dream of climbing. Lana, who was an amazing support while I was away, has been incredibly patient with me during my recent physical struggles and while writing this book. Thanks also go to my great work colleagues for their encouragement and friendship.

Without training at the gym under the careful eyes of Freya Thompson and Liam Barendsen there is no way I could have made it this far. A huge thank you goes out to these two, and especially Freya, for all their hard work in getting me ready.

I am also indebted to the amazing and continued support of Macpac and MitoQ. Macpac has been a most generous sponsor, providing me with a good deal of gear, as has MitoQ, who supply me with an energy supplement that has helped me significantly, both while climbing and particularly during the writing of this book. In addition, I am deeply grateful for the support from Ask Design, Auckland Camera

Centre, Avalanche Coffee, Bushnell, Goodbye Sandfly, New World Aokautere, Skinnies Sungel, SteriPen and Whittaker's Chocolate.

Finally, I would like to acknowledge the help and support of Multiple Sclerosis New Zealand. Philippa Russell from MS Central Districts deserves a huge thank you for her tireless work, and for her help in getting Mastering Mountains started. I would also like to thank Amanda Keefe and the board of MSNZ for their support of Mastering Mountains Charitable Trust, and for helping to set up the scholarship programme.

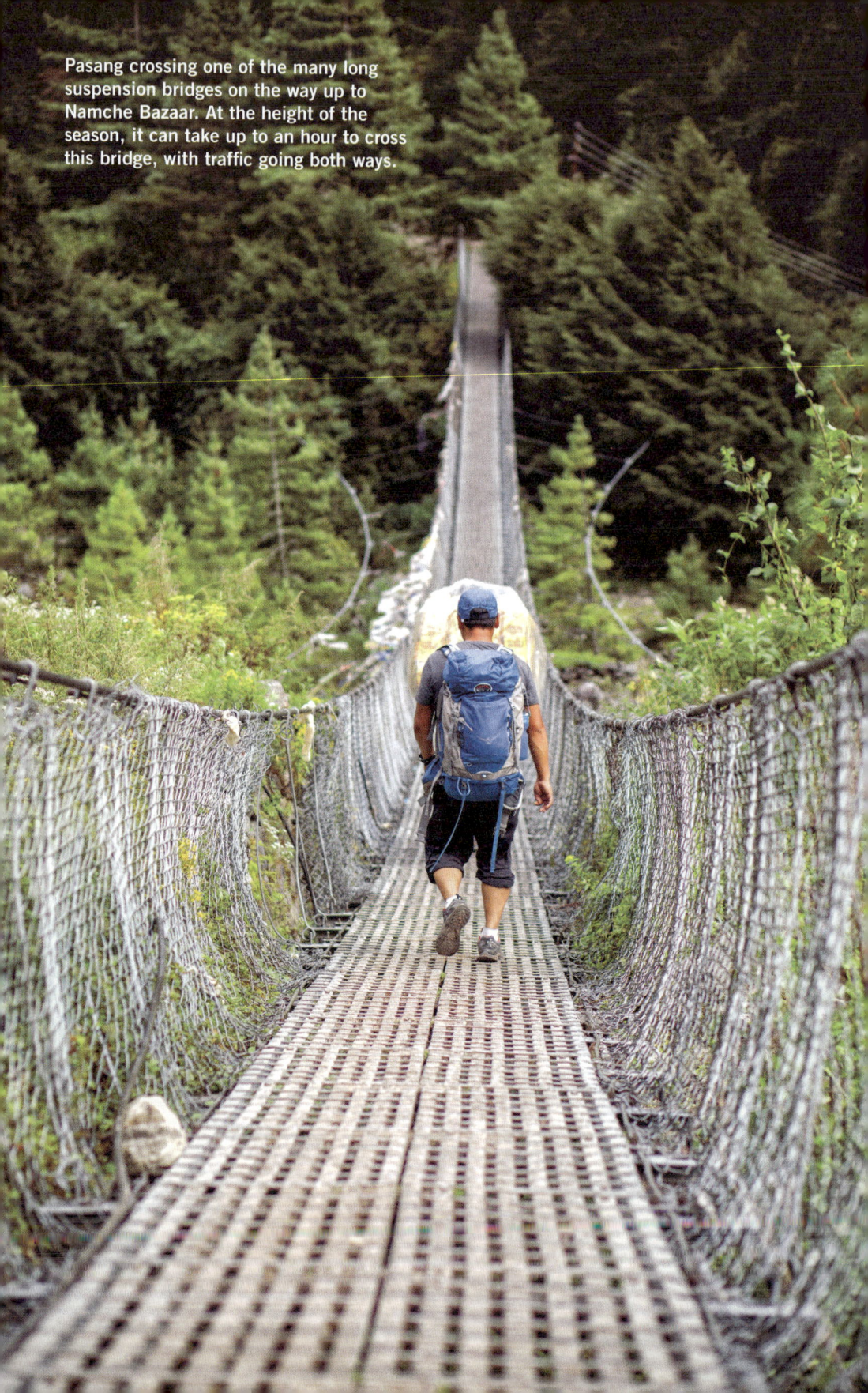

Pasang crossing one of the many long suspension bridges on the way up to Namche Bazaar. At the height of the season, it can take up to an hour to cross this bridge, with traffic going both ways.

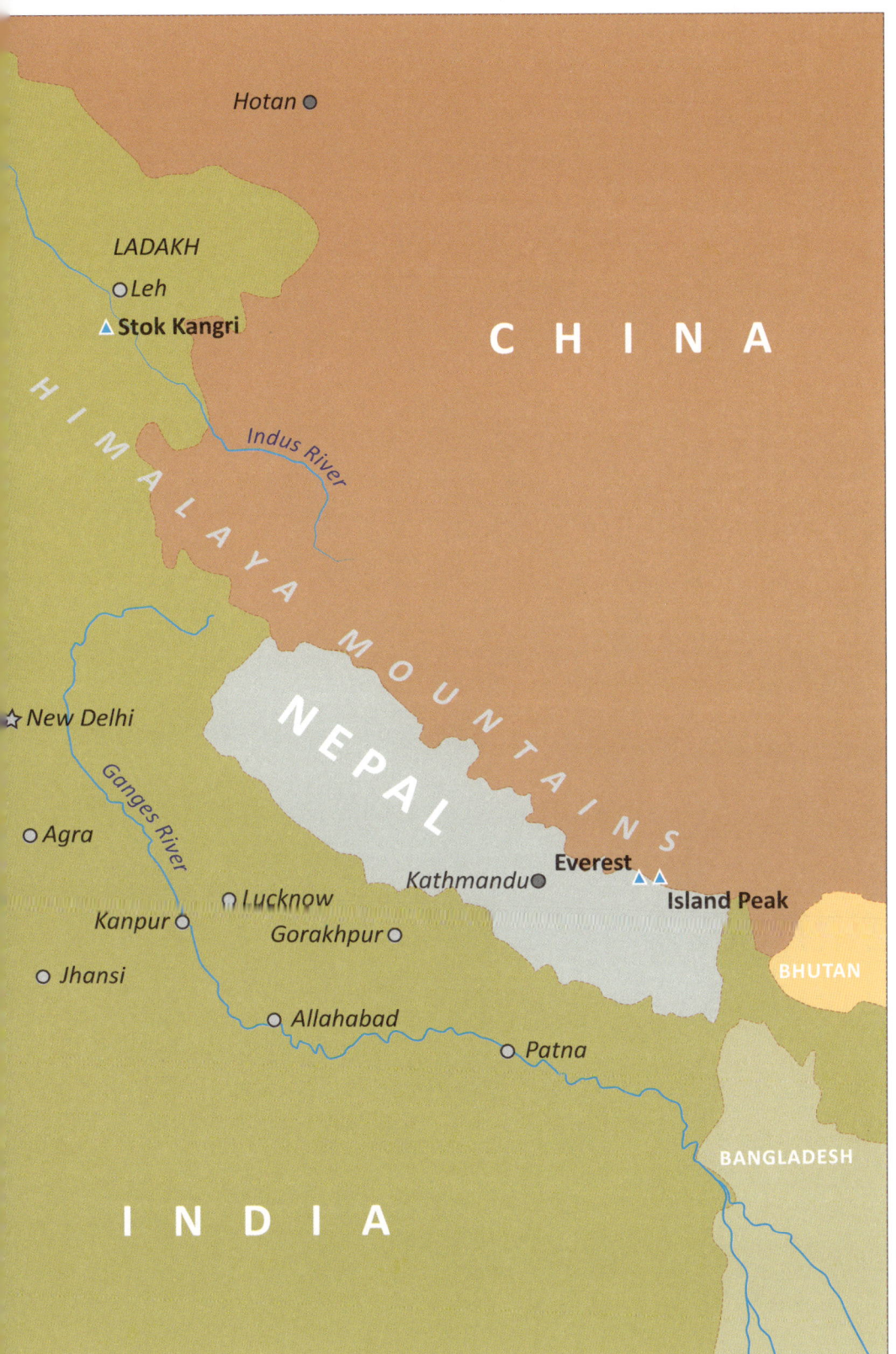

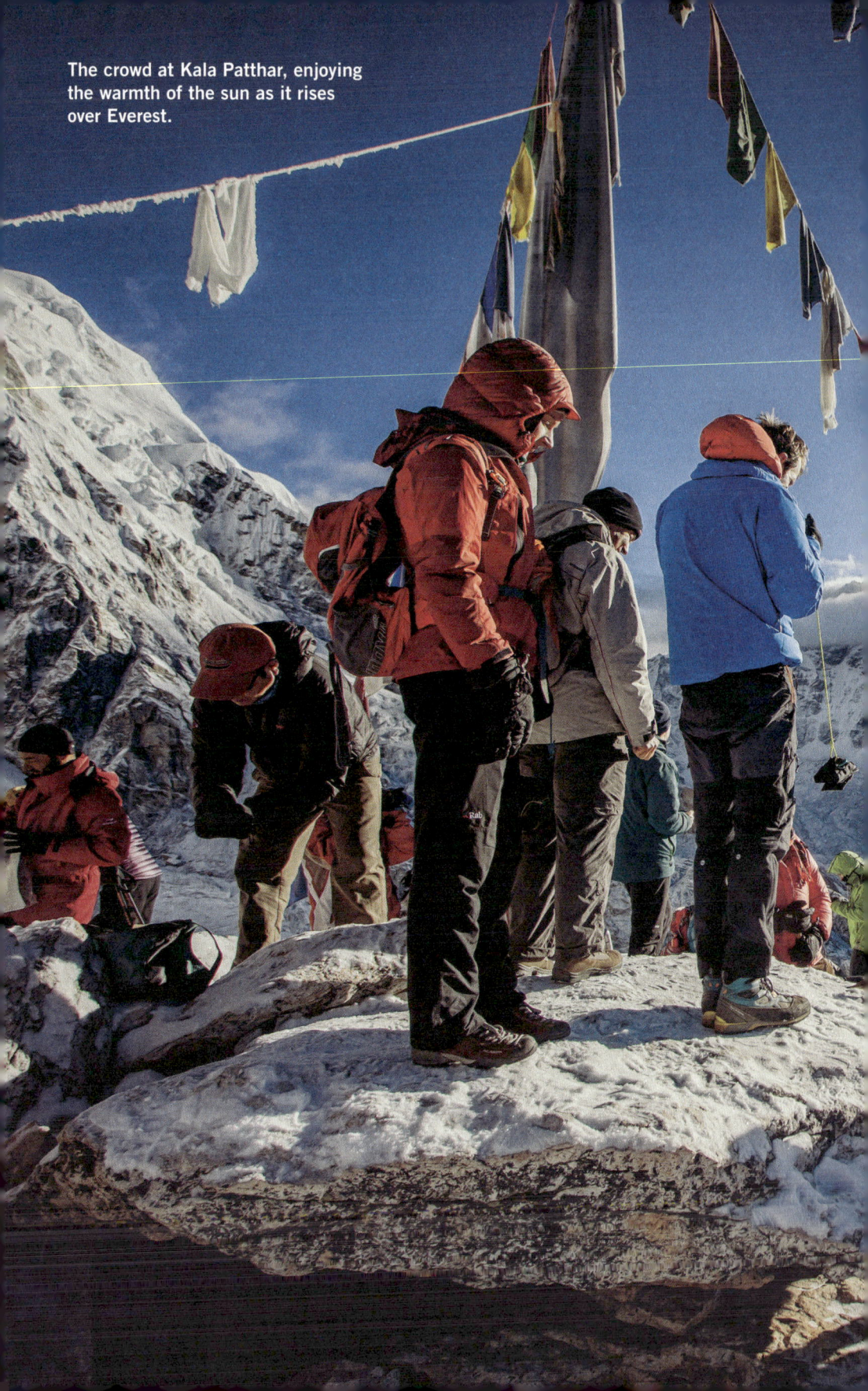
The crowd at Kala Patthar, enjoying the warmth of the sun as it rises over Everest.

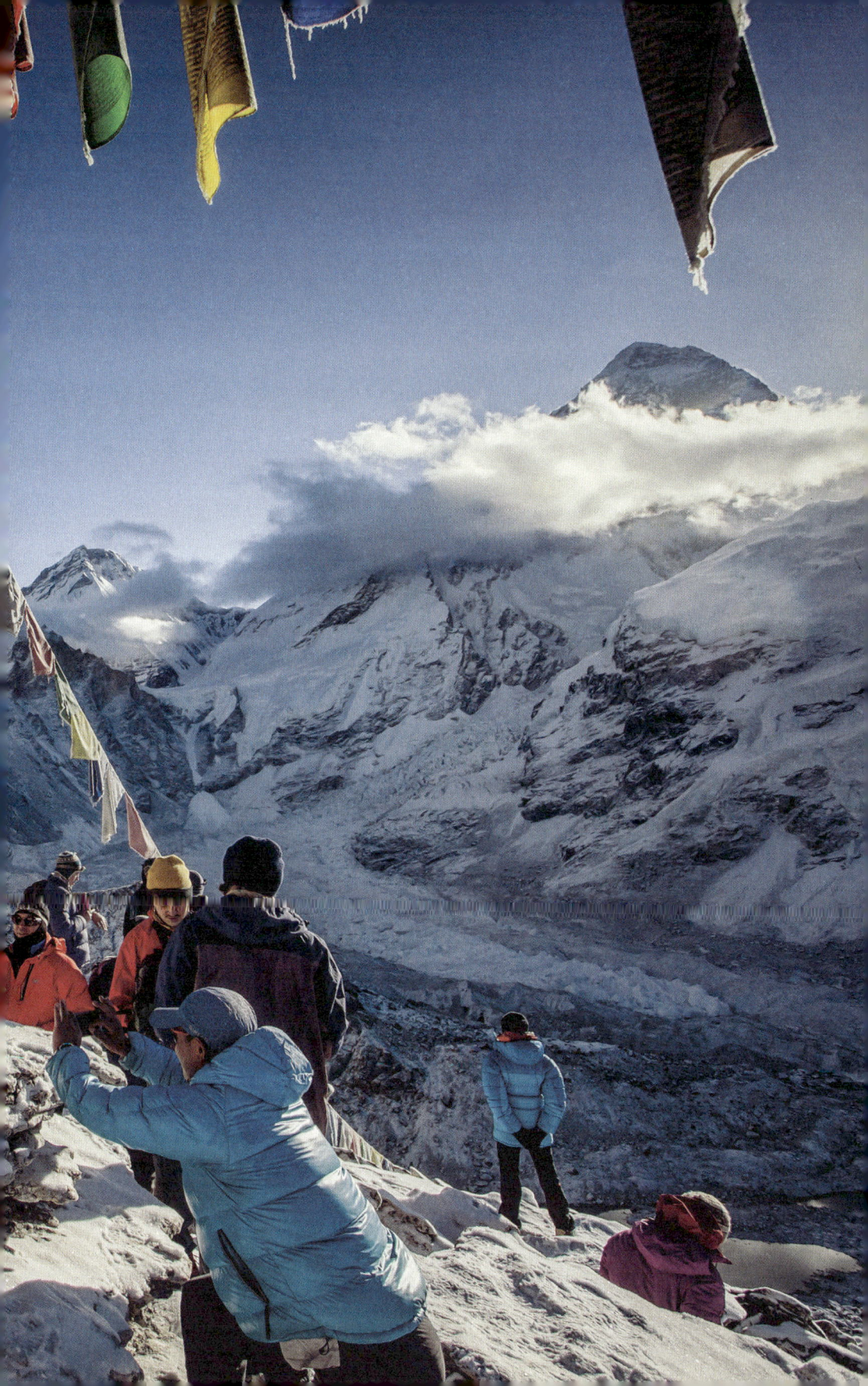

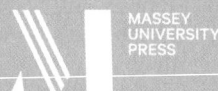

First published in 2016 by Massey University Press

Massey University Press, Private Bag 102904
North Shore Mail Centre, Auckland 0745, New Zealand
www.masseypress.ac.nz

Text and images copyright © Nicholas Allen, 2016

Design by Kate Barraclough
Map on page 301 by Janet Hunt

The moral right of the author has been asserted

The publisher is grateful to the following for permission to reproduce material in this book: Jenny Bornholdt and Victoria University Press, extracts from 'Instructions for how to get ahead of yourself while the light still shines' on page 50; Stephanie de Montalk and Victoria University Press, extract from 'Violinist at the edge of an ice field' on page 108; and Brian Turner, 'Place' on page 180.

All rights reserved. Except as provided by the Copyright Act 1994, no part of this book may be reproduced, stored in or introduced into a retrieval system or transmitted in any form or by any means (electronic, mechanical, photocopying, recording or otherwise) without the prior written permission of both the copyright owner(s) and the publisher.

A catalogue record for this book is available from the National Library of New Zealand

Printed and bound in China by Everbest

ISBN: 978-0-9941300-4-4
eISBN: 978-0-9941325-7-4